Anxiety is a complex experience, with psychological, physiological, behavioral and cognitive manifestations. It is a universal part of the human condition, but becomes abnormal when its intensity and duration grow disproportionate, or when it occurs without recognizable threat. First described in a Sumerian epic of the third millennium BC, new categories of anxiety disorder have been described only in recent years.

This comprehensive text covers all the anxiety disorders found in the latest DSM and ICD classifications. Written by two internationally recognized authorities in the field, it provides detailed information about eight principal disorders, including anxiety disorders due to medical conditions and substances. For each, it covers diagnostic criteria, epidemiology, etiology and pathogenesis, clinical features, natural history and differential diagnosis, and describes treatment approaches, both psychological and pharmacological. The scientific literature of the past two decades is thoroughly surveyed, with added insights from history, philosophy and the arts.

At once scholarly and clinically to the point, this is a definitive reference for psychiatrists at all levels. It will also be of interest to other mental health professionals, and to physicians in other specialties.

RUSSELL NOYES, JR is Professor of Psychiatry at the University of Iowa College of Medicine and Director of the Anxiety Clinic at the University of Iowa Hospitals and Clinics. RUDOLF HOEHN-SARIC is Professor of Psychiatry at the Johns Hopkins University School of Medicine and Director of the Outpatient Services and Anxiety Disorders Clinic at the Henry Phipps Psychiatric Service of the Johns Hopkins Medical Institutions.

T0275735

Publisher's Note

The Publishers acknowledge their debt to the late George Winokur, MD, who in the last years of his life worked with them to develop this book, and three further volumes, as the first titles in a new series under his editorship, to be called *Concepts in Clinical Psychiatry*. Dr Winokur was not, unfortunately, able to see any of these works in their final form.

Dr Winokur's contribution to contemporary psychiatry – in particular his dedication to the medical model – was distinctive, and his editorial style was inimitable. These four volumes are a tribute to his vision for psychiatry as a clinical discipline founded on the principles of scientific evidence.

The Anxiety Disorders
Russell Noyes, Jr and Rudolf Hoehn-Saric

Delusional Disorder
Paranoia and related illnesses
Alistair Munro

Schizophrenia
Concept and clinical management
Eve C. Johnstone, Martin Humphreys, Fiona Lang, Stephen Lawrie and Robert Sandler

Somatoform and Dissociative Disorders
William R. Yates, Carol S. North and Richard D. Wetzel

THE ANXIETY DISORDERS

RUSSELL NOYES, Jr
University of Iowa College of Medicine

and

RUDOLF HOEHN-SARIC
Johns Hopkins University School of Medicine

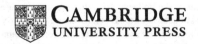

CAMBRIDGE
UNIVERSITY PRESS

CAMBRIDGE UNIVERSITY PRESS
Cambridge, New York, Melbourne, Madrid, Cape Town, Singapore, São Paulo

Cambridge University Press
The Edinburgh Building, Cambridge CB2 2RU, UK

Published in the United States of America by Cambridge University Press, New York

www.cambridge.org
Information on this title: www.cambridge.org/9780521552073

© Cambridge University Press 1998

First published 1998
This digitally printed first paperback version 2006

A catalogue record for this publication is available from the British Library

Library of Congress Cataloguing in Publication data
Noyes, Russell
    The anxiety disorder/Russell Noyes, Jr. and Rudolf Hoehn-Saric.
        p.   cm.
    Includes index.
    ISBN (invalid) 0 521 55207 9 (hb)
    1. Anxiety.   I. Hoehn-Saric, Rudolf.   II. Title.
    [DNLM: 1. Anxiety Disorders.   WM 172 N957a   1998]
    RC531.N69   1998
    616.85′223–dc21   97–42566 CIP
    DNLM/DLC
    for Library of Congress

ISBN-13 978-0-521-55207-3 hardback
ISBN-10 0-521-55207-9 hardback

ISBN-13 978-0-521-03048-9 paperback
ISBN-10 0-521-03048-X paperback

Contents

Preface

Anxiety has proven a challenging and rewarding field of inquiry, one that begins with normal anxiety. Normal anxiety signals danger and readies the individual for action. While psychologists have explored the mechanisms of this adaptive response, philosophers and theologians have sought to give it meaning and to offer guidance for dealing with it. The biology of anxiety is complex and includes arousal with its physiological changes, learning and the acquisition of skills for dealing with dangerous situations, as well as cognitive elaborations. Recently, our understanding of the biology has been enriched by animal models that have permitted study of stress-related changes in the nervous system. Also, new pharmacological probes and imaging techniques have opened windows to the human brain.

Anxiety disorders represent deviations from the normal. Although these disorders can be explained in psychological terms, they are rooted in distinct nervous system abnormalities that distort the normal response. Thus, the exploration of psychological and biological differences between normal and pathological anxiety encompasses most areas of human knowledge.

The idea for this book on anxiety and its disorders originated with George Winokur, MD, who envisioned a series of volumes based on the medical model. For this champion of data-based psychiatry, psychiatric illnesses are like other medical conditions. They have distinctive clinical features and are separable from other disorders on the basis of characteristic epidemiological factors, biological abnormalities, family and genetic features, course and outcome, and response to treatment. This book examines the anxiety disorders within the framework of this model. Chapters dealing with individual disorders contain information about definition, epidemiology, etiology and pathogenesis, clinical picture, natural history, differential diagnosis, and treatment. Included are all of the disorders found in the most recent DSM-IV and ICD-10 classifications and all aspects that are of importance to clinicians are covered. The material is clearly written and presented in a consistent format so as to be readable and informative. The book is intended for psychiatrists at all levels from residents in training to practicing clinicians. It will also be of interest to nonpsychiatric physicians and other mental health professionals seeking basic information.

The anxiety disorders are perhaps the largest group of mental disturbances in terms of occurrence. Their 12-month prevalence is close to 15% of the population of the USA, and their importance extends beyond mere numbers. To begin with, they are associated with substantial impairment in functioning. Panic disorder, for example, causes distress and impairment equal to that from common physical illnesses, such as diabetes and heart disease, and mental illnesses such as major depression. Consequently, the costs to individuals and society are great. Also, because these disorders are chronic, their impact increases over time. They interfere with growth and development, undermine personality functioning, and increase vulnerability to other psychopathology. Finally, they are treatable. For each of the disorders covered in this book – generalized anxiety disorder, panic disorder, agoraphobia, social phobia, specific phobia, post-traumatic stress disorder, and anxiety disorders due to medical conditions and substances – there are proven pharmacological and psychological treatments.

The past two decades have seen remarkable professional and research interest in a group of disorders that had previously been neglected. Development of diagnostic criteria, beginning with DSM-III, and discovery of effective treatments, such as imipramine for panic disorder and exposure in vivo for agoraphobia, have created enormous enthusiasm for the field. Increasingly, persons with these otherwise debilitating conditions are being diagnosed and treated appropriately. It is to the furtherance of this medical triumph and to our increasingly hopeful patients that we dedicate this book.

Russell Noyes, Jr
Rudolf Hoehn-Saric

1

Normal anxiety and fear: psychological and biological aspects

Definition

Anxiety is a universal experience and, as such, is a part of the human condition. It serves as a biological warning system that is activated by danger. It may also occur following loss or may arise from intrapsychic conflict, as in conflict between inner drives and external demands or between conflicting value systems. Anxiety is a distressing emotion usually associated with bodily discomfort. In contrast to depression, which is a reaction to loss and is oriented toward the past, anxiety is a reaction to threat and is directed toward the future. The threat may involve danger, lack of support or what is unknown. Normal anxiety prepares the individual for a protective response. Low levels of anxiety are helpful in coping with adversity, but high levels cause impairment and can even be disorganizing. Anxiety becomes abnormal when its intensity and duration are disproportionate to the potential for harm, when it occurs in situations known to be harmless, or occurs without any recognizable threat.

Anxiety is a complex experience consisting of both psychic and somatic manifestations and hyperarousal. In addition, behavioral reactions are frequently present as well (Hoehn-Saric et al., 1995). Psychic manifestations consist of affective reactions ranging from tension to fear and, in the extreme, full-fledged panic. Cognitive aspects include uneasiness about how to deal with situations and uncertainty about the future. They also include worry, fear, anticipation of disaster, fear of being unable to cope with circumstances, and fear of developing anxiety and, as a result, embarrassing oneself in public. Anger is related to anxiety and a decrease in the former may result in a corresponding reduction in the latter (Deffenbacher et al., 1986). Transitory feelings of depression commonly occur when a person loses confidence in his or her ability to control anxiety.

1

Somatic manifestations of anxiety can be divided into muscular and autonomic. Muscular sensations range from barely perceived tension to tremor, spasms, and, sometimes, muscle weakness. Overall muscle tension reflects the level of central arousal (Hoehn-Saric et al., 1997). Not all muscle groups, however, respond equally to anxiety. Commonly, increased activity of head, neck and shoulder muscles causes discomfort and pain in these regions. Sometimes anxiety causes localized dysfunctions such as writer's cramp or laryngeal spasm.

Autonomic manifestations are common in severe anxiety but they vary in type and severity. Some individuals are constitutionally predisposed to certain autonomic responses, such as sweating or rapid heart beat, and experience autonomic symptoms even with mild anxiety. Autonomic symptoms include palpitations, flushing, feeling of heat, perspiration, clammy hands, dryness of the mouth, tightness in the chest, rapid breathing, shortness of breath, butterflies in the stomach, nausea and a need to urinate or defecate.

Hyperarousal ranges from heightened alertness to excessive vigilance and a feeling of excessive stimulation. During severe anxiety, hyperarousal causes distractibility and inability to focus attention. At night hyperarousal manifests itself in insomnia.

Behavioral manifestations of anxiety consist of flushing or palor, visible shaking, tense facial expression, strained voice, restlessness, immobilization, laughing or crying, and overtalkativeness. Depending on an individual's personality, anxiety may lead to avoidance, retreat into fantasy, dependence on others, seeking reassurance, soliciting others' advice, or search for distracting activities. It also may increase suspiciousness or lead to aggressive actions (Lader & Marks, 1971; Hoehn-Saric, 1979; Hoehn-Saric & McLeod, 1990).

Historical concepts

Ancient origins

The word anxiety derives from the Indogermanic root, Angh, meaning to press tight, to strangle, a burden, and trouble (Lewis, 1971). Change in the conceptualization of anxiety over the course of Western history has been reviewed by McReynolds (1975). The first written account of this emotion can be found in the Sumerian Epic of Gilgamesh, from the third millennium BC, in which Gilgamesh expresses concern about his mortality. Since antiquity men have sought to explain and cope with anxiety. It was often thought to be caused by gods, evil spirits or magic. The Greek god Pan, for example, frightened travelers into panic. Less superstitious early Greeks tried to control anxiety by achieving tranquility or ataraxia. According to Democritus of Abdera, the fifth century father of atomic theory, 'the end of action is tranquility, a state in which the soul continues calm and strong, undisturbed by any fear or superstition or any other emotion'. In the concept of responsibility for one's actions and the necessity to make choices among alternatives, Aeschylus anticipated today's conflict theory of anxiety. Plato emphasized the separation between reason and passion, while Aristotle wrote that 'fear may be defined as a pain or disturbance arising from a mental image of impending evil of a destructive or painful sort'. Cicero, anticipating Freud's separation of realistic fear from anxiety and Cattell's concept of state and trait anxiety, was the first to distinguish between 'angor', a transitory state, and 'anxietas', an abiding tendency. In subsequent centuries, Hellenistic and Roman thinkers tried to alleviate anxiety through Epicureanism, which taught that all behavior is directed toward reducing pain and fear, and through Stoicism, that espoused the belief that one should accede to life with equanimity.

Major religions

In the East, Buddhism tried to reduce anxiety by advocating the passive acceptance of one's fate in a state of indifference toward pain and pleasure, and Taoism counseled the maintenance of harmony with the universe. For Confucius, doing the right thing frees persons from anxiety (Chao, 1995). According to this religious leader, 'the wise men are free from doubts; the virtuous from anxiety; the brave from fear'. He felt men should simply carry out what had to be done, without concern about whether they would succeed or fail so long as their acts were morally correct. Christianity introduced the notion of sin; for Christians anxiety was due to failure to meet one's responsibilities or guilt. This view was contemplated in *The Confessions* of St. Augustine and recently reformulated as psychological theory by Mowrer (May, 1977).

Renaissance, enlightenment, and romanticism

The Renaissance placed the origin of anxiety within man himself, thereby encouraging self-examination. Montaigne said, 'The thing I fear most is fear', a phrase that, in modified form, became a slogan during World War II. Spinoza realized that fear is future directed and that destiny has not yet happened. According to this philosopher, 'There is no hope unmingled with fear, and no fear unmingled with hope'. In the eighteenth century, James Long introduced the idea that uncertainty can lead to anxiety. A century later, Kierkegaard distinguished two types of anxiety, namely apprehension associated with seeking after adventures and anxiety concerned with choices. Man is free in, and at the same time responsible for, his choices from a multitude of possibilities. Anxiety is, thus, a necessary accompaniment of increased individuation. Kierkegaard further described 'fear of nothingness', arising not only from dread of death but from meaninglessness of one's existence. He said, 'Truth exists for the particular individual only as he himself produces it in action. Selfhood depends upon the individual's capacity to confront anxiety and move ahead'. Other existential philosophers – amongst them Satre, Tillich and May – expressed similar thoughts (May, 1977).

Psychoanalytic theory

Early psychoanalytic theorists viewed anxiety as the consequence of conflict (Trautman, 1986). Like Cicero, Freud distinguished between fear, a response to a realistic threat, and anxiety, a response to inner danger. Anxiety was originally thought to arise when the psyche was unable to master endogenous sexual excitation. Repression of unconscious instinctual urges then gave rise to neurotic symptoms. Freud was not the first to believe in the unconscious (White, 1960), but he conceptualized it in such a way that anxiety played a crucial role. In his reformulation, Freud dropped the distinction between realistic and neurotic anxiety, and stated that the experience of helplessness is the essence of danger. Anxiety, then, is the response of the ego to the threat of helplessness. Melanie Klein (Trautman, 1986) extended Freud's idea of instinctual danger by arguing that aggressive rather than libidinal impulses are central to anxiety. In response to them, the psyche mobilizes defenses, using denial, which is common in children, and repression, which is similar to denial. Although these defenses make an individual unaware of emotions, these emotions continue to affect behavior. They lead to reaction formation (i.e., taking an attitude that contradicts the original), projection (i.e., seeing attributes in others without recognizing them in oneself), counterphobic behavior (i.e., seeking out feared situations instead of avoiding them), and regression (i.e., reverting to behavior that corresponds to earlier periods of life that were more pleasant) (Lader & Marks, 1971).

Anxiety was contained in Adler's central and inclusive concept of inferiority feelings (Ansbacher & Ansbacher, 1959). Jung regarded thoughts as well as feelings, including anxiety, as rational functions because they dealt with values. Both evaluate situations: thoughts in rational, analytic terms and feelings in global terms (Jacobi, 1951). Other analysts, notably Karen Horney, Erich Fromm and Harry Stack Sullivan (Munroe, 1958) saw anxiety arising out of disturbed interpersonal relationships. For them, neurotic needs were essentially security measures arising out of basic anxiety. Bowlby (1973) emphasized the importance of separation anxiety; he postulated that disturbances of infant–mother attachment may give rise to later anxiety reactions.

Behaviorist theory

Pavlov and subsequent behavioral psychologists took a different approach to explaining anxiety. Pavlov (1960) saw anxiety as a conditioned response, the consequence of pairing a previously neutral stimulus with an aversive one. After repeated co-occurrences of the two stimuli, the previously neutral stimulus acquires the affective and physiological attributes of the aversive stimulus. Watson, and later Skinner (Hall & Lindzey, 1957), explored contingencies that lead to and reinforced fear responses, and Mowrer (1951) formulated the stimulus–response theory of anxiety.

Cognitive theory

More recently, Clark & Beck (1989) merged psychoanalytic and behavioral concepts in formulating their cognitive behavioral therapy. They proposed that cognitive schemata, often formed during childhood, automatically trigger emotional responses. While appropriate schemata are necessary for spontaneous reaction, faulty schemata lead to inappropriate emotional reactions and need to be unlearned through cognitive and behavioral interventions.

Psychobiology of anxiety

Anxiety is a complex emotion which heightens arousal and focuses attention on the source of potential danger. It prepares the body to respond with flight and fight. Anxiety also leads to the induction of memories of fearful events, and through formation of conditioned responses and modification of cognitive structures, alters subsequent response to dangerous situations.

An early theory of emotion, the James–Lange theory, assumed that an

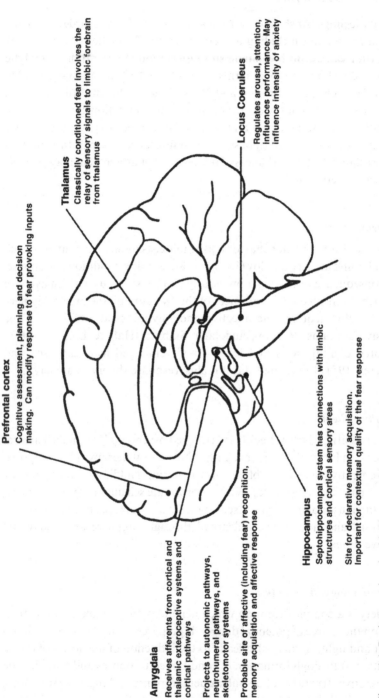

Prefrontal cortex

Cognitive assessment, planning and decision making. Can modify response to fear provoking inputs

Thalamus

Classically conditioned fear involves the relay of sensory signals to limbic forebrain from thalamus

Locus Coeruleus

Regulates arousal, attention, influences performance. May influence intensity of anxiety

Amygdala

Receives afferents from cortical and thalamic exteroceptive systems and cortical pathways

Projects to autonomic pathways, neurohumeral pathways, and skeletomotor systems

Probable site of affective (including fear) recognition, memory acquisition and affective response

Hippocampus

Septohippocampal system has connections with limbic structures and cortical sensory areas

Site for declarative memory acquisition. Important for contextual quality of the fear response

Figure 1.1 Brain areas involved in the neurobiology of anxiety. (From Pohl & Gershon, 1990. Reprinted with permission, © 1990, S. Karger, A. G.)

aroused individual first notices physical changes in his or her body (James, 1884). These changes, then, lead to awareness of a particular emotion. Thus, peripheral rather than central changes were seen as responsible for the identification of emotional states. Later, Cannon (1927) postulated that emotions arise from subcortical centers in the brain rather than changes in the periphery. Papez (1937) extended this theory by describing emotional circuits in the structures of the limbic system. More recently, Delgado (1960) concluded from animal studies that there are three types of brain structures: those unrelated to emotions, those related to behavioral mani-festations of emotions – such as the hypothalamus which when stimulated produces pseudoaffective reactions but not conditioned responses – and those related to both behavioral manifestations and the experience of emotions. The latter structures include the hippocampus, amygdala, thalamus, tectal area, central gray, and pallidum. Davis (1992) and LeDoux (1993) have demonstrated in animals the central role of the amygdala in the acquisition of fear responses.

Obviously no single system can be responsible for all manifestations of anxiety. Anxiety has to be seen as the end product of interactions between systems involving brain stem nuclei, limbic system, prefrontal cortex, and cerebellum. The brain stem is developmentally the oldest part of the brain and is partially responsible for controlling arousal. The limbic system, and within this system the amygdala, probably give rise to emotions and controls the emotional and autonomic response to stressors. Also, the hippocampus and the amygdala play an important role in cognitive and emotional learning and memory, including the acquisition, maintenance, and extinction of fear. The frontal lobes exercise overall executive function; they are involved in evaluating, planning, coordinating strategies and making decisions (Fuster, 1989). The differing contributions of these sys-tems shape the anxiety response to various internal and external stimuli. Differences in the function and dysfunction of these systems are likely to be responsible for the diversity of anxiety disorders (Figure 1.1).

Cerebral blood flow, metabolism, and hemispheric activity

Functional imaging in normal subjects suggests that anxiety initially in-creases cerebral blood flow and metabolism (Bryan, 1990; Harris & Hoehn-Saric, 1995). Beyond a certain point, however, other factors, such as hyperventilation and increased sympathetic vascular tone, lead to vasoconstriction that overrides the anxiety-induced increase in flow (Wilson & Mathew, 1993). Therefore, the effects of mounting anxiety on cerebral blood flow are not linear but follow an inverted U-shaped curve. Chronic stress may also reduce cerebral blood flow, possibly due to inhibition of glucose metabolism caused by glucocorticoids (Bryan, 1990).

Most electroencephalographic studies have found decreases in alpha activity, acceleration of alpha frequencies, and increases in beta activity associated with anxiety in both normal and neurotic individuals (Brazier et al., 1945; Faure, 1949; Ulett et al., 1953; Kennard et al., 1955; Johnson & Ulett, 1959; Gestaut et al., 1964; Earle, 1988). Frost et al. (1978), however, found no change in alpha production in normals who were anticipating an electric shock, in spite of increased heart rate and skin conductance. In addition, slow wave activity in the form of delta, theta and slow alpha has been observed in anxiety states (Earle, 1988).

Imaging as well as electroencephalographic studies suggest that the right frontal cortex may play a greater role in the perception of, and reaction to, negative emotions, including anxiety (Rodriguez et al., 1989). This corresponds with the observations of Davidson (1992) who, in normal volunteers, examined alpha asymmetry on the EEG. He found that subjects with higher activation in the left prefrontal region showed faster extinction of classically conditioned aversive responses and more effective inhibition of defensive reflexes than those with higher activation in the right prefrontal region. On the other hand, Carter et al. (1986) found that worry, the cognitive manifestation of anxiety, was associated with high overall cortical activity and with greater left hemispheric activation. Worry is not only a manifestation of anxiety, but an attempt to reduce it through language and logical reasoning. This factor may account for left hemispheric activation (Borkovec & Hu, 1990; Borkovec & Lyonfields, 1993).

Neuroanatomical regions and their functions

Brain stem nuclei: arousal, attention, and performance

Heightened arousal plays an important role in anxiety, leading to hypervigilance and insomnia. Moderate levels of arousal increase attention and, therefore, improve performance. High levels of arousal enhance conditioning but cause complex learning and performance to deteriorate. Anxious persons sleep less and lighter (Rosa et al., 1983). The variability of sleep disturbance in anxious individuals is great but, generally, they exhibit increased sleep latency (and often reduced sleep time), reduced slow wave sleep, greater tendency to arousal, and increased wakefulness.

Levels of arousal are, to a large extent, controlled by the same brain stem nuclei that are important in the biology of anxiety. These include the noradrenergic locus coeruleus, serotonergic raphe nuclei, and nucleus paragigantocellularis. An early biological theory of anxiety stated that the locus coeruleus plays a central role in anxiety. Stimulation with yohimbine, an antagonist of the alpha-2-noradrenergic autoreceptor, increases locus coeruleus activity and anxiety. Clonidine, an agonist to the autoreceptor, reduces locus coeruleus activity as well as anxiety (Hoehn-Saric et al., 1981). Anxiolytic effects are also obtained with other drugs that reduce locus coeruleus activity, such as benzodiazepines and opiates (Redmond, 1979). Thus, early studies suggested that anxiety is directly related to the level of locus coeruleus activity. Pohl et al. (1987), however, pointed out that buspirone, a drug that reduces anxiety, actually increases locus co-eruleus firing and that 3-methoxy-4-hydroxyphenyl glucol (MHPG), the central nervous system metabolite of norepinephrine, is not increased during lactate- or isoproterenol-induced panic attacks or caffeine-induced anxiety. Figure 1.2 depicts the effect of diverse inputs on the locus co-eruleus.

Recent studies have emphasized the role of the locus coeruleus in vigilance and signal processing. It is the nucleus paragigantocellularis, however, that first receives afferent information from a variety of sources. Therefore, it is in a unique position to integrate a broad range of data from internal and external sources and to coordinate the activity of the locus coeruleus as well as nuclei that control the sympathetic nervous system (Hsiao & Potter, 1990). The nucleus paragigantocellularis contains noradrenergic, serotonergic, cholinergic and excitatory amino acid receptors as well as chemoreceptors involved in monitoring carbon dioxide. Arousal is also modified by the serotonergic raphe nuclei, by corticotropin-releasing hormone, and by the limbic system and prefrontal cortex. The brain stem nuclei, particularly the locus coeruleus, do not appear to be the primary source of anxiety but serve as an amplification system (Hoehn-Saric et al., 1981). Consequently, an attenuation of locus coeruleus activity reduces surges of anxiety including panic attacks. Patients on clonidine often state that they continue to be anxious but that steady anxiety is more tolerable than attacks. Therefore, it is understandable that buspirone, an anxiolytic that increases locus coeruleus activity, is not useful in panic disorder (Sheehan et al., 1993). It lowers psychic rather than somatic anxiety (Rickels et al., 1982), and in accomplishing this, may act on other systems.

Some investigators have simplistically equated anxiety with arousal and have described all behavior in terms of intensity and approach/avoidance behaviors (Duffy, 1941; Malmo, 1957). Arousal should not be equated with

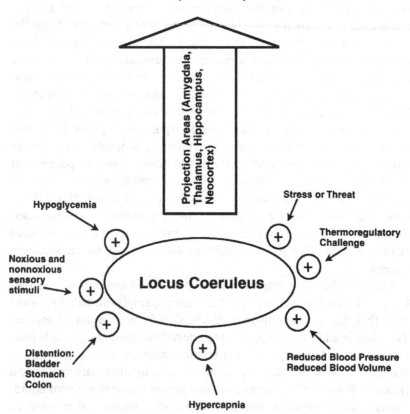

Figure 1.2 This figure depicts the activating effects of internal and external stimuli on the locus coeruleus–norepinephrine system. The system has a biologically integrative function which alerts the individual to stimuli important for survival. (From Pohl & Gershon, 1990. Reprinted with permission, © 1990, S. Karger, A. G.)

anxiety, as positive as well as negative affects are accompanied by heightened arousal. Anxiety is a state of heightened arousal with negative affective tone. The affective tone, however, derives from activity of the limbic system and possibly prefrontal cortex rather than brain stem nuclei.

Limbic system: site of emotions and learning

The limbic system, consisting of the amygdala, hippocampus, septal nuclei, and hypothalamus, is probably the seat of emotions. It also plays an important role in learning and memory. Gray (1982) developed a theory, based on animal data, in which the septo–hippocampal system plays a central role in anxiety. According to Gray, this system, with inputs from the noradrenergic and serotonergic systems, is crucial for induction and modification of anxiety. Stimuli coming from prefrontal and cingulate regions of the neocortex supply information to the septo–hippocampal system to generate predictions of expected events. These predictions are then matched against actual events. Aversive events or mismatches between internal predictions and events activate a hypothetical behavioral inhibition system that responds with arousal, attention, and anxiety. This theory has been questioned by LeDoux (1993), who found the amygdala, rather than the hippocampus, engaged in fear responses. Moreover, much of the animal behavior described in Gray's studies can also be attributed to arousal and attention rather than anxiety. While the hippocampus is predominantly involved in declarative memory, the amygdala is involved in the acquisition of emotional (including anxiety-related) memories. The amygdala also makes possible the identification of emotions. Patients who have had their amygdala surgically removed may recognize faces but be unable to identify the emotions they express (LaBar et al., 1995).

Present research findings suggest that the amygdala is the brain region of central importance in the biology of anxiety (Davis et al., 1994). It plays a crucial role in the acquisition, retention, and expression of conditioned fear. Information from all sensory modalities reaches the amygdala via projections from the cortex and a variety of subcortical structures, most notably the thalamus and parabrachial complex. Cortical projections which arise from secondary and polymodal association cortices probably relay affectively neutral information pertaining to sensory stimuli. Information concerning aversive properties is probably relayed separately via projections from the external lateral parabrachial complex, dysgranular insular cortex, and midline and intralaminar thalamic nuclei each of which receive nociceptive inputs and have output projections to the basolateral complex (Figure 1.3).

The four main output projections from the basolateral complex are (1) reciprocal projections back to the cortex, including frontal cortex that may involve conscious perception of fear, (2) projections to the ventral caudate-putamen, (3) the nucleus accumbens, which may transfer motivationally significant information to motor areas necessary for the avoidance of harmful stimuli, and (4) the central amygdaloid nucleus, critical for autonomic and somatic responses. The central nucleus of the amygdala projects to the lateral hypothalamus and periaqueductal gray, both key areas in the expression of conditioned emotional responses. These areas have major inputs into the nucleus paragigantocellularis and may transfer emotionally

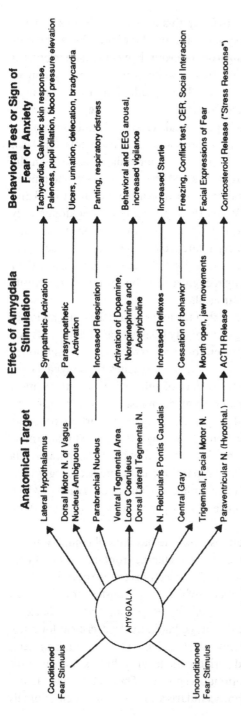

Anatomical Target

Lateral Hypothalamus

Dorsal Motor N. of Vagus
Nucleus Ambiguous

Parabrachial Nucleus

Ventral Tegmental Area
Locus Coeruleus
Dorsal Lateral Tegmental N.

N. Reticularis Pontis Caudalis

Central Gray

Trigeminal, Facial Motor N.

Paraventricular N. (Hypothal.)

**Effect of Amygdala
Stimulation**

Sympathetic Activation

Parasympathetic
Activation

Increased Respiration

Activation of Dopamine,
Norepinephrine and
Acetylcholine

Increased Reflexes

Cessation of behavior

Mouth open, jaw movements

ACTH Release

**Behavioral Test or Sign of
Fear or Anxiety**

Tachycardia, Galvanic skin response,
Paleness, pupil dilation, blood pressure elevation

Ulcers, urination, defecation, bradycardia

Panting, respiratory distress

Behavioral and EEG arousal,
increased vigilance

Increased Startle

Freezing, Conflict test, CER, Social Interaction

Facial Expressions of Fear

Corticosteroid Release ("Stress Response")

Conditioned
Fear Stimulus

AMYGDALA

Unconditioned
Fear Stimulus

Figure 1.3 Schematic diagram showing direct connections between the central nucleus of the amygdala and a variety of hypothalamic and brain stem target areas that may be involved in different animal tests of fear and anxiety. (From Aggleton, 1992. Reprinted with permission, © 1992 Wiley-Liss.)

important information to the locus coeruleus. Treatments that increase the excitability of amygdala output neurons in the basolateral nucleus, for example, by decreasing opiate and GABA transmission and increasing noradrenergic transmission, improve aversive conditioning; whereas treatments that decrease excitability, by increasing opiate or GABA transmission and decreasing glutaminergic or noradrenergic transmission, retard aversive conditioning and produce anxiolytic effects. As corticotropin-releasing hormone activates the locus coeruleus and the limbic system, it enhances the effect of punishment.

In this context, the theory of emotions by Lange and colleagues (1990) is of interest. They concluded that emotions are driven by two opposing motivation systems, the appetitive/pleasant and aversive/unpleasant systems of the brain. Arousal is not separate but reflects variation in metabolic activation of the brain. Aversive responses to stimuli are mediated through the amygdala. Somatic responses are mediated through other pathways, autonomic responses through lateral hypothalamus and central gray area. Thus, arousal, which is controlled by brain stem nuclei, is a component of emotions including anxiety but is independent of the emotional content set in the limbic system.

The association between anxiety and certain fearful situations has been the subject of intense study. It is now assumed that changes in synaptic function in the amygdala and hippocampus, known as long-term potentiation and long-term depression, are responsible for the acquisition of memories, including those associated with anxiety. The mechanism of these changes is discussed under Excitatory amino acids (pp. 17–18).

Prefrontal cortex: assessment, planning, and decision making

The frontal lobes integrate information from other parts of the brain and provide, as the executive part of the brain, the conscious experience of comprehending, planning, and decision-making. It is the only cortical area with a direct connection to the limbic system. Thus, the limbic system modifies the activity of the prefrontal cortex while the prefrontal cortex influences limbic system activity. A similar reciprocal relationship also exists with the locus coeruleus. The locus coeruleus alters levels of cortical arousal while the frontal cortex alters locus coeruleus activity. Frontal lobe activation is necessary for orienting behavior, planning and decision-making but not for automatic or conditioned behavior. For instance, the automatic reaction of a snake phobic to pictures of snakes does not increase frontal cerebral blood flow (Fredrikson et al., 1993), but thinking about snakes does so (Rauch et al., 1995).

The right prefrontal cortex is more engaged in emotional responses than the left. The left prefrontal cortex specializes in language and speech. It processes information in sequence (Davidson & Hugdahl, 1995; Fuster, 1989) and suppresses the amygdala (Davidson, 1995). Individuals with left-sided activation of the electroencephalogram exhibit more positive mood, extinguish aversive response more rapidly, and are more effective in inhibiting negative affect and defensive reflexes than those exhibiting heightened right-sided activation. The right prefrontal cortex specializes in spacial forms, tends to process incoming information in parallel, and makes judgments in a global, intuitive, and emotion-guided manner. The right hemisphere also generates physiological responses to distressing stimuli. Electroencephalographic and imaging studies suggest that anxiety, at least when cognitive components are present, activates the right prefrontal cortex (Harris & Hoehn-Saric, 1995; Hoehn-Saric & Greenberg, 1997).

Recent studies have shown that the cerebellum participates in frontal lobe functions and may modify anxiety responses. In animals, loss of fear response, disruption of habituation, and reduction of aggressive behavior have been observed after medial cerebellar lesions. In imaging studies, increased activity in vermal and paravermal structures was seen in patients with anxiety states and obsessive-compulsive disorder (Harris & Hoehn-Saric, 1995).

Neurotransmitters in anxiety

Many regions constantly interact in the brain. Therefore, few brain functions can be attributed to single regions. Certain ones, however, contribute in specific ways to the formation of anxiety. These are discussed under Neuroanatomical regions and their functions (pp. 8–14). Information is conveyed from one region to another by way of neurotransmitters. Some neurotransmitters are contained within anatomical units that carry messages to and modify the functions of distant brain regions. Other neurotransmitters affect primarily adjacent regions. As each region receives input from several neurotransmitters, the interaction between them is complex.

Some neurotransmitter systems, such as the GABA-ergic, glutamate, and adenosine systems, are widely distributed in the brain but generally affect only adjacent areas. Other systems, notably the norepinephrine, serotonin and dopamine systems, originate from specific nuclei and send their efferents to distant areas of the brain. Presently, the benzodiazepine–GABA, noradrenergic, and serotonergic neurotransmitter systems and the corticotropin-releasing hormone pathway are directly involved in the biology of anxiety. The scope of this book limits discussion of individual transmitter systems and brain regions. Articles containing comprehensive descriptions of these areas are referenced in the appropriate sections.

Benzodiazepine–GABA complex

Gamma aminobutyric acid (GABA) is the principal inhibitory neurotransmitter. It acts through the GABA-chloride ionophore which is a pentamer surrounding the chloride channel. Subtypes of the receptor have varying combinations of alpha, beta and gamma subunits (McKernan & Whiting, 1996). The presence of GABA opens the channel which increases the influx of chloride ions into the neuron. This, then, leads to hyperpolarization of the nerve cell that, in turn, decreases responsiveness of the neuron to incoming stimuli. A subgroup of GABA receptors also contain benzodiazepine receptors which, when they are occupied by benzodiazepines, enhance the inhibitory effect of GABA (Gardner et al., 1993). Benzodiazepine receptors are found in many regions of the brain, including the cortex, limbic system, and certain brain stem nuclei such as the locus coeruleus and cerebellum, but the distribution differs between subtypes (Zezula et al., 1988). Variation in the composition of GABA-receptor subunits may explain the different effects of compounds that bind to the receptor. An unusual property of the benzodiazepine receptor is its response on the one hand to agonists that increase the chloride influx (causing sedation and anxiolysis) and on the other to inverse agonists that reduce the chloride influx (causing hyperarousal and anxiety) (Skolnick et al., 1984). As yet, no natural ligands to the benzodiazepine receptor have been identified. Thus, it is not known whether the biological function of this receptor is to increase the effects of GABA, thereby inducing relaxation and sedation, or is to inhibit the effects of GABA, thereby inducing heightened arousal.

Noradrenergic system

The noradrenergic system originates primarily in the locus coeruleus of the brain stem. The locus coeruleus and the sympathetic nervous system are closely linked; both receive inputs from the nucleus paragigantocellularis, a key area for the control of sympathetic activity. The locus coeruleus sends projections to the cerebral cortex, hippocampus, thalamus, midbrain, brain stem, cerebellum and spinal cord. Activity of this nucleus increases the level of arousal and enhances the signal-to-noise ratio. Thus, relevant signals are strengthened while irrelevant neural activities are suppressed in pertinent areas of the brain. There is a definite relationship between the firing rate of the locus coeruleus and performance. Monkeys with slow firing rates are inattentive and drowsy, those with intermediate rates are attentive and perform tasks well, and those with high rates appear distracted and disorganized and perform poorly. Locus coeruleus activity is also reduced during active waking when animals are attending to tasks that do not require attention to the environment, such as grooming and eating. The highest level of activity is seen during orienting behavior or behavioral disruption.

Locus coeruleus neurons are easily conditioned and, then, respond to low intensity stimuli. While stimulation of the locus coeruleus leads to changes in many areas of the brain, these changes differ from one region to another, depending on local conditions. The noradrenergic system closely interacts with other, particularly the serotonergic, systems and changes in one alter function of the other. Thus, locus coeruleus activity is associated with arousal; it enhances attention and, when overactive, leads to disorganization (Aston-Jones et al., 1994). Abnormal paroxysmal activity of the locus coeruleus or of structures leading to it may cause panic attacks (Gorman et al., 1989).

Serotonergic system

The serotonergic system originates in the raphe nuclei and projects to the nigrostriatal and limbic systems and cortex. It is a highly complex system to which at least 14 different receptors and transporter sites contribute (Lucki, 1996). Depletion of serotonin produces large increases in the response to punishment in animals (Iversen, 1984). Serotonin reduction, however, may lessen response suppression rather than anxiolysis (Soubrie, 1986). Thus, serotonergic neurotransmission is a 'neurochemical break' on behavior and low brain levels of serotonin are associated with impulsivity (Benkelfat, 1993). In humans, blockade of serotonin receptors with metergoline induces anxiety (Graeff et al., 1985).

The animal literature suggests that different 5HT mechanisms, mediated by different receptor subtypes, are involved in the genesis of anxiety (Gribel, 1995). Similarly, in humans the $5HT_{1a}$ receptor has anxiolytic (Rickels et al., 1982) while the $5HT_{1c}$-$5HT_2$ (Katz et al., 1993) and $5HT_3$ receptors (Richardson & Engel, 1986) have anxiogenic properties. The $5HT_4$ receptor, which has the highest density in the limbic system, may be involved in anxiolysis (Eglen et al., 1995).

The $5HT_{1a}$ receptor has been most intensively studied. It is mainly found presynaptically in the dorsal and median raphe nuclei and postsynaptically in the limbic system and forebrain. Presynaptic receptors are autoreceptors that decrease activity of serotonergic neurons and have anxiolytic effects, while postsynaptic receptors cause anxiety-like behaviors in animals (File et al., 1996). Serotonin further alters noradrenergic and dopaminergic release in hippocampus and prefrontal cortex. Thus, serotonin reduces as well as enhances anxiety and increases impulsivity either directly or by altering functions of other neurotransmitter systems. Through its effect on the locus coeruleus, serotonin stabilizes arousal (Charney et al., 1990) and prevents uncontrolled anxiety or panic (Hoehn-Saric et al., 1993). Serotonin may also attenuate prefrontal activity, thus reducing psychic manifestations of anxiety (Hoehn-Saric et al., 1990; Harris & Hoehn-Saric, 1995).

Dopaminergic system

The dopaminergic system can be divided in four major subdivisions, the mesolimbic and mesocortical systems being of particular importance to psychiatry. The mesolimbic system originates in the midbrain tegmentum and innervates areas of the olfactory tubercles, nucleus accumbens, amygdala, and septum. The mesocortical system originates from the same area and projects to cortical areas including the prefrontal cortex. Stress causes release of dopamine in prefrontal cortex; however, this release is not necessarily associated with anxiety. Dopamine may have a role in increasing motivation and acquiring coping responses rather than affective states (Deutch & Young, 1995). Neuroleptics that block dopamine receptors are less anxiolytic than benzodiazepines (Hoehn-Saric, 1982).

Excitatory amino acids

Glutamate, a predominant excitatory neurotransmitter, is widely distributed throughout the brain. In interplay with the GABA-ergic system, it maintains a balance between excitatory and inhibitory states of the brain. This neurotransmitter may contribute to arousal and anxiety, because in animal studies, glutamate antagonists are anxiolytic (Stephens et al., 1991). Moreover, glutamate is necessary for the acquisition of memories and for the acquisition of conditioned emotional responses and, subsequently, their extinction (Davis et al., 1994). Glutamate's role in the acquisition of the fear response may result from its long-term potentiation of specific synapses in the amygdala. For this potentiation to occur, two conditions must be met: glutamate must be present at synapses and stimuli must partially depolarize postsynaptic cell membranes. Depolarization removes a magnesium block in the glutamate channel that impedes the entrance of calcium into the cell. Once it enters, calcium initiates a cascade of reactions leading to long-term potentiation of synapses. Even weak stimuli that are incapable of sustaining potentiation by themselves become effective when activated concurrently by stronger inputs from other, converging pathways (Dudai, 1989). Such temporary association of diverse stimuli may form the basis for conditioned responses. In animals (Davis et al., 1994) as well as humans (R. Hoehn-Saric et al., unpublished results), pharmacological blockade of the N-methyl-D-aspartate (NMDA) receptor, a glutamate receptor associated with formation of long-term potentiation, prevents acquisition of the fear response. Figure 1.4 depicts neurophysiological pre- and postsynaptic changes leading to the formation of long-term potentiation.

Adenosine system

Adenosine is a neuromodulator that has calming effects in animals (Daval et al., 1991). Blocking adenosine receptors with a adenosine antagonist, caffeine, results in heightened arousal and anxiety-like behavior. The importance of adenosine in the psychobiology of anxiety is not known.

Histaminergic system

The histaminergic system plays an important role in arousal. Activity of histaminergic neurons is maximal during periods of wakefulness, and stress increases histamine levels in the brain. The arousing effect of histamine is mediated through the H_1 receptor (Schwartz et al., 1991). Antihistamines induce sedation and have anxiolytic effects (Rickels et al., 1970).

Corticotropin-releasing hormone

Corticotropin-releasing hormone is associated with the stress response. From hypothalamic centers, it stimulates the secretion of ACTH and activates the hypothalamic–pituitary–adrenal axis. Central effects of corticotropin-releasing hormone include stimulation of the noradrenergic locus coeruleus and limbic system. Corticotropin-releasing hormone causes behavioral and physiological reactions in animals that resemble anxiety. These effects are attenuated by benzodiazepines (Pihoker & Nemeroff, 1993). In animals, corticotropin-releasing hormone antagonists appear to have anxiolytic properties (Baldwin et al., 1991). As functions of the hypothalamic–pituitary–adrenal axis are disturbed in major depres-

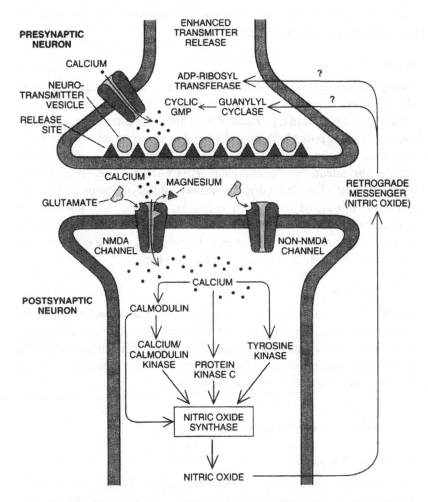

Figure 1.4 In long-term potentiation the postsynaptic membrane is depolarized by the actions of the non-NMDA receptor channels. The depolarization relieves the magnesium blockade of the NMDA channel, allowing calcium to flow through the channel. The calcium triggers calcium-dependent kinases that lead to the induction of LTP. The postsynaptic cell is thought to release a retrograde messenger capable of penetrating the membrane of the presynaptic cell. This messenger, which may be nitric oxide, is believed to act in the presynaptic terminal to enhance transmitter (glutamate) release, perhaps by activating guanylyl cyclase or ADP-ribosyl transferase. (From Kandel & Hawkins, 1992. Reprinted courtesy of I. Worpole/*Sci. Amer.*, 1992.)

sion, corticotropin-releasing hormone is a possible link between the pathobiology of anxiety and depression.

Opiate system

Endogenous opiates consist of beta endorphines, enkephalines and dynorphines. Stress alters their concentration in the hypothalamus, striatum, pituitary, and midbrain tegmental areas. This suggests that they modulate stress responses, possibly through fine-tuning the secretion of other neuropeptides, including corticotropin-releasing hormone (Stout et al., 1995). Opiates also attenuate locus coeruleus activity and norepinephrine release (Gold et al., 1979). Anecdotally, opioids have anxiolytic properties. Blockade of the mu opiate receptor by naloxone, however, does not increase anxiety during stressful laboratory tasks (Hoehn-Saric & Masek, 1981). Thus, endogenous opioids do not seem to play a major role in the biology of anxiety, although they modify some of its effects.

Cholecystokinin

Cholecystokinin, a neuropeptide found in the cerebral cortex, amygdala and hippocampus, can elicit anxiety and panic-like attacks that are prevented by benzodiazepines. The locus of these angiogenic effects may be the posteromedial aspect of nucleus accumbens. The role of cholecystokinin in anxiety is unknown (Ravard & Dourish, 1990).

Autonomic and neuroendocrine responses to anxiety

Physiological responses

Anxiety induces physiological changes that prepare the body to respond to danger. The response may be immobilization or flight or fight. During acute fear, individuals become momentarily immobile, experience a slowing of heart rate, a lowering of blood pressure and weakening of muscular tone. Uncontrolled micturition and defecation sometimes occur. Soon, sweating, pupillary dilatation, and increases in heart rate and blood pressure set in. Thus, symptoms of fright suggest an initial sharp increase in parasympathetic activity followed by sympathetic activation (Gellhorn, 1965). Subacute fear involves both autonomic systems with greater predominance of sympathetic tone (Hoehn-Saric & McLeod, 1988). While the physiology of acute fright is difficult to study in humans, fright-induced immobility in rabbits is associated with slow waves in the neocortex and hippocampus. Recovery occurs with an abrupt burst of activity (Marks, 1987).

Endocrine changes in acute anxiety consist of increase in epinephrine and norepinephrine, cortisol, growth hormone, and prolactin, and decreased testosterone in men (Ursin et al., 1978). The degree of endocrine response depends not only on the level of anxiety but on the novelty of the situation and constitutional factors.

In non-anxious individuals, stressors cause strong autonomic responses that normalize after the stress has passed. Increased muscular tension is the most common physiological response accompanying subacute or chronic anxiety, perhaps because it reflects central arousal (Hoehn-Saric et al., 1997). The autonomic response to stressors in persons with chronic anxiety differs from that of non-anxious persons; in chronic anxiety, one sees two types of reactions. Stressful tasks often evoke weaker but longer lasting autonomic responses. This is called diminished autonomic flexibility and indicates poor habituation (Hoehn-Saric et al., 1995). Such a response is less economical than that seen in non-anxious persons. Diminished autonomic flexibility has been observed in persons with all chronic anxiety disorders as well as poorly adjusted, anxious persons. It may represent a constitutional predisposition toward anxiety disorders; it may also represent a partial adjustment to chronic anxiety. For instance, when subjects with high and low anxiety traits viewed an unpleasant film, those with high anxiety responded with diminished salivary cortisol production (Hubert & de Jong-Meyer, 1992). Chronic posttraumatic stress disorder patients also exhibit reduced cortisol levels (Yehuda et al., 1990). Thus, diminished autonomic flexibility may also reflect an unsuccessful attempt to regain homeostasis. Finally, it also may reflect a diminished involvement in tasks that are not perceived as central to one's anxiety (Shapiro & Crider, 1969). Individuals with diminished autonomic flexibility, however, may still have excessive physiological reactions when faced with situations related to their psychopathology.

It has been assumed that physiological change is necessary for the acquisition and maintenance of a fear response. Acute stress is always associated with heightened central arousal as well as autonomic and endocrine changes, although the intensity varies among individuals (Ursin et al., 1978). However, once acquired, a fear may be accompanied by mostly muscular and few autonomic changes. Even panic attacks, the most dramatic eruptions of anxiety, can occur without measurable physiological change. Recently, Lenz et al. (1995) provoked panic without concomitant physiological changes in a patient by stimulating a region of the thalamus electrically. This suggests that, once an anxiety response has been established, the subjective perception of anxiety corresponds to the memory rather than the reality of the original physiological manifestations. Sensory feedback of peripheral changes contributes to the perception of anxiety. Hochmann (1966) found that adult males with spinal cord injuries experienced weaker feelings of anger, sexual arousal and fear. In shy persons, body changes like blushing may signal the beginning of anxiety that contributes to further anxiety. On the other hand, patients with pheochromocytoma – a tumor that produces epinephrine and, therefore, many bodily changes associated with anxiety – rarely display an anxiety disorder (Starkman et al., 1990). As Schachter and Singer (1962) demonstrated, arousal and concomitant physiological changes need cognitive input to induce specific emotions, including anxiety.

While emotions are readily distinguished through self-reports and facial expressions, they are difficult to distinguish on physiological measures alone (Hoehn-Saric & McLeod, 1993). Wolf & Wolff (1947) observed the stomach of a laboratory employee with a gastric fistula. The mucosa became pale when he was apprehensive or frightened and engorged with blood when angry. Ax (1953) claimed to have obtained 'epinephrine-like' physiological changes with anxiety, and 'norepinephrine-like' changes with anger. Most studies could not distinguish emotions through such physiological means. Recent studies suggest that some physiological measures, such as skin conductance, measure general arousal, while others, such as the startle reflex, are more specifically associated with emotions (Lang et al., 1990). Physiological responses also vary in individuals because of differences in age, sex, race, inheritance, constitution, and acquired physiological response patterns.

Perception of physiological responses

It is well known that people are poor judges of bodily reactions. Subjective estimations of physiological states and changes in them are poorly correlated with those obtained by objective measures, although they can improve with biofeedback training. For instance, veteran parachutists report little subjective fear despite marked physiological reactivity (Epstein, 1967). On the other hand, phobic subjects sometimes report high levels of fear without displaying physiological disturbances (Hoehn-Saric & McLeod, 1993). In one study, individuals were able during acute stress to state correctly the direction of physiological changes but not the degree (McLeod et al., 1986). Successfully treated patients with generalized anxiety disorder, however, rated changes in somatic symptoms according to their mental rather than physiological state. Patients who felt improved rated themselves to having less palpitations or muscle tension in spite of having higher heart rate, blood pressure and electromyographic activity (McLeod et al., 1990). This discrepancy between body changes and their perception shows that perceptions are modified by expectations and attention. Anxious individuals direct their attention inwardly while non-anxious individuals are more focused on external events and ignore body sensations. Finally, perception of bodily states is influenced by past experiences and this can lead to excessive attention to, and misinterpretations of, bodily states.

Genetic and evolutionary theories

Trait anxiety, namely the tendency to respond to stressors with anxiety, is, at least in part, inherited. The level of trait anxiety is normally distributed in the general population. Therefore, Eysenck (1975) suggested that intermediate levels of neuroticism, which corresponds roughly to trait anxiety, has been favored by natural selection and constitutes the population optimum for this particular trait. He speculated that during the stone age, excessively brave persons may have been killed before they could procreate, while overly anxious persons had diminished opportunities to procreate. Therefore, most of us are decendents of individuals whose anxiety levels were moderate.

Twin studies found greater similarity in emotional responses, including tension and shyness, in monozygotic than dizygotic twins (Kendler, 1986; Marks, 1987). Recently, Lesch and colleagues (1996) found neuroticism to be associated with a short variant of the serotonin transporter gene regulatory region, confirming the genetic basis of trait anxiety on a molecular basis. Certain populations, reviewed in subsequent chapters, have a greater tendency to develop specific anxiety disorders (Skre et al., 1993).

Psychological and social functions of anxiety

Anxiety and development

During development, children go through several stages with respect to fears (Campbell, 1986). These fears can be conceptualized as biologically determined response tendencies that lead to the avoidance of environmental hazards and the approach of protective figures. For the first few months, an infant responds with startle to loud noises and changes of position but not to changes in its environment. Only with the development of recall and discrimination do differentiated responses become possible. During the first 6 months, infants respond to all comforting strangers. However, as they learn to discriminate between people, they begin to fear strangers. The intensity of fear varies from infant to infant and is influenced by the approach of a stranger. Women generally induce less fear in infants than men. During the same time – between the ages of 6 to 18 months – infants also develop separation anxiety, or intense distress whenever they are separated from familiar adults. While these reactions are universal, the intensity varies greatly and has, at least in primates, a strong hereditary component (Suomi, 1986).

As children widen their experience, their fears also change. While fear of strangers diminishes, other more realistic fears, such as fears of certain animals, emerge. Later, in school, fears of performing inadequately scholastically as well as socially make their appearance. Thus, fears are common in childhood but in healthy children they are transitory and not disabling. Of particular importance for normal development is what Thomas & Chess (1984) called 'goodness of fit', namely the congruence between expectations of adults and temperament of the child. Congruence leads to healthy development with natural resolution of fears while dissonance leads to tension, anxiety and, if persistent, to developmental difficulties, separation anxiety, shyness, and simple or social phobias (Marks, 1987).

The role of anxiety in conditioning

The simplest model of fear acquisition is classical conditioning. Pairing of a fear-inducing, unconditioned stimulus and a previously neutral, conditioned stimulus, leads to a conditioned response. For instance, if a child is slapped each time it reaches for a toy, it will eventually fear and avoid the toy (Shaffer, 1986). Some fears – for instance, fear of touching a hot stove – can be acquired in this way; however, anxieties are frequently acquired in more complex ways (Marks, 1987). Rachman (1978) pointed out that conditioning theory provides only a partial explanation for the genesis of fears. It cannot explain the observed distribution of fears (for instance, the more frequent fear of snakes than of dentists), the uncertain origin of phobias (many start without apparent trauma), the indirect transmission of fears (in children of anxious mothers), and the failure of fears to arise in situations demanded by conditioning theory (for example, the failure to acquire fears during airplane rides). Individuals learn the relationship between response patterns and the probability of an adverse event through operant conditioning and social learning (by observing the reactions of others to fear-producing situations). Moreover, Mowrer (1951), in his two-stage theory of fear and avoidance, concluded that fear can energize behavior. Anxiety can, therefore, be regarded as a secondary drive to lessen or avoid threatening stimuli and the distress they engender. Any behavior leading to a reduction of anxiety, then, acts as a reinforcer.

Effect of anxiety on cognition, performance, and mastery

Effect on cognitive functioning

Anxiety alters the quality of cognitive performance. Individuals high on trait anxiety differ from those low on trait anxiety in their cognitive appraisal of threatening stimuli. High anxiety subjects have a selective bias favoring processing of threat-related stimuli, whereas low anxiety subjects have the opposite. High anxiety subjects are more likely to perceive ambiguous situations as threatening (Eysenck, 1991). Thus, individuals with high trait anxiety have maladaptive cognitive schemata (Clark & Beck, 1989). Such schemata are the organizational structure for the cognitive system. Anxious persons develop schemata with the theme of danger or harm. Their thinking contains cognitive distortions, task-irrelevant thoughts, self-absorption, automatic processing, and cognitive asymmetry (Ingram & Kendall, 1987). Such distortions, while of minor importance in healthy persons, are of pathological significance in patients with anxiety disorders, because they connect external and internal events to physical or psychological threats. This gives them an exaggerated sense of vulnerability.

Effect on performance

According to the Yerkes–Dobson law (Yerkes & Dobson, 1908), performance is influenced by the level of arousal. Mild anxiety improves, and high anxiety worsens, performance. Highly anxious individuals are vigilant and pick up information outside of their normal attentional focus. While such a strategy alerts them to potential threats from the environment, it also makes them more prone to distraction (Mathews et al., 1990). The effect of anxiety on performance depends on the complexity of a task and the degree to which a response has been learned. When overlearned, responses become automatic and less affected by anxiety. To minimize disorganization, the military overtrains soldiers for combat.

Worry

One of the most prominent characteristics of anxiety is worrying. As anxiety deals with uncertainties, anxious individuals worry and form anxious expectations. Expectancy, however, is a double-edged sword. As individuals expand their awareness of potential danger, they become more anxious but are less likely to be taken by surprise or overwhelmed by anxiety (Epstein, 1972). Such observations led Roemer & Borkovec (1993) to hypothesize that worry, a constant state of negative expectancy, is used by anxious individuals to suppress affective and physiological responses. Worry is perceived by the worrier as an attempt to avoid further danger (Borkovec & Hu, 1990).

Mastery

While avoidance leads to reduction of anxiety, mastering a feared situation provides a sense of control that not only lowers anxiety but increases self-confidence (Liberman, 1978). Mastery is a subjective perception. A person's sense of whether he or she can control a situation is a more important determinant of fear than the actual likelihood of controlling it. Loss of control causes fear only if the outcome is expected to be aversive. As controllability is related to predictability, individuals have since antiquity sought to control anxiety by reducing uncertainty.

With gradual mastery, the character of anxiety changes. Fenz & Epstein (1967) observed that, in novice parachutists, arousal peaks at the point of the jump while, in experienced parachutists, it peaks earlier but then goes down. In experienced jumpers, the mechanism of control is selective and cued specifically. For them, anxiety is highest when they have to make a decision about whether to jump on a particular day. This is usually done in the morning before reaching the airport. While novice jumpers ruminate about their fears and expend much energy controlling them, experienced jumpers become increasingly task-oriented and are more concerned about weather conditions, height, and terrain than personal feelings.

Trait anxiety and personality

Persons with high trait anxiety often are introverted. Extending Eysenck's theory of introversion and extroversion, Gray (1988) hypothesized a link between anxiety and personality traits. According to Gray, extroverts respond predominantly to positive, rather than to negative, reinforcers. Therefore, extroverts seek gratification but are insensitive to punishment.

On the other hand, introverts respond strongly to negative but weakly to positive reinforcers. Therefore, introverts take reprimands seriously but distrust praise. This reaction pattern makes introverts more anxiety prone than extroverts.

Heightened trait anxiety, however, can be found in all personality types (Hoehn-Saric, 1981). Anxiety interacts with personality traits and modifies them. A good example of such interaction is the relationship between trait anxiety and impulsivity. By studying only these two traits, Barratt (1972) demonstrated that anxiety improved the performance of impulsive persons. However, individuals with high anxiety and high impulsivity feared, but often could not control, their impulsivity and, therefore, had poorer interpersonal adjustments than those with high anxiety but low impulsivity. In another study, ship pilots who were impulsive and anxious had fewer accidents than non-anxious impulsive pilots because their greater cautiousness permitted timely correction of impulsive decisions (Hagart & Crawshaw, 1981).

Personality traits also modify a person's ability to cope with stress. For instance, under acute war stress, persons with 'normal' personalities – namely those who were flexible and adaptive – and persons with schizoid personalities – who emotionally isolated themselves – performed better than those with passive-dependent personalities (Ford, 1975). In addition, persons differ in their conception of what constitutes stress. Some individuals are more sensitive to interpersonal demands, others to physical danger and still others cannot tolerate ambiguity (Spielberger, 1975).

Finally, some persons do not seem to perceive anxiety even when it is present (Weinberger et al., 1979). Such persons are classified as 'repressors'. They deny feeling anxiety even though they respond non-verbally and on physiological measures like highly anxious individuals.

Social functions of anxiety

As safety lies in numbers, anxiety heightens social cohesiveness and emotional bonding in animals and humans; however, excessive anxiety may distort the bonding process. Mason (1970) has shown that monkey mothers who frequently punish or reject their offspring but, subsequently, provide an opportunity for them to cling, produce infants with unusual attachment. Similarly, excessive attachment also occurs in children of mothers who overreact in anger but afterwards feel guilty and comfort their just abused child. Thus, anxiety caused by frequent rejection, but followed by comforting, leads to pathological attachment.

Anxiety also contributes to the formation and maintenance of social bonds in adults. Aronson & Linder (1962) observed that a stranger finds another person more attractive if first rejected, then gradually accepted by the stranger, than when accepted from the beginning. As Festinger (1961) stated ' . . . rats and people come to love things for which they have suffered'. On a larger scale, anxiety induces bonding in religious and political groups (Frank, 1961). As Orwell (1996) recognized, external enemies bring cohesion to society.

Anxiety forces a person to develop strategies for dealing with threats. This often necessitates change in deeply ingrained attitudes that have outlived their usefulness (Hoehn-Saric, 1978). Attitudes have cognitive and affective components that are generally congruent. If an attitude has become incongruent or dissonant, it has to be corrected to become congruent again. Dissonance may occur because new cognitive information has been obtained or because of an emotional change (for instance, something previously liked has become disliked). Attitudes that are not deeply ingrained can be altered through cognitive means. When it comes to change of deeply ingrained attitudes, however, these means are often dismissed or rendered invalid unless they are preceded by emotional turmoil. Kurt Lewin (1958) stated that, to be changed, an attitude must first be unfrozen, then moved and, finally, refrozen in its new position. Political as well as religious leaders have known this for a long time. First they induce anxiety in their audience, usually fear of an economic or political, spiritual disaster or threat of hell. When the audience becomes sufficiently distressed, they proclaim salvation. At this stage, hyperaroused people are highly suggestible and ready to accept the words of the speaker. Psychotherapists also use emotional arousal with anxiety to unfreeze attitudes and move patients to healthier positions by evoking memories of past traumas or by heightening uncertainty about the solution of an emotional problem. Individuals are most susceptible to suggestion during the exhaustion that follows heightened arousal, the 'ultra-paradoxical inhibition' of Pavlov. The refreezing and maintenance of new attitudes, with all their social consequences, require regular reinforcement rather than strong arousal (Hoehn-Saric, 1978).

Summary

Anxiety is a biological warning system that alerts us to potential danger. It prepares us to cope mentally and physically with feared situations. Transitory fears during development protect children from separation or exposure to dangerous situations. In adults, anxiety not only alerts individuals to danger and motivates them, but it helps change attitudes that have lost their usefulness. In addition, anxiety has a social function, leading to greater cohesiveness. Anxiety also modifies personality traits; for example, it restrains impulsive individuals from acting precipitously. Anxiety responses are modified by hereditary and constitutional factors, personality traits, and age. To induce an optimal state of response, several regions of the brain must interact. They regulate the affective response, level of arousal and attention, physiological responses and mental coping mechanisms. For the latter, memories of past dangers are necessary as a blueprint for effective strategies. Severe anxiety, however, becomes disorganizing and loses its protective function. In anxiety disorders, pathological anxiety causes dysfunctions that need correction through psychological and pharmacological interventions.

References

Aggleton, V., ed. 1992. *The Amygdala*. Wiley-Liss, New York.

Ansbacher, H. L. & Ansbacher, R. R. 1959. *The Individual Psychology of Alfred Adler*. Basic Books, New York.

Aronson, E. & Linder, D. 1962. Gain and loss of esteem as determinants of interpersonal attractiveness. In *The Social Animal*, ed. E. Aronson, pp. 342–358, W. H. Freeman, San Francisco.

Aston-Jones, G., Valentino, R. J., Van Bockstaele, E. J. et al. 1994. Locus coeruleus, stress, and PTSD: Neurobiological and clinical parallels. In *Catecholamine Function in Posttraumatic Stress Disorder*, ed. M. M. Murburg, pp. 17–62, American Psychiatric Press, Washington, DC.

Ax, A. F. 1953. The physiological differentiation between fear and anger in humans. *Psychosom. Med.* 25: 433–442.

Baldwin, H. A., Rassnick, S., Rivier, J. et al. 1991. CRF antagonist reverses the anxiogenic response to ethanol withdrawal in the rat. *Psychopharmacology* 103: 227–232.

Barratt, E. S. 1972. Anxiety and impulsiveness: Towards a neuropsychological model. In *Anxiety: Current Trends in Theory and Research*, Vol. 1, ed. C. D. Spielberger, pp. 195–222, Academic Press, New York and London.

Benkelfat, C. 1993. Serotonergic mechanisms in psychiatric disorders: New research tools, new ideas. *International Clinical Psychopharmacology* 8 (Suppl. 2): 53–56.

Borkovec, T. D. & Hu, S. 1990. The effect of worry on cardiovascular response to phobic imagery. *Behav. Res. Ther.* 28: 69–73.

Borkovec, T. D. & Lyonfields, J. D. 1993. Worry: Thought suppression of emotional processing. In *Attention and Avoidance*, ed. H. W. Krohme, Hogrefe and Huber Publishers, Gottingen.

Bowlby, J. 1973. *Attachment and Loss*, Vol. II: *Separation, Anxiety and Anger*. Basic Books, New York.

Brazier, M. A. B., Finesinger, J. E. & Cobb, S. A. 1945. A contrast between the electroencephalograms of 100 psychoneurotic patients and 500 normal adults. *Am. J. Psychiatry* 101: 443–448.

Bryan, R. M., Jr. 1990. Cerebral blood flow and energy metabolism during stress. *Am. J. Physiol.* 259: H269–H280.

Campbell, S. B. 1986. Developmental issues in childhood anxiety. In *Anxiety Disorders of Childhood*, ed. R. Gittelman, pp. 24–57, Guilford Press, New York.

Cannon, W. B. 1927. The James–Lange theory of emotion: A critical examination and an alternative theory. *Am. J. Psychol.* 39: 106–124.

Carter, W. R., Johnson, M. C. & Borkovec, T. D. 1986. Worry: An electrocortical analysis. *Adv. Behav. Res. Ther.* 8: 193–204.

Chao, Y. M. 1995. Nursing values from a Confucian perspective. *Int. Nurs. Rev.* 42: 147–149.

Charney, D. S., Woods, S. W., Krystal, J. H. et al. 1990. Hypotheses relating serotonergic dysfunction to the etiology and treatment of panic and generalized anxiety disorders. In *Serotonin in Major Psychiatric Disorders*, eds. E. F. Coccaro, D. L. Murphy, pp. 128–151, American Psychiatric Press, Washington, DC.

Clark, C. R. & Beck, A. T. 1989. Cognitive theory and therapy of anxiety and depression. In *Anxiety and Depression: Distinctive and Overlapping Features*, eds. P. C. Kendall, D. Watson, pp. 379–411, Academic Press, San Diego, CA.

Daval, J., Nehlig, A. & Nicolas, F. 1991. Physiological and pharmacological properties of adenosine: Therapeutic implications. *Life Sciences* 49: 1435–1453.

Davidson, R. J. 1992. Emotion and affective style: Hemispheric substrates. *Psychol. Sci.* 3: 39–43.

Davidson, R. J. 1995. Prefrontal and amygdala contributions to affect, affective style and affective disorders: EEG, PET and fMRI data. *Am. Coll. Neuropsychopharmacol.*, 17 (Abstract).

Davidson, R. J. & Hugdahl, K. 1995. *Brain Asymmetry*. MIT Press, Cambridge, MA.

Davis, M. 1992. The role of the amygdala in fear-potentiated startle: Implications for animal models of anxiety. *Trends Pharmacol. Sci.* 13: 35–41.

Davis, M., Rainnie, D. & Cassell, M. 1994. Neurotransmission in the rat amygdala related to fear and anxiety. *Trends Neurosci.* 17: 208–214.

Deffenbacher, J. L., Demm, P. M. & Brandon, A. D. 1986. High general anger: Correlates and treatment. *Behav. Res. Ther.* 24: 481–489.

Delgado, J. M. R. 1960. Emotional behavior in animals and humans. In *Explorations in the Physiology of Emotions*, eds. L. J. West, M. Greenblatt, pp. 259–266, American Psychiatric Press, Washington, DC.

Deutch, A. Y. & Young, C. D. 1995. A model of the stress-induced activation of prefrontal cortical dopamine systems. In *Neurobiological and Clinical Consequences of Stress: From Normal Adaptation to Post-Traumatic Stress Disorder*, eds. M. J. Friedman, D. S. Charney, A. Y. Deutch, pp. 163–175, Lippincott-Raven Publishers, Philadelphia.

Dudai, Y. 1989. *The Neurobiology of Memory: Concepts, Findings, Trends*. Oxford University Press, Oxford.

Duffy, E. 1941. An explanation of 'emotional' phenomena without the use of the concept 'emotion'. *J. Gen. Psychol.* 25: 283–293.

Earle, J. B. 1988. Task difficulty and EEG alpha asymmetry: An amplitude and frequency analysis. *Neuropsychobiology* 20: 96–112.

Eglen, R. M., Wong, E. H. F., Dumuis, A. & Bockaert, J. 1995. Central 5-HT4 receptors. *Trends Pharmacol. Sci.* 16: 391–397.

Epstein, S. 1967. Toward a unified theory of anxiety. In *Progress in Experimental Personality Research*, Vol. 4, ed. B. A. Macher, pp. 1–87, Academic Press, New York.

Epstein, S. 1972. The nature of anxiety with emphasis upon its relationship to expectancy. In *Anxiety: Current Trends in Theory*, Vol. 2, ed. C. D. Spielberger, pp. 291–337, Academic Press, New York.

Eysenck, H. J. 1975. A genetic model of anxiety. In *Stress and Anxiety*, Vol. 2, eds. I. G. Sarason, C. D. Spielberger, pp. 81–116, Hemisphere Publishing Corporation, Washington, DC.

Eysenck, M. W. 1991. Cognitive factors in clinical anxiety: Potential relevance to therapy. In *New Concepts in Anxiety*, eds. M. Briley, S. E. File, pp. 418–433, CRH Press, Boca Raton, FL.

Faure, J. 1949. Contribution to the EEG in anxiety. *Electroencephalogr. Clin. Neurophysiol.* 1: 124–125.

Fenz, W. D. & Epstein, S. 1967. Gradients of physiological arousal in parachutists as a function of an approaching jump. *Psychosom. Med.* 24: 33–51.

Festinger, L. 1961. The psychological effects of insufficient rewards. *Am. Psychologist* 16: 1–11.

File, S. E., Gonzalez, L. E. & Andrews, N. 1996. Comparative study of pre- and postsynaptic 5-HT1A receptor modulation of anxiety in two ethological animal tests. *J. Neurosci.* 16: 4810–4815.

Ford, C. V. 1975. The Pueblo incident: Psychological response to sever stress. In *Stress and Anxiety*, Vol. 2, eds. I. G. Sarason, C. D. Spielberger, pp. 229–241, John Wiley, New York.

Frank, J. D. 1961. *Persuasion and Healing*. Johns Hopkins University Press, Baltimore.

Fredrikson, M., Wik, G., Greitz, T. et al. 1993. Regional cerebral blood flow during experimental phobic fear. *Psychophysiology* 30: 126–130.

Frost, R. O., Burish, T. G. & Holmes, D. S. 1978. Stress and EEG-alpha. *Psychophysiology* 15: 394–397.

Fuster, J. M. 1989. *The Prefrontal Cortex*. Raven Press, New York.

Gardner, C. R., Tully, W. R. & Hedgecock, C. J. R. 1993. The rapidly expanding range of neuronal benzodiazepine receptor ligands. *Prog. Neurobiol.* 40: 1–61.

Gellhorn, E. 1965. The neurophysiological basis of anxiety: A hypothesis. *Perspect. Biol. Med.* 8: 488–515.

Gestaut, H., Dongier, M., Broughton, R. et al. 1964. Electroencephalographic and clinical study of diurnal and nocturnal anxiety attacks. *Electroencephalogr. Clin. Neurophysiol.* 17: 475.

Gold, M. S., Redmond Jr, D.E. & Kleber, H. D. 1979. Noradrenergic hyperactivity in opiate withdrawal supported by clonidine reversal of opiate withdrawal. *Am. J. Psychiatry* 136: 100–102.

Gorman, J. M., Liebowitz, M. R., Fyer, A. J. et al. 1989. A neuroanatomical hypothesis for panic disorder. *Am. J. Psychiatry* 146: 148–161.

Graeff, F. G., Zuardi, A. W., Giglio, J. S. et al. 1985. Effect of metergoline on human anxiety. *Psychopharmacology* 86: 334–338.

Gray, J. A. 1982. *The Neuropsychology of Anxiety*. Oxford University Press, New York.

Gray, J. A. 1988. Anxiety and personality. In *Handbook of Anxiety*, Vol. 1: *Biological, Clinical and Cultural Perspectives*, eds. M. Roth, R. Noyes Jr, G. D. Burrows, pp. 231–257, Elsevier Science Publishers, New York.

Gribel, G. 1995. 5-Hydroxytryptamine-interacting drugs in animal models of anxiety disorders: More than 30 years of research. *Pharmacol. Ther.* 65: 319–395.

Hagart, J. & Crawshaw, C. M. 1981. Personality factors and ship handling behavior. *J. Navigation* 34: 202–207.

Hall, C. S. & Lindzey, G. 1957. *Theories of Personality*. John Wiley, New York.

Harris, G. J. & Hoehn-Saric, R. 1995. Functional neuroimaging in biological psychiatry. In *Advances in Biological Psychiatry*, ed. J. Panksep, pp. 113–160, JAI Press, Greenwich, CN.

Hazlett, R. L., McLeod, D. R. & Hoehn-Saric, R. 1994. Muscle tension in generalized anxiety disorder: Elevated muscle tonus or agitated movement? *Psychophysiology* 31: 189–195.

Hochmann, G. W. 1966. Some effects of spinal cord lesions on experienced emotional feelings. *Psychophysiology* 3: 143–156.

Hoehn-Saric, R. 1978. Emotional arousal, attitude change, and psychotherapy. In *Effective Ingredients of Successful Psychotherapy*, eds. J. D. Frank, R. Hoehn-Saric, S. D. Imber, B. L. Liberman, A. R. Stone, pp. 73–106, Brunner Mazel, New York.

Hoehn-Saric, R. 1979. Anxiety: Normal and abnormal. *Psychiat. Ann.* 9: 11–24.

Hoehn-Saric, R. 1981. Characteristics of chronic anxiety patients. In *Anxiety: New Research and Changing Concepts*, eds. D. F. Klein, J. Rabkin, pp. 399–409, Raven Press, New York.

Hoehn-Saric, R. 1982. Neurotransmitters in anxiety. *Arch. Gen. Psychiatry* 39: 735–742.

Hoehn-Saric, R., Borkovec, T. D. & Nemiah, J. C. 1995. Generalized anxiety disorder. In *Treatments of Psychiatric Disorders*, Second Edition, ed. G. O. Gabbard, pp. 1537–1567, American Psychiatric Press, Washington, DC.

Hoehn-Saric, R. & Greenberg, B. D. 1997. Psychobiology of obsessive compulsive disorder: Anatomical and physiological considerations. *Int. Rev. Psychiatry* 9: 15–29.

Hoehn-Saric, R., Hazlett, R. L., McLeod, D. R. et al. 1997. Muscle tension as measure of arousal. *Psychiatry Res.*, in Press.

Hoehn-Saric, R., Lipsey, J. R. & McLeod, D. R. 1990. Apathy and indifference in patients on fluvoxamine and fluoxetine. *J. Clin. Psychopharmacol.* 10: 343–345.

Hoehn-Saric, R. & Masek, B. J. 1981. Effects of naloxone on normals and chronically anxious patients. *Biol. Psychiatry* 16: 1041–1050.

Hoehn-Saric, R. & McLeod, D. 1988. The peripheral sympathetic nervous system: Its role in normal and pathologic anxiety. *Psychiat. Clin. N. Am.* 11: 375–386.

Hoehn-Saric, R. & McLeod, D. R. 1990. Generalized anxiety disorder in adulthood. In *Handbook of Child and Adult Psychopathology*, eds. M. Hersen, C. G. Last, pp. 247–260, Pergamon Press, New York.

Hoehn-Saric, R. & McLeod, D. R. 1993. Somatic manifestations of normal and pathological anxiety. In *Biology of Anxiety Disorders*, eds. R. Hoehn-Saric, D. R. McLeod, pp. 177–222, American Psychiatric Press, Washington, DC.

Hoehn-Saric, R., McLeod, D. R. & Hipsley, P. A. 1993. Effect of fluvoxamine on panic disorder. *J. Clin. Psychopharmacol.* 13: 321–326.

Hoehn-Saric, R., Merchant, A. F., Keyser, M. L. et al. 1981. Effects of clonidine on anxiety disorders. *Arch. Gen. Psychiatry* 38: 1278–1282.

Hsiao, J. K. & Potter, W. Z. 1990. Mechanisms of action of antipanic drugs. In

Clinical Aspects of Panic Disorder, ed. J. C. Ballenger, pp. 296–317, John Wiley, New York.

Hubert, W. & de Jong-Meyer, R. 1992. Saliva cortisol responses to unpleasant film stimuli differ between high and low trait anxious subjects. *Neuropsychobiology* 25: 115–120.

Ingram, R. E. & Kendall, P. C. 1987. The cognitive side of anxiety. *Cognitive Ther. Res.* 11: 523–536.

Iversen, S. D. 1984. 5-HT and anxiety. *Neuropharmacology* 23: 1553–1560.

Jacobi, J. 1951. *The Psychology of C. G. Jung*. Routledge and Kegan Paul, London.

James, W. 1884. What is an emotion ? *Mind* 9: 188–205.

Johnson, L. C. & Ulett, M. T. 1959. Stability of EEG activity and manifest anxiety. *J. Comp. Physiol. Psychol.* 52: 284–288.

Kandel, E. R. & Hawkins, R. D. 1992. The biological basis of learning and individuality. *Sci. Amer.*

Katz, R. J., Landau, P. S., Lott, M. et al. 1993. Serotonergic (5-HT$_2$) mediation of anxiety-therapeutic effects of serazepine in generalized anxiety disorder. *Biol. Psychiatry* 34: 41–44.

Kendler, K. S. 1986. Symptoms of anxiety and depression in a volunteer twin population. *Arch. Gen. Psychiat.* 43: 213–221.

Kennard, M. A., Rabinovitch, M. S. & Fister, W. P. 1955. The use of frequency analysis in the interpretation of the EEGs of patients with psychological disorders. *Electroencephalogr. Clin. Neurophysiol.* 7: 29–38.

LaBar, K. S., LeDoux, J. E., Spencer, D. D. et al. 1995. Impaired fear conditioning following unilateral temporal lobectomy in humans. *J. Neurosci.* 15: 6846–6855.

Lader, M. & Marks, I. M. 1971. *Clinical Anxiety*. William Heinemann, London.

Lang, P. J., Bradley, M. M. & Cuthbert, B. N. 1990. Emotions, attention, and the startle reflex. *Psychol. Rev.* 97: 377–395.

LeDoux, J. E. 1993. Emotional memory systems in the brain. *Behav. Brain Res.* 58: 69–79.

Lenz, F. A., Gracely, R. H., Romanoski, A. J. et al. 1995. Stimulation in the human somatosensory thalamus can reproduce both the affective and sensory dimensions of previously experienced pain. *Nature Med.* 1: 910–913.

Lesch, K. P., Bengel, D., Heils, A. et al. 1996. Association of anxiety-related traits with a polymorphism in the serotonin transporter gene regulatory region. *Science* 274: 1527–1531.

Lewin, K. 1958. Group decisions and social change. In *Reading in Social Psychology*, eds. E. E. Macoby, T. M. Newcomb, E. L. Hartley, pp. 197–211, Henry Holt, New York.

Lewis, A. 1971. The ambiguous word 'anxiety'. *Int. J. Psychiat.* 9: 62–110.

Liberman, B. L. 1978. The role of mastery in psychotherapy: Maintenance of improvement and prescriptive change. In *Effective Ingredients of Successful Psychotherapy*, eds. J. D. Frank, R. Hoehn-Saric, S. D. Imber. B. L. Liberman, A. R. Stone, pp. 35–72, Brunner Mazel, New York.

Lucki, I. 1996. Serotonin receptor specificity in anxiety disorders. *J. Clin. Psychiat.* 57 (Suppl. 6): 5–10.

Malmo, R. B. 1957. Anxiety and behavioral arousal. *J. Psychol. Rev.* 64: 276–287.

Marks, I. M. 1987. *Fears, Phobias and Rituals*. Oxford University Press, New York.

Mason, W. A. 1970. Motivational factors in psychological development. In

Nebraska Symposium on Motivation, eds. W. J. Arnold, M. M. Page, pp. 35–67, University of Nebraska Press, Lincoln.

Mathews, A. M., May, J., Mogg, K. et al. 1990. Attentional bias in anxiety: Selective search or defective filtering. *J. Abn. Psychol.* 99: 166–173.

May, R. 1977. *The Meaning of Anxiety.* W. W. Norton, New York.

McKernan, R. M. & Whiting, P. J. 1996. Which GABAa-receptor subtypes really occur in the brain? *Trends Neurosci.* 19: 139–143.

McLeod, D. R., Hoehn-Saric, R. & Stefan, R. L. 1986. Somatic symptoms of anxiety: Comparison of self-report and physiological measures. *Biol. Psychiatry* 21: 301–310.

McLeod, D. R., Hoehn-Saric, R., Zimmerli, W. D. et al. 1990. Treatment effects of alprazolam and imipramine: Physiological versus subjective changes in patients with generalized anxiety disorder. *Biol. Psychiatry* 28: 849–861.

McReynolds, P. 1975. Changing conceptions of anxiety: A historical review and a proposed integration. In *Stress and Anxiety*, Vol. 2, eds. I. G. Sarason, C. D. Spielberger, pp. 3–26, Hemisphere Publishing Corporation, Washington, DC.

Mowrer, O. H. 1951. Two-factor learning theory: Summary and comment. *Psychol. Rev.* 58: 350–354.

Munroe, R. L. 1958. *Schools of Psychoanalytic Thoughts.* Drydeen Press, New York.

Orwell, G. 1996. 1984. Viking Penguin, New York.

Papez, J. W. 1937. A proposed mechanism of emotions. *Arch. Neurol. Psychiatry* 38: 725–743.

Pavlov, I. P. 1960. *Conditioned Reflexes.* Dover Publications, New York.

Pihoker, C. & Nemeroff, C. B. 1993. The role of corticotropin-releasing factor in the pathophysiology of anxiety disorders. In *Biology of Anxiety Disorders*, eds. R. Hoehn-Saric, D. R. McLeod, pp. 109–128, American Psychiatric Press, Washington, DC.

Pohl, R. & Gershon, S., eds. 1990. *The Biological Basis of Psychiatric Treatment. Prog. Basic Clin. Pharmacol.* Karger, Basel.

Pohl, R., Rainey, J. M., Ortiz, A. et al. 1987. Locus coeruleus and anxiety. *Biol. Psychiatry* 22: 116–117.

Rachman, S. J. 1978. *Fear and Courage.* W. H. Freeman, San Francisco.

Rauch, L. S., Savage, C. R., Alpert, N. M. et al. 1995. A positron emission tomography study of simple phobic symptom provocation. *Arch. Gen. Psychiatry* 52: 20–28.

Ravard, S. & Dourish, C. T. 1990. Cholecystokinin and anxiety. *Trends Pharmacol. Sci.* 11: 271–273.

Redmond, D. E., Jr. 1979. New and old evidence for involvement of a brain norepinephrine system in anxiety. In *Phenomenology and Treatment of Anxiety*, eds. W. E. Fann, I. Karacan, A. D. Pokorny, R. L. Williams, pp. 153–203, Spectrum Publications, New York.

Richardson, B. P. & Engel, G. 1986. The pharmacology and function of 5-HT$_3$ receptors. *Trends Neurosci.* 9: 424–428.

Rickels, K., Gordon, P. E., Zamostien, B. B. et al. 1970. Hydroxyzine and chlordiazepoxide in anxious neurotic outpatients: A collaborative controlled study. *Compr. Psychiatry* 11: 457–474.

Rickels, K., Wiseman, K., Norstad, N. et al. 1982. Buspirone and diazepam in anxiety: A controlled study. *J. Clin. Psychiatry* 43: 81–86.

Rodriguez, G., Cogorno, P., Gris, A. et al. 1989. Regional cerebral blood flow and anxiety: A correlational study in neurologically normal patients. *J. Cerebral Blood Flow Metab.* 9: 410–416.

Roemer, L. & Borkovec, T. D. 1993. Worry: Unwanted cognitive activity that controls unwanted somatic experience. In *Handbook of Mental Control*, eds. D. W. Wegner, J. Pennebaker, pp. 220–238, Prentice Hall, Englewood Cliffs, NJ.

Rosa, R. R., Bonnet, M. H. & Kramer, M. 1983. The relationship of sleep and anxiety in anxious subjects. *Biol. Psychol.* 16: 119–126.

Schachter, S. & and Singer, J. E. 1962. Cognitive, social and psychological determinants of emotional state. *Psychol. Rev.* 69: 379–399.

Schwartz, J.-C., Arrang, J.-M., Garbarg, M. et al. 1991. Histaminergic transmission in the mammalian brain. *Physiol. Rev.* 71: 2–51.

Shaffer, D. 1986. Learning theories of anxiety. In *Anxiety Disorders of Childhood*, ed. R. Gittelman, pp. 157–167, Guilford Press, New York.

Shapiro, D. & Crider, A. 1969. Psychophysiological approaches in social psychology. In *The Handbook of Social Psychology*, Second Edition, eds. G. Lindzey, E. Aronson, pp. 1–49, Addison-Wesley Publishing, Reading.

Sheehan, D. V., Raj, A. B., Harnett-Sheehan, K. et al. 1993. The relative efficacy of high-dose buspirone and alprazolam in the treatment of panic disorder: A double-blind placebo-controlled study. *Acta Psychiatrica Scand.* 88: 1–11.

Skolnick, P., Crawley, J. N., Glowa, J. R. et al. 1984. Beta-carboline-induced anxiety states. *Psychopathology* 17 (Suppl. 3): 52–60.

Skre, I., Onstad, S., Torgersen, S. et al. 1993. A twin study of DSM-III-R anxiety disorders. *Acta Psychiatrica Scand.* 88: 85–92.

Soubrie, P. 1986. Reconciling the role of central serotonin neurons in human and animal behavior. *Behav. Brain Sci.* 92: 319–364.

Spielberger, C. D. 1975. Anxiety: State-trait process. In *Stress and Anxiety*, Vol. 1, eds. C. D. Spielberger, I. G. Sarason, pp. 115–143, John Wiley, New York.

Starkman, M. N., Cameron, O. G., Nesse, R. M. et al. 1990. Peripheral catecholamine levels and the symptoms of anxiety: Studies in patients with and without pheochromocytoma. *Psychosom. Med.* 52: 129–142.

Stephens, D. N., Andrews, J. S., Turski, L. et al. 1991. Excitatory amino acids and anxiety. In *New Concepts in Anxiety*, eds. M. Briley, S. E. File, pp. 366–381, CRH Press, Boca Raton, FL.

Stout, S. C., Kilts, C. D. & Nemeroff, C. B. 1995. Neuropeptides and stress. In *Neurobiological and Clinical Consequences of Stress: From Normal Adaptation to Post-Traumatic Stress Disorder*, eds. M. J. Friedman, D. S. Charney, A. Y. Deutch, pp. 103–123, Lippincott-Raven Publishers, Philadelphia.

Suomi, S. J. 1986. Anxiety-like disorders in young nonhuman primates. In *Anxiety Disorders in Childhood*, ed. R. Gittelman, pp. 1–23, Guilford Press, New York.

Thomas, A. & Chess, S. 1984. Genesis and evolution of behavioral disorders: From infancy to early adult life. *Am. J. Psychiatry* 141: 1–9.

Trautman, P. D. 1986. Psychodynamic theories of anxiety and their application to children. In *Anxiety Disorders of Childhood*, ed. R. Gittelman, pp. 168–187, Guilford Press, New York.

Ulett, G. A., Gleser, G., Winokur, G. et al. 1953. The EEG and reaction to photic stimulation as an index of anxiety proneness. *Electroencephalogr. Clin. Neurophysiol.* 5: 23–32.

Ursin, H., Baade, E., and Levine, S. 1978. *Psychobiology of Stress: A Study of*

Coping Men. Academic Press, New York.

Weinberger, D. A., Schwartz, G. E. & Davidson, R. J. 1979. Low-anxious, high-anxious, and repressive coping styles: Psychometric patterns and behavioral and physiological responses to stress. *J. Abn. Psychol.* 88: 369–380.

White, L. L. 1960. *The Unconscious before Freud.* Basic Books, New York.

Wilson, W. H. & Mathew, R. J. 1993. Cerebral blood flow and metabolism in anxiety disorders. In *Biology of Anxiety Disorders,* eds. R. Hoehn-Saric, D. R. McLeod, pp. 1–59, American Psychiatric Press, Washington, DC.

Wolf, S. & Wolff, H. G. 1947. *Human Gastric Function: An Experimental Study of a Man and his Stomach.* Oxford University Press, New York.

Yehuda, R., Southwick, S. M., Nussbaum, G. et al. 1990. Low urinary cortisol excretion in patients with post-traumatic stress disorder. *J. Nerv. Ment. Dis.* 178: 366–369.

Yerkes, R. M. & Dobson, J. D. 1908. The relation of strength of stimulus to rapidity of habit-formation. *J. Comp. Neurol. Psychol.* 18: 459–482.

Zezula, J., Cortes, R., Probst, A. et al. 1988. Benzodiazepine receptor sites in the human brain: Autoradiographic mapping. *Neuroscience* 25: 771–795.

2

Generalized anxiety disorder

Definition

Generalized anxiety disorder is a chronic disturbance characterized by excessive anxiety and worry. It is a newly described disorder about which much uncertainty exists. Its resemblance to normal anxiety and lack of distinctive features have contributed to poor diagnostic reliability. The relative mildness of symptoms and high rates of comorbidity have caused some to view it as an associated feature of other disorders. Nevertheless, depending upon where the threshold is set, generalized anxiety disorder is common, and its chronicity and comorbidity add to its overall impact. Most persons with the disorder are seen by primary care practitioners and, partly for this reason, it remains the least studied of the anxiety disorders.

Generalized anxiety disorder first appeared in DSM-III as a residual category, although chronic free-floating anxiety was described as early as 1895 by Freud. Also, the description in DSM-III bore a resemblance to trait anxiety, conceptualized by Speilberger (1972) and others. When panic disorder was removed from the earlier diagnostic category, anxiety neurosis (DSM-II), what remained was labeled generalized anxiety disorder (American Psychiatric Association, 1968). The observation by Klein & Fink (1962) of two anxiety syndromes that were differentially responsive to drugs was important in defining the new category. They observed that imipramine blocked panic attacks but that benzodiazepines might be more effective for anticipatory anxiety (Klein, 1981).

Diagnostic criteria

Generalized anxiety disorder first appeared in DSM-III (American Psychiatric Association, 1980). As initially defined, its essential feature was one of generalized, persistent anxiety manifested by symptoms grouped under

37

four headings. Two of them – apprehensive expectation and vigilance and scanning involved psychological symptoms, and two – motor tension and autonomic hyperactivity – involved somatic symptoms. The criteria called for at least one symptom from each category and a duration of at least 1 month. Consistent with its residual status the diagnosis could only be made if symptoms were not due to another disorder.

The disorder was first given independent status in DSM-III-R (American Psychiatric Association, 1987). Its essential feature – excessive worry – was shifted to the cognitive sphere. Characteristic worry had to be present more days than not, had to involve two or more areas of activity (i.e., work, finances, health, etc.), and could not be focused exclusively on the features of another disorder. In the revised criteria, 18 symptoms were grouped under three headings, including vigilance and scanning, motor tension, and autonomic hyperactivity. In order to separate generalized anxiety from adjustment disorders, a duration of 6 months was specified and the hierarchical exclusions in DSM-III were removed.

Further refinements in the criteria appeared in DSM-IV shown in Table 2.1 (American Psychiatric Association, 1994). These were intended to improve reliability and sharpen the distinction between generalized anxiety and other anxiety disorders. The essential feature remains excessive worry, but to separate this from normal worry, it is described as uncontrolled and having multiple foci (Abel & Borkovec, in press). As autonomic symptoms are less frequent in generalized anxiety disorder than in panic disorder, these symptoms were dropped and more distinctive symptoms were retained (Starcevic et al., 1994). Three of six symptoms are now required during periods of excessive worry. Also, the disorder must be associated with significant distress or impairment.

The definition of generalized anxiety disorder in ICD-10 differs somewhat from that in DSM-IV (Table 2.2) (World Health Organization, 1993). The primary symptoms are those of anxiety and the duration is several weeks to months. Symptom categories are the same as those found in DSM-IV except for vigilance and scanning, but symptoms from that grouping are found under the heading of apprehension. Certain hierarchical exclusions not found in DSM-IV exist in ICD-10; thus, a patient does not meet criteria for generalized anxiety disorder if he or she meets criteria for some other anxiety or depressive disorders.

Conceptualizations of generalized anxiety disorder

Authors writing about generalized anxiety disorder have referred to the disturbance as anything from anxious temperament to an independent

Table 2.1. *DSM-IV Criteria for generalized anxiety disorder*

A. Excessive anxiety and worry (apprehensive expectation), occurring more days than not
   for at least 6 months, about a number of events or activities (such as work or school
   performance)
B. The person finds it difficult to control the worry
C. The anxiety and worry are associated with three (or more) of the following six symptoms
   (with at least some symptoms present for more days than not for the past 6 months)
   (1) restlessness or feeling keyed up or on edge
   (2) being easily fatigued
   (3) difficulty concentrating or mind going blank
   (4) irritability
   (5) muscle tension
   (6) sleep disturbance (difficulty falling or staying asleep, or restless unsatisfying sleep)
D. The focus of the anxiety and worry is not confined to features of an axis I disorder, e.g.,
   the anxiety or worry is not about having a panic attack (as in panic disorder), being
   embarrassed in public (as in social phobia), being contaminated (as in
   obsessive-compulsive disorder), being away from home or close relatives (as in
   separation anxiety disorder), gaining weight (as in anorexia nervosa), having multiple
   physical complaints (as in somatization disorder), or having a serious illness (as in
   hypochondriasis), and the anxiety and worry do not occur exclusively during
   posttraumatic stress disorder
E. The anxiety, worry, or physical symptoms cause clinically significant distress or
   impairment in social, occupational, or other important areas of functioning
F. The disturbance is not due to the direct physiological effects of a substance (e.g., a drug
   of abuse, a medication) or a general medical condition (e.g., hyperthyroidism) and does
   not occur exclusively during a mood disorder, a psychotic disorder, or a pervasive
   developmental disorder

disorder. Some are inclined toward a dimensional view. One such possibility is that generalized anxiety is a personality trait (Rapee, 1991a). The disorder's early and gradual onset, as well as its long-term stability, fit this conceptualization (Nisita et al., 1990). Another possibility is that generalized anxiety is a variable dimension of other psychopathology. In accord with this view, the separation from normal anxiety appears to be a gradual one (Hoehn-Saric & McLeod, 1990). Also, anxiety symptoms accompany many psychiatric disorders, and their occurrence is, in most cases, a matter of degree (Sanderson & Wetzler, 1991).

Some who take a categorical approach are likewise reluctant to grant generalized anxiety independent status. For Tyrer (1986) generalized anxiety disorder may simply be a less severe form of panic disorder. From a longitudinal perspective, it may, in some cases, be a prodromal or residual form of other disorders (Uhde et al., 1985; Garvey et al., 1988). For instance, some patients with panic disorder experience generalized anxiety symptoms for lengthy intervals before or after the occurrence of panic attacks

Table 2.2. *ICD-10 Criteria for Generalized Anxiety Disorder*

A. There must have been a period of at least 6 months with prominent tension, worry, and feelings of apprehension about every day events and problems
B. At least four of the symptoms listed below must be present, at least one of which must be from item (1) to (4):

Autonomic arousal symptoms
(1) palpitations or pounding heart, or accelerated heart rate
(2) sweating
(3) trembling or shaking
(4) dry mouth (not due to medication or dehydration)

Symptoms involving chest and abdomen
(5) difficulty breathing
(6) feeling of choking
(7) chest pain or discomfort
(8) nausea or abdominal distress (e.g., churning in stomach)

Symptoms involving mental state
(9) feeling dizzy, unsteady, faint or light-headed
(10) feelings that objects are unreal (derealization), or that the self is distant or "not really here" (depersonalization)
(11) fear of losing control, "going crazy", or passing out
(12) fear of dying

General symptoms
(13) hot flushes or cold chills
(14) numbness or tingling sensations

Symptoms of tension
(15) muscle tension or aches and pains
(16) restlessness and inability to relax
(17) feeling keyed up, on edge, or mentally tense
(18) a sensation of a lump in the thoat, or diffculty in swallowing

Other non-specific symptoms
(19) exaggerated response to minor surprises or being startled
(20) difficulty in concentration, or mind "going blank", because of worrying or anxiety
(21) persistent irritability
(22) difficulty in getting to sleep because of worrying

C. The disorder does not meet the criteria for panic disorder, phobic anxiety disorders, obsessive–compulsive disorder, or hypochondriacal disorder
D. The anxiety disorder is not due to a physical disorder, such as hyperthyroidism, an organic mental disorder, or a psychoactive substance-related disorder, such as excess consumption of amphetamine-like substances or withdrawal from benzodiazepines

(Fava & Kellner, 1991). Other reasons to withhold independent status include a high rate of comorbidity, lack of distinctive features, and the relative mildness of symptoms. When generalized anxiety disorder coexists with other disorders, it may sometimes be an associated feature of those disorders (Barlow & DiNardo, 1991; Wittchen et al., 1994).

Reliability and validity

Reliability

On the whole, the reliability of generalized anxiety disorder has proven only fair, lower than other anxiety disorders, and not clearly improved by revisions in the classification (DiNardo et al., 1983; Barlow, 1985; Riskind et al., 1987a; Mannuzza et al., 1989; Onstad et al., 1991; Williams et al., 1992; DiNardo et al., 1993; Wittchen et al., 1995). There has been considerable variability, however, with kappas for interrater agreement ranging from 0.27 to 0.95 for the DSM-III-R disorder. Mannuzza et al. (1989) obtained unacceptable agreement for the current diagnosis (0.27), but good agreement for the lifetime diagnosis (0.60). The highest kappas were obtained in studies that used rating of recorded interviews, a procedure that eliminates subject variability (Riskind et al., 1987a; Onstad et al., 1991). Apart from these more extreme values, most studies reported fair agreement (kappas of 0.47 to 0.60). Disagreement in studies involved the distinction between what is normal versus abnormal anxiety and that between an associated feature and a separate disorder, in this case generalized anxiety disorder (DiNardo et al., 1993; Wittchen et al., 1995).

As attempts have been made to refine the criteria for generalized anxiety disorder, the reliability of individual symptoms has been examined. Using the Schedule of Affective Disorders and Schizophrenia, Lifetime Anxiety Version, Fyer et al. (1989) found low kappas for persistent anxiety (0.42) and for individual generalized anxiety symptoms (0.08 to 0.54). Similarly, Barlow & DiNardo (1991) found the reliability of criterion symptoms (DSM-III-R) variable and generally low (0.05 to 0.63). Recent studies have been more encouraging. For example, Craske et al. (1989) reported 82% agreement between raters asked to determine foci of worry, Sanderson & Barlow (1990) reported a kappa of 0.90 for excessive worry, and Marten et al. (1993) reported agreement of more than 70% for DSM-IV criterion symptoms. However, none of these studies called for the usual kind of diagnostic discrimination.

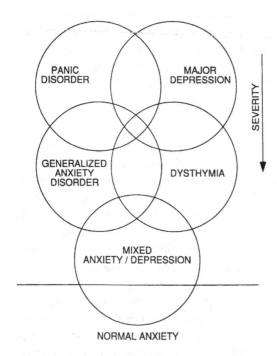

Figure 2.1 Schematic representation of the relationship between generalized anxiety disorder and other anxiety and mood disorders.

Validity

As generalized anxiety disorder was created by dividing DSM-II, anxiety neurosis, most of the evidence for validity comes from studies comparing patients with generalized anxiety disorder and panic (Hoehn-Saric, 1982; Raskin et al., 1982; Anderson et al., 1984; Rapee, 1985; Thyer et al., 1985; Cameron et al., 1986; Torgersen, 1986; Noyes et al., 1992; Clark et al., 1994). Research in this area has been reviewed by Weissman (1990), Andrews (1993), and by Brown et al. (1994). As is shown in Figure 2.1, the disorder must also be distinguished from mood disorders (i.e., dysthymia and major depressive disorder) and from normal anxiety. Studies have consistently shown an age of onset in the mid-teens for generalized anxiety disorder compared to the mid to late 1920s for panic disorder (Thyer et al., 1985). Also, the symptoms of autonomic hyperactivity that characterize panic are relatively infrequent in generalized anxiety disorder (Anderson et al., 1984; Hibbert, 1984; Rapee, 1985; Noyes et al., 1987, 1992; Holt & Andrews, 1989; Clark et al., 1994). Among patients with generalized anxiety, symptoms of vigilance and scanning and, to a lesser extent, motor tension predominate (Marten et al., 1993).

Family and twin studies have involved small samples and yielded inconsistent results. A preliminary family study showed an increase of generalized anxiety disorder among the relatives of probands with generalized anxiety but not among the relatives of panic subjects (Noyes et al., 1987). Other family and twin studies have found no such increase (Torgersen, 1983; Andrews et al., 1990; Mendlewicz et al., 1993; Skre et al., 1993). In two family studies, relatives of patients with panic disorder and agoraphobia had no greater risk for generalized anxiety disorder than relatives of controls (Crowe et al., 1983; Noyes et al., 1986). Andrews et al. (1990), however, reported that relatives of probands with neurotic symptoms were more likely to have neuroses but not necessarily of the same type as the proband.

Differences in the natural course and treatment response of generalized anxiety and panic disorder support validity (Rickels & Schweizer, 1990). Two follow-up studies found a less favorable outcome in patients with generalized anxiety disorder than patients with panic disorder (Woodman et al., 1995; Yonkers et al., 1996). Among the former, impairment remained greater, and fewer had experienced remission in 3–5 years. With respect to treatment, Klein's original observation concerning a differential response to drugs has not received support (Klein & Fink, 1962; Klein, 1964). Benzodiazepines are effective for panic disorder as are tricyclic antidepressants for generalized anxiety disorder (Ballenger et al., 1988; Schweizer & Rickels, 1991; Rickels et al., 1993). Some drugs used to treat generalized anxiety (e.g., buspirone, propranolol) appear ineffective for panic, but they may simply be weaker anxiolytics.

Diagnostic validity also depends upon evidence of separation from depressive disorders. Questions about the distinction between generalized anxiety and both major depressive disorder and dysthymia have been raised because of overlapping symptoms and frequent comorbidity (Angst et al., 1990). Although some studies have found high rates of comorbid major depression, examination of temporal relationships has often shown that generalized anxiety existed long before the onset of depression (Brown et al., 1994). Also, differences in clinical characteristics have emerged in recent studies (Beck et al., 1987; Riskind et al., 1987a; Shores et al., 1992). For instance, Nisita et al. (1990) found that patients with generalized anxiety disorder had an earlier onset and fewer depressive symptoms than patients with major depressive disorder. Likewise, Clark et al. (1994) reported that patients with anxiety were distinguished by symptoms of autonomic arousal, threat-related cognitions, and subjective anxiety and

tension; whereas patients with depression were distinguished by anhedonia, cognitions of loss or failure, and dysphoric mood.

The only comparison of generalized anxiety disorder and dysthymia was
undertaken by Riskind et al. (1991). The distinction between these disorders is of interest because both are chronic and are highly comorbid with
other anxiety and depressive disorders. Riskind et al. (1991) showed that,
despite overlap, patients with these disorders exist and can be distinguished
on the basis of symptoms and cognitions. While both anxious and depressive symptoms were important, depressive cognitions (i.e., hopelessness)
were the ones that separated the groups.

Measurement

Structured interviews

Several structured interviews are available for screening clinical and non-
clinical populations. They yield DSM-IV, and in some cases ICD-10,
diagnoses. Two were designed specifically for anxiety disorder populations.
One of these, the Anxiety Disorders Interview Schedule, Revised Version
(ADIS-IV) focuses on pathological worry and its distinguishing characteristics (Brown et al., 1994). It also elicits information about important
clinical features of generalized anxiety disorder, including the history of the
disorder, extent of avoidance, situational and cognitive cues, etc. Global
ratings of severity on nine-point linear scales are made, and these are used
to determine the predominant disturbance when more than one disorder
exists. The ADIS-IV was developed for use in anxiety clinic populations,
but it includes screening for other important disorders.

Another structured interview developed specifically for anxiety disorders is the Schedule for Affective Disorders and Schizophrenia-Lifetime
Anxiety Version (SADS-LA) (Manuzza et al., 1986). A DSM-IV revision of
this instrument is in progress. The SADS-LA includes detailed assessment
of many individual symptoms and yields diagnoses according to several
classification systems. It elicits information about subthreshold symptoms
and syndromes and about relationship between coexisting disorders. The
SADS-LA provides coverage of most psychiatric disorders but is lengthy.
It was designed for use in research involving anxiety disorders and the
relationships between them. Other structured interviews are briefly described in Chapter 4.

Symptom rating scales

A great number of instruments have been developed for the measurement
of anxiety. Although some were designed for screening, most are used to

measure the level of symptoms and change that occurs with treatment. The scales that have been used most frequently in studies of generalized anxiety disorder are the State-Trait Anxiety Inventory, Trait Version (STAI-T) and the Hamilton Anxiety Scale (HAS) (Hamilton, 1959; Speilberger, 1983).

The STAI consists of two self-rated measures, one for trait anxiety (i.e., tendency to react in an anxious manner in stressful situations) and the other for state anxiety (i.e., current level of anxiety). The STAI-T contains 20 statements to which patients respond by indicating how they generally feel on four-point scales (1 almost never to 4 almost always). Items include worry, tension, and psychological symptoms typical of generalized anxiety disorder. The STAI-S also contains 20 items about how patients feel at the moment. The trait version (STAI-T) is a brief measure that is widely used. It has undergone extensive psychometric testing and normative data are available.

The Hamilton Anxiety Scale (HAS) is an observer-rated scale used to measure the severity of anxiety symptoms in clinical populations. It consists of 14 items rated on five-point scales (0 not present to 4 very severe). Many items correspond to groupings of symptoms (e.g., gastrointestinal, cardiovascular) which makes for awkward administration. Factor analyses have identified psychic and somatic dimensions which can be scored separately. A score of 18 is indicative of clinically significant anxiety. The HAS, like the STAI-T, is sensitive to change, and these instruments are commonly used in treatment studies (Maier et al., 1988; Durham & Allan, 1993). A reconstructed scale has been developed to better discriminate between anxiety and depression (Riskind et al., 1987b). Also, the Clinical Anxiety Scale is a refinement of the HAS developed by Snaith et al. (1982).

Recently, an instrument was developed to measure worry, now the essential feature of generalized anxiety disorder (Meyer et al., 1990). The Penn State Worry Questionnaire (PSWQ) is a 16-item self-rated scale. The items, shown in Table 2.3, are rated on five-point linear scales. The scale has shown excellent psychometric properties in student and clinical populations (Brown et al., 1992). It measures a single cognitive dimension that is correlated with other psychological constructs related to worry (e.g., self-esteem, perfectionism) but is not correlated with other measures of anxiety. The scale has proven sensitive to change with treatment (Meyer et al., 1990).

Other commonly used scales include the Symptom Checklist-90 (SCL-90) and the Beck Anxiety Inventory (BAI) (Derogatis, 1983; Beck et al., 1988). The SCL-90 is a 90-item, multidimensional self-report inventory designed to measure symptomatic distress. It has an anxiety subscale. The BAI is a 21-item self-report instrument for measuring the severity of

Table 2.3. *Penn State Worry Questionnaire*

Please indicate the extent to which each of the following statements is typical or not typical
of you

	Not at all typical of me				Very typical of me
	1	2	3	4	5
1. If I do not have enough time to do everything, I do not worry about it.	1	2	3	4	5
2. My worries overwhelm me.	1	2	3	4	5
3. I do not tend to worry about things.	1	2	3	4	5
4. Many situations make me worry.	1	2	3	4	5
5. I know I should not worry about things, but I just cannot help it.	1	2	3	4	5
6. When I am under pressure I worry a lot.	1	2	3	4	5
7. I am always worrying about something.	1	2	3	4	5
8. I find it easy to dismiss worrisome thoughts.	1	2	3	4	5
9. As soon as I finish one task, I start to worry about everything else I have to do.	1	2	3	4	5
10. I never worry about anything.	1	2	3	4	5
11. When there is nothing more I can do about a concern, I do not worry about it any more.	1	2	3	4	5
12. I have been a worrier all my life.	1	2	3	4	5
13. I notice that I have been worrying about things.	1	2	3	4	5
14. Once I start worrying, I cannot stop.	1	2	3	4	5
15. I worry all the time.	1	2	3	4	5
16. I worry about projects until they are all done.	1	2	3	4	5

Source: Meyer et al. (1990). © Elsevier Science Ltd. Reprinted with permission.

anxiety symptoms. It was designed to minimize overlap with depression.
Reviews of the assessment of anxiety and the scales used for that purpose
are available (Beck et al., 1986; Nietzel et al., 1988; Walker,1990).

Epidemiology

Prevalence

Estimates of the prevalence of generalized anxiety disorder in the general
population have varied due to changes in diagnostic criteria (Oakley-
Browne & Joyce, 1992; Brawman-Mintzer & Lydiard, 1996). For example,
when Breslau & Davis (1985) lengthened the duration requirement from 1
month, as in DSM-III, to 6 months, as in DSM-III-R, the lifetime prevalence fell from 45% to 9% in the mothers of chronically ill children. Despite
this, generalized anxiety is one of the more prevalent anxiety disorders.
Prevalence rates from the National Comorbidity Survey (NCS), using

DSM-III-R criteria, were 1.6% for current, 3.1% for 12-month, and 5.1% for lifetime generalized anxiety disorder, higher than the rates for panic disorder (Wittchen et al., 1994). Estimates from the Epidemiologic Catchment Area (ECA) study were similar but excluded persons with comorbid disorders (Blazer et al., 1991). As might be expected, the broader definition of generalized anxiety disorder in ICD-10 produced a higher, 8.9%, lifetime estimate (Wittchen et al., 1994). The prevalence of overanxious disorder, a childhood forerunner of generalized anxiety disorder, averaged 6.9% in a series of epidemiologic studies (Rey et al., 1992).

Generalized anxiety disorder is perhaps the most common anxiety disorder in primary care settings. Current prevalence was estimated at 7.9% in the World Health Organization collaborative study (Sartorius et al., 1996). This is in contrast to the rarity with which the disorder is seen by mental health professionals. Barlow (1986a) and Noyes (1988a) estimated that only about 10% of anxiety clinic referrals are for generalized anxiety disorder. Perhaps because the disorder lacks distinctly abnormal or alarming features (e.g., panic attacks), relatively few persons seek specialist attention.

Risk factors

As with most anxiety disorders, women are more often affected than men. The female-to-male ratio for generalized anxiety disorder is roughly 2 to 1 (Wittchen et al., 1994). The prevalence is relatively low in adolescence and early adulthood, much higher rates being found in women age 45 years and older (current 3.5% and lifetime 10.3%) (Whitaker et al., 1990). In the ECA study, correlates of the disorder were living in a large city, had lower occupational status, having lower income, being financial dependent, and being unmarried, all potential indicators of social stress (Blazer et al., 1991). Risk factors that emerged from the NCS study were being female, being older than 24 years, being previously married, being unemployed, being a homemaker, and living in the Northeastern United States (Wittchen et al., 1994).

Comorbidity

Data from community and clinical samples show extremely high rates of comorbidity in persons with generalized anxiety disorder (Brawman-Mintzer & Lydiard, 1996). As may be seen in Table 2.5, 90.4% of persons with this disorder in the National Comorbidity Survey had at least one lifetime disorder, and 66.3% had at least one additional current disorder. The strongest links were with major depression and dysthymia followed by

Table 2.4. *Lifetime comorbidity in persons with generalized anxiety disorder in the National Comorbidity Survey*

	Percentage	Odds ratio
Major depression	62.4	9.7
Dysthymia	39.5	13.5
Mania	10.5	9.9
Panic disorder	23.5	12.3
Agoraphobia	25.7	5.8
Simple phobia	35.1	4.9
Social phobia	34.4	3.8
Alcohol use disorders	37.6	2.0
Substance use disorders	27.6	3.1
Any disorder	90.4	11.6

Source: Modified from Wittchen et al. (1994). © 1994, American Medical Association. Reprinted with permission.

panic disorder. Among the anxiety disorders, simple and social phobia also showed high rates of coexistence. For 9.6% of persons, however, generalized anxiety disorder was the only lifetime disorder, and for 12.2% the onset of generalized anxiety was earlier than that of any other disorder. Thus, 21.8% of cases met one or another criteria for primary generalized anxiety disorder.

High rates of comorbidity also exist in clinical samples. For example, Brawman-Mintzer et al. (1993) found that 74% of patients with generalized anxiety disorder had at least one additional lifetime diagnosis. Thirty-seven percent had one, 20% had two, and 17% had three additional diagnoses. The most frequent comorbid anxiety disorders were simple and social phobia, consistent with earlier studies (Sanderson & Wetzler, 1991). Variation in the rates of major depressive disorder (6–46%) and dysthymia (6–33%) among studies probably reflect differing methods of subject recruitment (Riskind et al., 1991; Brown et al., 1994). The early onset of generalized anxiety suggests that this disorder may confer vulnerability to later-developing disorders (Brown et al., 1994; Wittchen et al., 1994).

There has been little study of the relationship between generalized anxiety disorder and personality (Mauri et al., 1992). As has been mentioned, clinical studies have found generalized anxiety associated with the dimension of neuroticism and anxious (cluster C) personality disorders (Koenigsberg et al., 1985; Gasperini et al., 1990). Similar findings in patients with panic disorder suggest that the association may be non-specific

(Mavissakalian et al., 1993). Data from the Epidemiological Catchment Area Study showed a strong association between generalized anxiety disorder and compulsive personality traits (Nestadt et al., 1992). Further discussion of the relationship to personality is found on pp. 53–4.

Family and twin studies

Early family and twin studies suggested that anxiety neurosis (DSM-II and before) might be familial, and that hereditary factors might be important in its transmission. Recent studies involving generalized anxiety disorder have been inconclusive and are difficult to interpret because of small sample sizes, variable diagnostic criteria, and other methodologic problems (Woodman, 1993; Brown et al., 1994). One preliminary study showed a higher prevalence of generalized anxiety disorder in the relatives of persons with generalized anxiety than in the relatives of controls or persons with panic disorder (Noyes et al., 1987). A family history study supported these findings (Noyes et al., 1992). Another study found no excesses of anxiety disorders in relatives of probands with a syndrome resembling generalized anxiety disorder (Cloninger et al., 1981). Also, Breslau et al. (1987) did not find the children of mothers with generalized anxiety any more anxious than the children of normal mothers.

With respect to twin studies, the results have also been inconsistent. Studies by Torgersen (1983) and Andrews et al. (1990) found no significant difference in concordance for generalized anxiety among monozygotic and dizygotic twins. On the other hand, Skre et al. (1993) found an increase in concordance rates for generalized anxiety disorder among monozygotic compared to dizygotic twins but only for those with a history of a mood disorder. Kendler et al. (1992a) reported results from a sample of over 1000 female twin pairs among whom 23.5% had 1-month generalized anxiety disorder and 5.9% had the 6-month disorder. The tetrachoric correlations were + 0.35 for monozygotic and + 0.12 for dizygotic twins for the 1-month disorder. The authors concluded that generalized anxiety disorder is moderately familial and that the tendency for the disorder to run in families is largely due to genetic factors. They estimated the heritability of the disorder at a modest 30%, and indicated that the remaining variance in liability resulted from environmental factors not shared by the twins. According to Kendler (1996), generalized anxiety disorder and major depression share a genetic predisposition (at least in women), but the environmental risk factors for these disorders may be relatively distinct.

Etiology and pathogenesis

Biological factors

Cerebral metabolism

Functional scans, examining cerebral blood flow and metabolism, have found no specific regional differences between patients with generalized anxiety disorder and normals (for detailed reviews see Wilson & Mathew, 1993; Harris et al., 1995). Only one study, using positron emission tomography, reported lower absolute metabolic rates in basal ganglia and white matter (Wu et al., 1991). In several studies, using 133-xenon inhalation, anxiety correlated negatively with cerebral blood flow, but this finding was not limited to patients with generalized anxiety (Wilson & Mathew, 1993). Vasoconstriction secondary to hyperventilation and increased sympathetic tone might explain lower blood flow and metabolic rates observed in individuals with high anxiety. Wu et al. (1991) reported that change in the anxiety levels of generalized anxiety patients correlated with change in the limbic system and basal ganglia glucose metabolism, which suggests that these structures may be involved in the psychobiology of anxiety.

Grillon & Buchsbaum (1987) found that patients with generalized anxiety disorder have a lesser decrease in alpha activity on the electroencephalogram (EEG) when exposed to light stimuli than normal controls. Also, less variability in the EEG of generalized anxiety patients under task demands was reported by Inz (1990).

Neuroendocrine systems

No neuroendocrine abnormalities have been demonstrated conclusively in generalized anxiety disorder patients. Corticotropin-releasing hormone levels in cerebrospinal fluid were shown to be in the normal range (Fossey et al., 1996). Studies also failed to show increased resting plasma or urinary cortisol levels (Rosenbaum et al., 1983; Hoehn-Saric et al., 1991). Two studies found 27% rates of non-suppression after dexamethasone challenge (Schweizer et al., 1986; Tiller et al., 1988). In one of these, the response normalized after successful behavioral therapy, indicating that, in some patients, non-suppression may have been induced by high levels of anxiety (Tiller et al., 1988).

No abnormalities have been found in cerebrospinal fluid thyrotropin-releasing hormone or in plasma thyroid hormone in generalized anxiety disorder patients (Munjack & Palmer, 1988; Fossey et al., 1993). Serum prolactin levels also have been within the normal range and have not changed with anxiety reduction induced by relaxation (Mathew et al., 1979).

The blockade of opiate receptors by naloxone did not affect the generalized anxiety of these patients to a greater degree than placebo (Hoehn-Saric & Masek, 1981). Also, Khan et al. (1986) found no difference in platelet MAO-B activity. Rocca et al. (1991) reported a reduction in lymphocyte peripheral benzodiazepine receptors that normalized after treatment with a benzodiazepine. Increased urinary tribulin, a non-peptide inhibitor of benzodiazepine binding and of monoamine oxidase activity, was observed to be high in generalized anxiety patients but remained so after successful behavior therapy (Clow et al., 1988).

Generalized anxiety disorder patients appear to be more prone to upper respiratory infections. Among these patients, decreased expression of interleukin 2 receptors correlated linearly with stress intrusion scores and with the number of sick days related to upper respiratory infections (Laria et al., 1996).

Neurotransmitter systems

The central noradrenergic system, when challenged by the alpha-2-noradrenergic antagonist, yohimbine, did not appear to be hypersensitive (Charney et al., 1987); however, Abelson et al. (1991) reported blunted growth hormone response to challenge by clonidine, an alpha-2-agonist, which suggests a downregulation of post-synaptic alpha-2-receptors. Such downregulation, however, is non-specific and occurs in other psychiatric conditions. The same group also reported a reduction in platelet alpha-2-adrenergic binding sites, using tritiated clonidine as a marker (Cameron et al., 1990). Prior exposure to psychotropic drugs may have influenced the results. Mathew et al. (1981) reported increased plasma epinephrine and norepinephrine levels in one study but were unable to reproduce these findings in another (Mathew et al., 1982). They attributed positive results in the first study to premature withdrawal of blood samples after venipuncture. Munjack et al. (1989) found no differences in plasma levels of epinephrine, norepinephrine, or MHPG between generalized anxiety patients and normal controls, while Sevy et al. (1989) found increased plasma norepinephrine and MHPG levels and a decreased number of alpha-2-adrenoreceptors in patients with generalized anxiety disorder.

Only few studies examined the serotonergic system in patients with generalized anxiety. Ritanserin, a serotonin-2 (5-HT$_2$) receptor antagonist, produced the same amount of slow wave sleep in generalized anxiety patients as in healthy controls. Thus, generalized anxiety disorder does not appear to be associated with a hypersensitivity of brain 5-HT$_2$ receptors (Davis, 1992). Schneider et al. (1987) found no differences in platelet imipramine binding sites, or consequently, in the density of serotonin transporters between patients and controls; however, Garvey et al. (1995) found urinary 5-HIAA and VMA levels associated with several anxiety symptoms measured on the Hamilton Anxiety Scale. The same authors also reported an increase of the lysosomal enzyme, N-acetyl-beta-glucosaminides, which could be a marker for serotonin metabolism in generalized anxiety disorder patients (Garvey et al., 1993).

Adenosine has been found to have an inhibiting effect on the central nervous system, an effect antagonized by caffeine. Bruce et al. (1992) found generalized anxiety patients more sensitive to a caffeine challenge in terms of self-reported anxiety and sweating, and in skin conductance, alpha activity, auditory evoked potentials, and critical flicker fusion. A second caffeine challenge study showed no such oversensitivity (Mathew & Wilson, 1990).

Physiological reactivity

In the laboratory, Hoehn-Saric et al. (1989b) and Hazlett et al. (1994) observed that muscle tension but not skin conductance, respiration, heart rate or blood pressure was greater in generalized anxiety disorder patients than in non-anxious controls. During the performance of stressful mental tasks, patients and controls showed similar physiological response, except that skin conductance and heart rate changes were smaller in patients. The smaller changes indicate a narrower range of autonomic reactivity during laboratory stress. These investigators obtained similar results in patients wearing ambulatory monitors and responding to everyday stressors. Birket-Smith et al. (1993) found fluctuations of electrodermal activity and its habituation to be similar in generalized anxiety disorder patients and controls. Others, however, have reported increased heart rate, lower heart rate variability, and lower cardiac vagal tone in patients at rest and during worrisome thinking (Lyonfields et al., 1995; Thayer et al., 1996). On the other hand, still others have not found differences in vagal tone between patients and normals (R. Hoehn-Saric et al., unpublished resuslts; Kollai & Kollai, 1992). Munjack et al. (1993) found a higher mean respiration rate and lower mean venous carbon dioxide pressure in generalized anxiety patients than in controls.

An interesting observation made in several laboratories is that of decreased physiological flexibility among generalized anxiety patients during arousal and psychological stress. Such reduced variability was found in

EEG recordings, forehead muscle tension, heart rate, and skin conductance (Grillon & Buchsbaum, 1987; Hoehn-Saric et al., 1989b; Inz, 1990; Hazlett et al., 1994; Lyonfields et al., 1995; Thayer et al., 1996); however, diminished physiological flexibility is not disorder specific. It may represent a predisposition for developing an anxiety disorder, a partial physiological adaptation to chronic stress, or diminished attention to stimuli that are not specific to the patient's anxiety.

Patients with generalized anxiety disorder frequently complain of sleep disturbances. Sleep studies have shown that these patients have longer sleep latency, shorter duration of sleep, reduced slow wave sleep, but no REM sleep disturbances of the kind seen in major depression (Reynolds et al., 1983; Papadimitrious et al., 1988; Arriaga et al., 1990).

In summary, in spite of their intense anxiety and numerous somatic complaints, patients with generalized anxiety disorder show no specific changes in imaging studies, and to a large extent, appear physiologically similar to non-anxious persons when they are at rest. Only muscle tension and sleep disturbances have consistently been altered. Under laboratory stress, the degree of response in generalized anxiety patients is comparable to that of normal controls, except that the range of responsivity is narrower.

Generalized anxiety disorder patients do not form a homogeneous group, and subgroups may differ in their response to stress. Some studies show increased noradrenergic tone, lower cardiac vagal activity, and hyperventilation in these patients. We found that generalized anxiety patients with prominent cardiovascular symptoms not only needed higher doses of benzodiazepines but also exhibited greater cardiac lability (Hoehn-Saric et al., 1989a). Stress hormone levels appear within the normal range, although subgroups may have higher catecholamine outputs. Differences in methodology, for instance, a shorter rest period before recording or different preparation for the study, as well as differences in physiological characteristics of certain subgroups may explain discrepancies in laboratory findings.

Psychological factors

Personality

The notion that anxiety proneness may arise from personality is contained in the formulations of Spielberger (1972), Eysenck & Eysenck (1985), Gray (1987), and Cloninger (1988). Yet, evidence of a personality vulnerability to generalized anxiety disorder is indirect because few studies have examined

Table 2.5. *Family problems in childhood and adolescence*

	Longitudinal diagnosis				
	Pure depression $N = 137$ (%)	Pure anxiety $N = 29$ (%)	Depression + anxiety $N = 82$ (%)	Controls $N = 207$ (%)	p^*
Conflict between parents	29	38	41	21	0.006
Conflict with parents	38	41	41	23	0.004
Sexual trauma	14	17	20	7	0.03
Lack of attention	30	31	27	14	0.002
Low prestige of family	17	10	18	6	0.01
More severely punished	25	7	27	9	0.0001

*Contingency tables: chi-square with 3 df. *Source*: From Angst and Vollrath (1991). © 1991, Munksgaard International Publishers Ltd. Reprinted with permission.

this disorder apart from others. Early studies of anxious patients found high levels of neuroticism (Kerr et al., 1970; Hoehn-Saric, 1982), and Roth et al. (1972) described premorbid social anxiety, hypersensitivity to criticism, dependence, immaturity, hysteria, and anergia among anxious patients. Prospective studies have also linked preexisting personality traits to the later development of anxiety. Specifically, Nyström & Lindegård (1975) found traits of anxiety and asthenia, and Angst & Vollrath (1991) reported nervousness, depressiveness, instability (low frustration tolerance), inhibition, neuroticism, and autonomic lability. Although, as noted elsewhere, recent studies have found an association between generalized anxiety and anxious personality traits, it is unclear whether these traits are premorbid or reflect the influence of chronic anxiety on personality (Nestadt et al., 1992).

Childhood environment

Evidence for the importance of adverse early environmental factors is accumulating, but these factors may not be specific for generalized anxiety disorder. In an epidemiologic study, Angst & Vollrath (1991) found more family problems during childhood among subjects with anxiety than among controls. As is shown in Table 2.6, more subjects with anxiety reported conflict between parents, conflict with parents, lack of attention from parents, distressing sexual experiences, and low prestige of the family.

These factors were also reported with greater frequency by depressed than by control subjects. Studies comparing patients with generalized anxiety and panic disorder have not found consistent differences in childhood environment (other than separation from a parent) based on small samples (Hoehn-Saric, 1982; Raskin et al., 1982; Torgersen, 1986; Noyes et al., 1992).

The finding of an increased prevalence of generalized anxiety among the adult children of alcoholics suggests that early adversity may be a factor. Data from the ECA study showed that 17.9% of women who had alcoholic fathers had lifetime generalized anxiety disorder compared to 9.7% of women who had not had such fathers (Mathew et al., 1993). In addition to generalized anxiety disorder these women had an increased prevalence of panic disorder, agoraphobia, simple phobia, and dysthymia. It is unclear whether the increase in anxiety disorders was due to an adverse childhood environment or genetic transmission. There is a causal link between certain anxiety and alcohol disorders, and genetic factors may be important (Kushner et al., 1990).

Evidence for the role of adverse childhood environment also comes from studies of the impact of parental loss, although the evidence is conflicting. Kendler et al. (1992b), in a large twin sample, reported that the rates of most psychiatric disorders were increased among persons who had experienced the loss of a parent before age 17 years. In this study, the risk of generalized anxiety disorder was increased by separation from, but not the death of, a parent, a pattern similar to that observed in major depressive disorder. Also, in this study, separation from a mother influenced risk more than separation from a father. In the ECA study, the risks of panic disorder and agoraphobia were increased by parental loss but not generalized anxiety disorder (Tweed et al., 1989). As described elsewhere, parental loss may have a direct effect or an indirect effect, mediated by certain antecedents (e.g., parental conflict) or consequences (e.g., lack of care) of the loss (Kendler et al., 1992b).

Among clinical populations, childhood sexual and physical abuse is associated with anxiety disorders as with other psychopathology (Mancini et al., 1995). Patients with a history of abuse have more severe anxiety disorders and more coexisting depression.

Life events

Stressful life events have long been viewed as having an important role in the generation of anxiety, and evidence of their importance for generalized anxiety disorder is beginning to accumulate (Ifeld, 1979). In the ECA study, information about stressful life events was gathered for the year prior to interview (Blazer et al., 1987). Generalized anxiety disorder was more frequent in men (but not women) who reported four or more events in the previous year. The disorder was also more frequent among persons who reported at least one unexpected, negative, or very important event. In a similar Canadian study, persons with generalized anxiety disorder had higher life event scale scores in the past year than those without the disorder (Newman & Bland, 1994). Such data suggest that adverse events are important but do not indicate whether they are the cause or result of anxiety.

Further evidence for the importance of life events comes from the study of disaster victims. Prevalence rates for generalized anxiety disorder were 10.9% in survivors of the Mount St. Helens' eruption, 16.3% in persons exposed to dioxin and floods, 29% in survivors of a plane crash, and 34.5% in persons exposed to the Exxon Valdez oil spill (Shore et al., 1989; Smith et al., 1986, 1990; Palinkas et al., 1993). Compared to unexposed persons, those with high exposure to the oil spill were 3.6 times as likely to have generalized anxiety disorder in the year after the disaster (Palinkas et al., 1993). Also, generalized anxiety disorder was experienced by 27% of those who lost their retirement savings compared to 10% of control subjects (Ganzini et al., 1990). Consistent with data linking depression to losses and anxiety to threats, the association with major depression was stronger than with generalized anxiety (Finlay-Jones & Brown, 1981). Of course, loss of retirement savings involves both.

Cognitive factors

Cognitive factors may be important in developing and maintaining generalized anxiety disorder. This has been considered in detail by Rapee (1991b). Persons with this disorder appear to have a biased perception of threat as well as a sense of uncontrollability. They focus more attention on detecting potential threats, more readily interpret ambiguous stimuli as threatening, and automatically view threats as greater than non-anxious persons. In addition, they see themselves as lacking control of events which further increases the perception of threat. Worry, which is triggered by such perceptions, may, by reducing anxiety and preventing complete emotional processing, actually reinforce itself and perpetuate the maladaptive response (Borkovec & Inz, 1990).

Clinical picture

Clinical characteristics

Psychological symptoms

Patients with generalized anxiety disorder experience psychological symptoms that are both affective and cognitive in nature. Their mood is often anxious, and they are troubled by a sense of uneasiness or anxious foreboding. Such an affective state is often accompanied by an unpleasant feeling of arousal such that patients feel keyed-up or on-edge. In this state of preparedness, they are unusually sensitive to sensory stimuli (i.e., noise, light, etc.) and experience irritability and a tendency to startle. Patients report that sleep is difficult to initiate because their minds will not turn off, and they are unable to relax their bodies. These symptoms, originally listed under the heading of vigilance and scanning (DSM-III), appear more prominent in generalized anxiety than panic disorder (Noyes et al., 1992).

The defining characteristic of generalized anxiety disorder (DSM-IV) is worry. Patients report that their minds are filled with thoughts and images of what could go wrong and of what might be done to forestall disaster. They recognized that this worry is excessive or unrealistic. Their thinking is ruminative, repetitious and uncontrollable; hence it is unproductive and diverts attention from other activities. While some dwell on possible physical harm (e.g., death of a family member, serious illness in self), others worry about possible social misfortune (e.g., personal failure, criticism from others) (Beck et al., 1974; Zwemer & Diffenbacher, 1984; Borkovec et al., 1991). The thinking of patients tends to be catastrophic, overgeneralized and absolute (i.e., black or white) in nature. They see unlikely dangers as probable and unfortunate consequences as devastating (Beck et al., 1974). Many patients have high standards and demand perfection of themselves or insist upon control when neither is realistic.

Somatic symptoms

Somatic symptoms accompany the apprehension and worry just described, and musculoskeletal symptoms are often prominent (Hazlett et al., 1994). Patients experience tightness in their muscles, especially across their shoulders and in the back of the neck. This tension is often associated with muscle aching and fatigue, and tension headaches are common. Patients also report that they feel restless and are unable to relax. Lack of movement may increase their discomfort and patients with more severe anxiety may be unable to sit, instead pacing to relieve painful inner tension. This motor aspect of anxiety reaches its height in agitation seen in the most severely anxious patients.

Symptoms of autonomic arousal also accompany apprehension and worry (Hoehn-Saric & McLeod, 1993). Patients often experience rapid or forceful heartbeat, sweating, and a sinking sensation in the stomach. The pattern of autonomic symptoms varies from one individual to the next. Parasympathetically mediated gastrointestinal symptoms may be more frequent in generalized anxiety than panic disorder (Cameron et al., 1986; Hoehn-Saric et al., 1989b). Some patients experience dry mouth, abdominal distress, nausea, and diarrhea. Others experience sweaty or cold clammy hands, frequent urination, and ringing in the ears. Sympathetically-mediated symptoms are less prominent than in panic disorder but many patients experience cardiovascular symptoms (Noyes et al., 1992). They report tightness in the chest, shortness of breath, feelings of dizziness, and parasthesias in addition to rapid and irregular heartbeat.

Vegetative disturbances may also be part of the clinical picture. Patients may experience changes in sex drive and appetite. Some find that sexual activity and eating relieve tension while others lose interest in food and sex with increased anxiety (Hoehn-Saric & McLeod, 1990). In addition to initial insomnia, patients find their sleep restless and their dreams filled with disasters of one kind or another.

Avoidant behavior

Generalized anxiety disorder does not have the obvious avoidance seen with phobic disorders. Still, avoidance of a more subtle kind is an important clinical feature (Gelder, 1991). Patients have a dislike for situations and people that are new or unfamiliar, hence they avoid them. They tend to avoid social situations where they fear embarrassment or physical environments where they fear physical injury. In such situations they are often reticent or timid, avoiding confrontation or risk of injury, however remote. Many are unassertive and defer to others, showing anxious personality traits in the interpersonal sphere. Avoidance may extend to anxious thoughts and feelings, the internal representations of the disorder. Such diversion of attention prevents reappraisal of danger and interferes with finding solutions to problems (Gelder, 1991).

Subtypes

Those who write about generalized anxiety disorder frequently comment on the heterogeneity of the category. There have, however, been few suggestions concerning possible subtypes. Various investigators have observed interacting dimensions of anxiety and suggested that patients might be categorized according to predominant symptomatology. Following this notion, patients were separated into those with predominantly psychic versus those with somatic symptoms and their response to medication examined (Tyrer, 1976). Also, based upon an extensive review of the literature, Cloninger (1986) identified prototypic psychic and somatic forms of anxiety associated with contrasting personality traits, learned response styles, physiological reactivity, and response to psychoactive drugs.

In an effort to distinguish a characterological subtype from a more discrete syndrome, Hoehn-Saric et al. (1993) compared patients with early and late onset (before or after age 20 years). Early-onset patients were younger and less likely to report precipitating events. During childhood the early-onset patients were exposed to more domestic disturbances, had more fears, were more inhibited, and were more socially maladjusted. As adults they had higher trait anxiety, higher neuroticism, more interpersonal sensitivity, and more obsessional traits. The authors concluded that early-onset patients might have greater constitutional vulnerability to stressors, more adverse early environment, or a more severe anxiety disorder. Late-onset patients appeared to have been better adjusted until unfavorable events precipitated anxiety symptoms.

Pattern of morbidity

The notion that generalized anxiety disorder is a mild disturbance with little impairment has been challenged by recent studies. In the National Comorbidity Survey (NCS), subjects meeting DSM-III-R criteria (impairment not required) were asked if the disorder had ever interfered a lot with their life and activities, if they had ever sought professional help for it, and if they had ever taken medication for the disorder (Wittchen et al., 1994). As is shown in Table 2.7, 82.0% of those with lifetime generalized anxiety disorder endorsed at least one of these indicators of significant impairment. The results also show that, while comorbidity was associated with higher endorsement, 59.2% of those without comorbidity reported at least one indicator.

Data from a large clinical sample, show that, for persons who become psychiatric patients, generalized anxiety disorder is associated with significant impairment. Among the patients studied by Massion et al. (1993) only 52% were employed full-time and 25% were receiving disability payments.

Table 2.6. *Indicators of impairment reported by persons meeting criteria for lifetime Generalized Anxiety Disorder*

GAD	Interference (%)	Help seeking (%)	Medication (%)	Any indicator (%)
Without comorbidity	28.1	48.2	24.1	59.2
With comorbidity	51.2	67.9	46.2	84.4
All subjects	49.0	66.0	44.0	82.0

GAD: Generalized Anxiety Disorder. *Source*: Wittchen et al. (1994). © 1994, American Medical Association. Reprinted with permission.

About a third reported missing more than a week of work in the past year due to emotional problems. Of those who were married, a quarter rated their relationship as fair or poor. About a quarter rated their physical health as fair or poor and three-quarters gave their emotional health a similar rating. Of course, most of these patients had comorbid disorders contributing to overall disability.

Natural history

Onset

Generalized anxiety disorder may begin at any age, but the peak period appears to be the mid-teens (Raskin et al., 1982; Anderson et al., 1984; Rapee, 1985, 1991a; Thyer et al., 1985; Barlow et al., 1986a; Blazer et al., 1991). Up to 30% of persons experience an onset in childhood before the age of 11 (Rapee, 1989). This is consistent with the high prevalence of overanxious disorder (eliminated from DSM-IV) that may persist into adulthood (Rey et al., 1992). Many persons describe lifelong symptoms or find it difficult to be precise about when symptoms first began. Persons with a childhood onset appear to have a more severe disorder (Hoehn-Saric et al., 1993).

The onset of generalized anxiety disorder is gradual and is frequently associated with stressful life events (Barrett, 1979; Anderson et al., 1984; Rapee, 1985; Angst & Vollrath, 1991). Treatment seeking for generalized anxiety disorder is often delayed many years. Rapee (1991a) noted that, for a particular clinical population, nearly 25 years had elapsed between the onset and presentation for treatment. This delay is likely due to the insidious onset, misinterpretation of symptoms, and barriers to treatment (Nisita et al., 1990). Also, persons with generalized anxiety disorder are more likely to seek help from alternative sources, such as acupuncture, self-help books, etc. (Rapee, 1985).

Course and outcome

By definition generalized anxiety disorder has a duration of at least 6 months. The data with respect to course are limited but indicate that, as defined, it has greater chronicity than panic disorder (Rickels & Schweizer, 1990). Much of this data was collected prior to DSM-III and deals with anxiety states or neuroses. This literature, reviewed by Greer (1969), Marks & Lader (1973), and Angst & Vollrath (1991), tends to combine the now separated categories of generalized anxiety and panic. Across studies, the recovery rates for anxiety disorders (generalized anxiety and panic disorder) vary between 12 and 25%. As Angst & Vollrath (1991) stated, even after many years, most subjects still suffer from at least mild symptoms, and about half have more severe symptoms with impairment in work and social functioning.

Clinical samples of patients with generalized anxiety disorder are notable for their chronicity (Anderson et al., 1984). For instance, Barlow et al. (1986) reported that patients in their early 40s had had continuous symptoms for an average of over 20 years. Also, Noyes et al. (1987) described uninterrupted symptoms in 75% of patients. In a follow-up of patients with generalized anxiety disorder 1 year after they had taken part in a treatment study, Mancuso et al. (1993) found that 50% still met criteria for the disorder despite having received additional treatment. Longer follow-ups of treated samples have found low rates of remission and less favorable outcomes compared to patients with panic disorder (Woodman et al., 1995; Yonkers et al., 1996). The waxing and waning course of generalized anxiety disorder is influenced by the level of stressful events or difficulties (Rickels & Schweizer, 1990; Leenstra et al., 1995).

Follow-ups of treated samples show that psychological therapy favorably influences long-term course. Based on their review of recent studies, Durham & Allan (1993) concluded that generalized anxiety patients who had benefited from newly developed psychological methods maintained their improvement for 6–12 months afterward. There is little evidence of long-term benefit from pharmacological therapy once discontinued, however. High relapse rates (63% and 81%) have been reported 1 year after acute treatment with benzodiazepines (Rickels et al., 1980, 1986). In one study, 47% of patients who received 6 months of anxiolytic therapy still had moderate to severe anxiety after 40 months (Rickels & Schweizer, 1990).

Complications

Alcohol and drug dependence

The prevalence of alcohol and drug use disorders is higher among persons in the community with generalized anxiety disorder than those with no disorder. According to the National Comorbidity Survey (NCS), 37.6% of those with the lifetime disorder had an alcohol disorder and 27.6% had a drug use disorder. Kushner et al. (1990) stated that generalized anxiety often results from alcohol use and may be a manifestation of alcohol withdrawal. Of course, generalized anxiety symptoms accompany the alcohol withdrawal syndrome and are difficult to distinguish from it (Brown & Barlow, 1992). As with other anxiety disorders, alcohol or drugs may be used to self-medicate, and this may result in dependence. The finding of a high rate of generalized anxiety disorder among the children of alcoholics suggests a possible genetic component (Mathew et al., 1993).

Major depressive disorder

Epidemiologic and clinical studies indicate that major depressive disorder is a frequent complication of generalized anxiety disorder. The rate of lifetime major depression was 62.4% in the NCS study (Wittchen et al., 1994). Similar rates have been found in clinical samples (Brown & Barlow, 1992). The onset of generalized anxiety disorder usually precedes the onset of depression (Brawman-Mintzer et al., 1993). Other comorbid disorders, either mental or physical, increase the likelihood of depression (Noyes et al., 1992). Comorbid depression is an important factor in treatment-seeking (Wittchen et al., 1994).

Suicide

Generalized anxiety disorder does not appear to be associated with suicidal behavior. One study of psychiatric outpatients found suicidal ideation (ever) in 18% and suicide attempts (ever) in 17% of patients with this disorder (Asnis et al., 1993). However, the rate of suicidal ideation was significantly less than that found in patients with depression, substance use, and adjustment disorders.

Predictors of course and outcome

Although some prognostic factors have been identified for anxiety disorders in general, it is unclear how they apply to generalized anxiety disorder. In their review, Angst & Vollrath (1991) found no evidence that demographic factors, such as age and gender, have prognostic value. Other variables, such as social class and marital status, may be important. The general rule that future course is best predicted by the past probably applies to generalized anxiety disorder, and a duration of less than 3 years may be more favorable than longer (Noyes et al., 1980).

Comorbidity appears to have prognostic significance (Angst & Vollrath, 1991). In a retrospective study, Mancuso et al. (1993) found more personality disorders among subjects who still met criteria for generalized anxiety disorder after 1 year, and Mann et al. (1981), in a prospective study, found some effect of premorbid personality on outcome of neurotic outpatients after 1 year. There is also some evidence that chronic physical illness and depression worsen the prognosis of anxious patients (Giel et al., 1978; Huxley et al., 1979; Murphy et al., 1986). Also, Mancuso et al. (1993) found coexisting dysthymia and social phobia associated with a worse prognosis.

The influence of life events on course is unclear (Angst & Vollrath, 1991). Mancuso et al. (1993) found no difference in the number of life events reported by good and poor prognosis patients 6 months prior to follow-up. Some studies have found that life events influence the course and outcome of anxiety disorders but others have not (Giel et al., 1978; Davies et al., 1983; Wittchen & von Zerssen, 1987). One study suggests that different types of events may be associated with recovery from anxiety and depression (Brown, 1991). Similarly, the influence of social support on outcome remains unknown (Wittchen & von Zerssen, 1987).

Differential diagnosis

To begin with, generalized anxiety disorder must be distinguished from anxiety disorders due to general medical conditions and substances (see Chapter 7). The diagnosis of anxiety disorder due to a general medical condition is reserved for patients whose symptoms are a direct biological consequence of a specific condition. Many medical conditions are associated with anxiety syndromes and, for some, the typical clinical picture is one of generalized anxiety (e.g., hyperthyroidism, pheochromocytoma) (Table 7.6). Where a medical condition exists, a temporal relationship between anxiety symptoms and the illness should be present. Evidence from the literature of an association between anxiety symptoms and the existing condition supports such a diagnosis. Also, features that are atypical for a primary anxiety disorder (e.g., unusual age of onset, absence of family history) support the diagnosis of an anxiety disorder due to a medical condition (American Psychiatric Association, 1994).

Generalized anxiety disorder must also be distinguished from a substance-induced anxiety disorder. Anxiety disorders can occur during intoxication with some substances and withdrawal from others. Generalized anxiety commonly follows intoxication with stimulants (e.g., amphetamines, cocaine, caffeine), sympathomimetics (e.g., ephedrine, theophylline) and withdrawal from alcohol, sedative hypnotics (e.g., barbiturates) and benzodiazepines. The list of substances and medications that may cause anxiety symptoms is long (Table 7.7). Generalized anxiety symptoms should alert the clinician to substance use disorders and to toxicity of certain therapeutic drugs (e.g., theophylline, thyroxine). Blood levels of agents known to cause anxiety may be useful. A detailed history of drug administration, including relationships between anxiety symptoms and initiation of treatment, dose changes, etc., may also be helpful.

Generalized anxiety is commonly associated with mood and psychotic disorders, and according to DSM-IV, should not be diagnosed separately if it occurs exclusively during the course of such conditions (American Psychiatric Association, 1994). It may be diagnosed in the presence of other anxiety disorders providing the focus of worry is not the other disorder. For instance, excessive worry should not be restricted to having a panic attack or its feared consequences, such as having a heart attack or losing one's mind. Similarly, worry should not be focused exclusively on embarrassment in public situations as in social phobia or on obsessions (e.g., fear of contamination, fear of harming someone) as in obsessive-compulsive disorder.

The worry of generalized anxiety disorder must be distinguished from obsessional thoughts and from worry about health that is characteristic of hypochondriasis. Obsessional thoughts are not simply exaggerated worries about everyday problems but are ego-dystonic intrusions upon an individual's mental life (American Psychiatric Association, 1994). Also, they may take the form of images, urges, or impulses, whereas the worry of generalized anxiety is almost exclusively thoughts (Brown et al., 1993b). Persons with generalized anxiety disorder may worry excessively about their health as part of a pattern of anxious preoccupation about many areas of life; however, if fear of serious disease, despite lack of evidence, is the dominant and exclusive focus of worry, then a diagnosis of hypochondriasis may be warranted (American Psychiatric Association, 1994).

Generalized anxiety disorder must also be distinguished from adjustment disorder with anxious mood. Stressful life events are commonly associated with the onset or exacerbations of generalized anxiety disorder, and the diagnosis of an adjustment disorder should only be made when the criteria for generalized anxiety disorder are not met. Adjustment disorder is a residual category reserved for patients who do not have sufficient generalized anxiety symptoms and whose disturbance does not last 6 months or after termination of the stressor or its consequences. Adjustment disorders may become chronic in reaction to continuing stressors or stressors with enduring consequences.

Finally, generalized anxiety disorder must also be distinguished from normal worry and anxiety. This is difficult because there is no clear point of demarcation. Several factors are important to consider. In DSM-IV an impairment criterion has been added; the anxiety, worry, or physical symptoms must cause significant distress or impairment (American Psychiatric Association, 1994). Also, the worry of generalized anxiety disorder, in addition to being excessive, is difficult to control, and this characteristic is important in separating abnormal from normal worry (Sanderson & Barlow, 1990; Marten et al., 1993). In addition, normal worry is less likely than that of generalized anxiety disorder to be accompanied by physical symptoms. In general, the worry of generalized anxiety disorder is more pervasive, pronounced, distressing, longer lasting, and more likely to occur without provocation. Also, it involves more life circumstances than does normal worry (Borkovec et al., 1993).

Treatment

Management

Most patients with generalized anxiety disorder present to, and are managed by, primary physicians, although some with more severe symptoms and comorbid disorders are referred to psychiatrists or other mental health professionals. Psychological and pharmacological treatments are both effective, but residual symptoms and stress-related vulnerability commonly persist. Most patients should receive some form of psychological intervention, and some, but not all, may benefit from medication (Andrews et al., 1994). Education and supportive counseling, conducted by the primary physician, is all that many patients require. Cognitive behavioral therapy has proven beneficial and is the treatment of choice where trained professionals are available. With respect to drug therapy, benzodiazepines have a long-established place in the treatment of anxiety and are the drugs of choice for rapid control of symptoms, but because of their dependence potential, short-term administration is usually advised. For long-term administration an antidepressant, such as imipramine, is perhaps the treatment of choice.

Patients with generalized anxiety disorder should first have a thorough physical examination and routine laboratory testing to rule out a physical cause of symptoms. Additional screening is usually not necessary, but where symptoms of a particular organ system are prominent, testing directed toward that system (e.g., electrocardiogram for chest tightness, palpitations) may be considered. The most common physical cause is hyperthyroidism, but routine thyroid tests are not usually necessary. Patients with prominent somatic symptoms are concerned about their health, so appropriate reassurance can relieve this added source of worry. Also, inquiry should be directed towards use of caffeine, alcohol, and illicit drugs, and where use is associated with symptoms, discontinuation should be advised.

Most patients with mild generalized anxiety can be treated in the primary care setting by supportive counseling without resort to medication (Shapiro et al., 1983; Catalan et al., 1984). In addition to providing emotional support, brief counseling focuses on sources of anxiety that can be modified. Patients are helped to identify problems, then make changes by confronting them directly or altering their lifestyle in some manner. Also, many will benefit from being taught problem-solving skills and stress-management techniques. Counseling may be supplemented by self-help materials (Marks, 1989; Sorby et al., 1991; Lader, 1994). For patients with more severe anxiety, specific psychological techniques and medication may be helpful.

Psychological treatment

Research examining psychological treatment for generalized anxiety disorder is recent (Barlow et al., 1992; Hoehn-Saric et al., 1995; Barlow & Lehman, 1996). Early studies focused on the physiologic manifestations of anxiety and evoking the relaxation response to control them. Later studies added behavioral and cognitive interventions. These included imaginal exposure to anxiety cues coupled with relaxation, anxiety management training, and modification of dysfunctional cognitions. Current approaches combine these procedures and often include training in coping more effectively with anxiety as well as problem-solving strategies to deal with interpersonal sources of anxiety, time management, etc. Reviews of controlled trials indicate that such therapy is effective and superior to analytically-oriented psychotherapy (Hunt & Singh, 1991; Rapee, 1991a; Durham & Allan, 1993; Andrews et al., 1994; Durham et al., 1994; Borkovec & Whisman, 1996).

Borkovec & Whisman (1996) reviewed controlled studies that met stringent methodologic criteria. The average duration of symptoms in the nearly 600 subjects treated was more than 5 years. In these studies, psychological treatments were more effective than no treatment and produced significant change. Also, improvement was maintained for 6–12 months, and in two studies, further improvement was observed (Butler et al., 1988; White & Keenan, 1992). Evidence favoring specific interventions over nonspecific therapies is only suggestive. Several studies compared cognitive behavioral therapies in this regard. Of these, four found no difference, but two found cognitive behavioral therapy superior (Borkovec et al., 1988; Butler et al., 1991).

In their review, Durham & Allan (1993) agreed with these conclusions but noted that, overall, psychological treatment had resulted in only modest improvement. They found the mean reduction in Hamilton Anxiety Scale scores across studies was only about 50%, similar to that observed in studies employing benzodiazepines (Barlow, 1988). The average reduction in these drug studies to be 47.5% compared to 30% with placebo. In studies that included criteria for a favorable response, about half returned to normal functioning. Durham & Allan (1993) noted that the best results are obtained in primary care patients not on anxiolytic medication. Patients seen in psychiatric facilities appear less responsive to psychological therapy.

Cognitive behavioral therapy, designed to correct maladaptive responding to threats, has been described by Borkovec & Whisman (1996). This therapy focuses upon worrisome thinking, catastrophic imagery, autonomic activation, behavioral avoidance, and external threats. As anxious patterns of responding are identified, efforts are made to replace them with adaptive coping strategies. Applied relaxation methods relieve somatic manifestations of anxiety (especially muscle tension) and reduce the intrusion of worrisome thoughts (e.g., initial insomnia). Patients are instructed to practice applied relaxation twice a day and are taught derivative techniques (e.g., differential relaxation, cue-controlled relaxation) for coping with stressors and developing a relaxed lifestyle (Öst, 1987).

Patients with generalized anxiety use repetitious thoughts to avoid fear-evoking imagery (Borkovec & Lyonfields, in press). To counteract this, patients are taught to generate fear-producing images, and at the same time, elicit relaxation to reduce associated anxiety. This technique is called self-control desensitization and is used to extinguish aversive responses (Brown et al., 1993b). Cognitive therapy methods, based on techniques outlined by Beck & Emery (1985), include logical analysis of probability, development of adaptive thoughts, behavioral testing of predictions, and decatastrophizing, all by the Socratic method. Using these methods, patients learn more adaptive and flexible methods of coping that can be sustained over time. Many mental health professionals are trained in such cognitive behavioral methods.

Psychopharmacological treatment

A number of medications, including tricyclic antidepressants, benzodiazepines, azopriones, beta-blocking drugs, and antihistaminics are efficacious in generalized anxiety disorder (reviewed by Hoehn-Saric et al., 1995). The benzodiazepines are widely prescribed, and an extensive literature supports their use; however, the role of these and other drugs in the treatment of generalized anxiety disorder remains unclear. The literature examining efficacy is extensive, but most of it appeared before generalized anxiety disorder appeared in DSM-III. Studies before and since have had methodological problems and inconsistent findings (Solomon & Hart, 1978; Perry et al., 1990; Swinson et al., 1993). In a recent review, Perry et al. (1990) noted that, although the benzodiazepines appear to be effective, differences between drug and placebo are not always strong. Indeed, the placebo response rate of 40% for generalized anxiety disorder is perhaps the highest among the anxiety disorders (Fossey & Lydiard, 1990). Consequently, nonspecific factors are important in the treatment of this disorder.

Few comparisons of pharmacological and psychological treatments, either alone or in combination, have been made. Shapiro et al. (1983) found little effect of diazepam over placebo in anxious psychiatric outpatients when these agents were added to brief psychotherapy. Diazepam was superior in patients with medium or high levels of anxiety but not those with lower levels. Power et al. (1990a, b, 1991) found that primary care patients who received cognitive behavioral therapy plus diazepam did better than those who received cognitive behavioral therapy plus placebo. Seventy-six percent of patients receiving the combined treatment were very much improved.

Short-term efficacy, however, is only part of the issue. Relapse rates are high for patients who discontinue benzodiazepines, whereas patients who received cognitive behavioral treatment characteristically maintain therapeutic gains (Rickels et al., 1986; Borkovec & Whisman, 1996). For example, Rickels et al. (1986) observed that 63% of general practice patients who had been treated with diazepam relapsed within 1 year. Also, the question of whether drug therapy diminishes or enhances the effectiveness of psychological treatments remains unsettled (Hoehn-Saric et al., 1995).

Benzodiazepines

The short-term anxiolytic effects of benzodiazepines are well documented (Shader & Greenblatt, 1983; Hollister et al., 1993). These drugs have their most pronounced effects on arousal and somatic anxiety (Hoehn-Saric et al., 1988; Rickels et al., 1993). They also reduce hypervigilance, induce muscle relaxation and, in higher doses, cause sedation; however, their effect on psychic symptoms is less, so the tendency to worry and feel anxious may be only slightly affected. Whether benzodiazepines maintain their effectiveness long-term is less clear. Although tolerance develops to sedative and other effects, it does not appear to develop to the anxiolytic effects. Most patients receive the same benefit for months or years without having to increase the dose (Uhlenhuth et al., 1988).

The various benzodiazepines are similar in their therapeutic properties but differ in terms of pharmacokinetics (e.g., rate of absorption, elimination half-life) (Greenblatt et al., 1981). Drugs that are rapidly absorbed, such as diazepam, may have greater abuse potential. Drugs with long elimination half-lives, such as clonazepam, give a more even effect and require less frequent administration. The main side-effect is sedation, but this often subsides with time or dose reduction. Mild cognitive and memory impairment may occur with therapeutic doses but this is rarely of clinical significance except in the elderly (Pomara et al., 1984). Likewise, slight psychomotor impairment is rarely important except in the elderly or persons using alcohol. The drugs are safe in overdose, but combined with other substances, may contribute to successful suicide.

The greatest drawback to the benzodiazepines is their dependence potential. Psychological dependence (i.e., craving, drug-seeking behavior, increasing the dose for the same effect) is rare and is usually associated with abuse of multiple drugs. Physical dependence (i.e., rebound anxiety, discontinuation symptoms) occurs in nearly half of persons who use therapeutic doses for a year or more (Noyes et al., 1988). The severity of withdrawal symptoms is influenced by the dose, duration of use, rate of discontinuation, and elimination half-life of the drug. Discontinuation of benzodiazepines, even if accomplished slowly (e.g., over 6–10 weeks), may be associated with rebound anxiety that can be difficult to distinguish from symptoms of the original disorder.

Tricyclic antidepressants

Several studies have examined the efficacy of imipramine in generalized anxiety disorder. Three were controlled trials in which imipramine was compared to a benzodiazepine or another tricyclic (Kahn et al., 1986; Hoehn-Saric ct al., 1988; Rickels et al., 1993). In these trials, the benzodiazepine showed the earliest effects and was superior to tricyclics during the first 2 weeks. Beginning with the second or third week, imipramine showed comparable efficacy and, in one study, became superior to chlordiazepoxide (Kahn et al., 1986). Imipramine proved more effective in relieving psychic symptoms of worry, apprehension, and tension whereas the benzodiazepines (i.e., alprazolam and diazepam) had more effect on somatic symptoms (Hoehn-Saric et al., 1988; Rickels et al., 1993). In one study, moderate to marked improvement was reported by 73% of patients on imipramine compared to 66% on diazepam and 47% on placebo (Rickels et al., 1993). The mean daily dose of imipramine was 91 mg in one study and 143 mg in the other, which suggests that patients with generalized anxiety disorder may respond to lower doses than patients with panic or major depressive disorder. Such drugs may be especially useful in patients with coexisting depression (Rickels et al., 1993).

Azapirone

Azapirones are partial agonists of the serotonin receptor that are pharmacologically unrelated to benzodiazepines (Cadieux, 1996). Buspirone, the only currently available azapirone, has been shown to have anxiety-reducing properties comparable to those of benzodiazepines; however, unlike the benzodiazepines, it does not have muscle relaxant or sedative properties. Also, it appears to have no dependence potential or discontinuation symptoms. Buspirone does not act immediately and must be taken regularly for 2 weeks or more to be effective. Also, like the tricyclic antidepressants, it has more effect upon psychic than somatic symptoms. Patients taking buspirone may also report less anger and interpersonal sensitivity (Rickels et al., 1982). Side-effects include nausea, headaches and, in higher doses, jitteriness and dysphoria. The drug does not potentiate the effects of alcohol and is compatible with most medications.

Beta-blocking drugs

Beta-adrenergic blocking drugs inhibit the effects of epinephrine and norepinephrine on beta-adrenergic receptors (Noyes, 1988b). Drugs like propranolol appear to block the peripheral manifestations of anxiety, especially rapid heart rate and tremor, thereby reducing the somatic symptoms. Some beta-blockers cross the blood–brain barrier while others do not, but for the most part, their anxiety-reducing effects are peripheral.

Beta-blockers have no dependence potential and are generally well-tolerated. Side-effects include dizziness, fatigue, and trouble sleeping; also, depressed mood may occur in persons with a history of depression. The drugs should be avoided in patients with asthma, heart block, bradycardia, or cardiac failure. Abrupt discontinuation may be dangerous in patients with coronary artery disease due to rebound effects. The anxiolytic effects of drugs such as propranolol, atenolol, etc., appear to be less potent than those of the benzodiazepines and are of little benefit in more severe anxiety (e.g., panic disorder).

Antihistamines

Antihistamines, such as benadryl, also have anxiolytic effects. These drugs block the H receptor that mediates the level of arousal. They decrease vigilance and hyperalertness but appear to have little effect on psychic anxiety. The anxiolytic effects are weaker than those of benzodiazepines, and in effective doses, may be quite sedating (Rickels et al., 1970). The antihistaminic effects of sedating tricyclic antidepressants (e.g., doxepin, amitriptyline) may explain their immediate anxiolytic effects. Antihistamines may be administered in single doses or on a regular basis because of their rapid action. In spite of their relatively weak anxiolytic action, they remain popular because they are not habit-forming.

Treatment guidelines

Generalized anxiety disorder is a variable and complex disturbance. Treatment must be approached individually, taking into account the type and severity of symptoms, factors that elicit or aggravate symptoms, life stressors, coping ability, personality traits, and motivation for change (reviewed by Hoehn-Saric et al., 1995). In the majority of cases, generalized anxiety is chronic, but the severity of symptoms may be influenced by stressful circumstances.

The first decision has to do with whether a patient needs psychotherapy, pharmacotherapy, or both. Often patients request a certain type of therapy, and their wishes should be considered. Mild forms of anxiety respond well to simple psychological interventions and usually do not require medications (Catalan et al., 1984). More severe generalized anxiety usually requires pharmacological treatment. For reduction of general tension, hyperalertness, insomnia, and physical symptoms, benzodiazepines are the most effective medications. They should be given on a regular basis for several weeks to provide steady relief. During this time, the physician should initiate supportive therapy or make arrangements for cognitive behavioral therapy.

Patients who have a history of substance abuse or who have unstable personality disorders should not receive benzodiazepines. When alcohol or drug abuse coexists with anxiety symptoms, steps must be taken to discontinue the abused substances including substance abuse treatment, if necessary (Brawman-Mintzer & Lydiard, 1997). Once this is accomplished, the patient's symptoms should be reevaluated. Treatment with drugs lacking abuse potential (e.g., tricyclic antidepressants, buspirone) may be advisable. Tollefson et al. (1992) found that buspirone reduced both anxiety and craving for alcohol in alcoholics with generalized anxiety disorder.

For regular administration, benzodiazepines with longer half-lives are generally preferable because they have a more even effect than those with short half-lives. Drugs with short half-lives may cause rebound anxiety between doses, especially early morning anxiety (Kales et al., 1983). On the other hand, elderly patients and those with liver disease should receive benzodiazepines with short half-lives (e.g., lorazepam) to avoid accumulation and excessive sedation.

An important question is how long a patient should remain on a benzodiazepine. The data reviewed above indicate that many patients need long-term or intermittent psychological treatment or medication. A substantial minority require only short intervention. For such patients, a few weeks or months of drug treatment may suffice (Brawman-Mintzer & Lydiard, 1997). Thereafter, attempts should be made to reduce the dose. When a benzodiazepine has been given for long periods, Rickels et al. (1990) negotiates an agreement with patients to reduce the dose to the point of complete withdrawal, but promises to reinstitute medication should significant anxiety persist 4 weeks after discontinuation. Otto et al. (1993) have had success with a cognitive behavioral intervention designed to help patients discontinue medication, and Chiaie et al. (1995) found that buspirone reduced rebound anxiety and withdrawal symptoms on discontinuation.

Patients with intense psychic symptoms may profit from antidepressants or buspirone. The disadvantage of these medications is that they have little immediate effect and thus have to be taken regularly. While no controlled studies exist, clinical experience suggests that antidepressants are more potent than buspirone. As neither of these medications has strong effects on the autonomic system, a combination with a benzodiazepine or beta-blocker may be useful in patients with prominent somatic symptoms.

Regardless of what medication is used or how it is prescribed, it is important to tell patients that a drug is a helpful adjuvant in the effort to acquire better techniques for reducing anxiety and coping with life's stressors. The message is that medication is not an end in itself. Patients should be constantly encouraged to develop more effective approaches that will permit them to live without medication, or if medication is necessary, with the smallest possible dose.

References

Abel, J. L., Borkovec, T. D. In Press. Generalizability of DSM-III-R generalized anxiety disorders to proposed DSM-IV criteria and cross-validation of proposed changes. *J. Affect. Dis.*

Abelson, J. L., Glitz, D., Cameron, O. G. et al. 1991. Blunted growth hormone response to clonidine in patients with generalized anxiety disorder. *Arch. Gen. Psychiat.* 48:157–162.

American Psychiatric Association 1968. *Diagnostic and Statistical Manual of Mental Disorders,* Second Edition, American Psychiatric Association, Washington, DC.

American Psychiatric Association 1980. *Diagnostic and Statistical Manual of Mental Disorders,* Third Edition, American Psychiatric Association, Washington, DC.

American Psychiatric Association 1987. *Diagnostic and Statistical Manual of Mental Disorders,* Third Edition, Revised, American Psychiatric Association, Washington, DC.

American Psychiatric Association 1994. *Diagnostic and Statistical Manual of Mental Disorders,* Fourth Edition, American Psychiatric Association, Washington, DC.

Anderson, D. J., Noyes, R. & Crowe, R. R. 1984. A comparison of panic disorder and generalized anxiety disorder. *Am. J. Psychiatry* 141: 572–575.

Andrews, G., Stewart, G., Allen, R. et al. 1990a. The genetics of six neurotic disorders: A twin study. *J. Affect. Dis.* 19: 23–29.

Andrews, G., Crino, R., Hunt, C. et al. 1994. *The Treatment of Anxiety Disorders: Clinicians Guide and Patient Manuals,* Cambridge University Press, Cambridge, pp. 307–318.

Angst, J. & Vollrath, M. 1991. The natural history of anxiety disorders. *Acta Psychiatrica Scand.* 84: 446–452.

Angst, J., Vollrath, M., Merikangas, K. et al. 1990. Comorbidity of anxiety and depression in the Zurich Cohort Study of Young Adults. In *Comorbidity of Mood and Anxiety Disorders,* eds. J. D. Maser, C. R. Cloninger, pp. 123–137, American Psychiatric Press, Washington, DC.

Arriaga, F. & Paiva, T. 1990. Clinical and EEG sleep changes in primary dysthymia and generalized anxiety: A comparison with normal controls. *Neuropsychobiology* 24: 109–114.

Asnis, G. M., Friedman, T. A., Sanderson, W. C. et al. 1993. Suicidal behavior in adult psychiatric outpatients. I. Description and prevalence. *Am. J. Psychiatry* 150: 108–112.

Ballenger, J. C., Burrows, G., DuPont, R. L. et al. 1988. Alprazolam in panic
    disorder and agoraphobia: Results of a multicenter trial. I. Efficacy in
    short-term treatment. *Arch. Gen. Psychiatry* 45: 413–422.
Barlow, D. H. 1985. The dimensions of anxiety disorders. In *Anxiety and the
    Anxiety Disorders*, eds. A. H. Tuma, J. D. Maser, pp. 479–500, Lawrence
    Erlbaum Association, Hillsdale, NJ.
Barlow, D. H. 1988. *Anxiety and Its Disorders: The Nature and Treatment of
    Anxiety and Panic*, Guilford Press, New York.
Barlow, D. H., Blanchard, E. B., Vermilyea, J. A. et al. 1986. Generalized anxiety
    and generalized anxiety disorder: Description and reconceptualization. *Am.
    J. Psychiatry* 143: 40–44.
Barlow, D. H. & DiNardo, P. A. 1991. The diagnosis of generalized anxiety
    disorder: Development, current status, and future directions. In *Chronic
    Anxiety: Generalized Anxiety Disorders and Mixed Anxiety-Depression*, eds.
    R. M. Rapee, D. H. Barlow, pp. 95–118, Guildord Press, New York.
Barlow, D. H. & Lehman, C. L. 1996. Advances in the treatment of anxiety
    disorders. Implications for psychological national health care. *Arch. Gen.
    Psychiatry* 53: 727–735.
Barlow, D. H., Rapee, R. M. & Brown, T. A. 1992. Behavioral treatment of
    generalized anxiety disorder. *Behav. Ther.* 23: 551–570.
Barrett, J. E. 1979. The relationship of life events to the onset of neurotic
    disorders. In *Stress and Mental Disorder*, eds. J. E. Barrett et al., Raven Press,
    New York.
Barrett, J. E., Barrett, J. A., Oxman, T. E. et al. 1988. The prevalence of psychiatric
    disorders in a primary care practice. *Arch. Gen. Psychiatry* 45: 1100–1106.
Beck, A. T., Apstein, N., Brown, G. et al. 1988. An inventory for measuring
    clinical anxiety: Psychometric properties. *J. Consult. Clin. Psychol.* 56:
    893–897.
Beck, A. T., Brown, G., Steer, R. A. et al. 1987. Differentiating anxiety and
    depression: A list of the content-specific hypotheses. *J. Abn. Psychol.* 96:
    179–183.
Beck, A. T. & Emery, G. 1985. *Anxiety Disorders and Phobias: A Cognitive
    Perspective*. Basic Books, New York.
Beck, A. T., Laude, R. & Bohnert, M. 1974. Ideational components of anxiety
    neurosis. *Arch. Gen. Psychiatry* 31: 319–325.
Beck, P., Kastrup, M. & Rafaelsen, O. J. 1986. Mini-compendium of rating scales
    for states of anxiety, depression, mania, schizophrenia with corresponding
    DSM-III syndromes. *Acta Psychiatrica. Scand.* 73 (Suppl. 326): 6–13.
Birket-Smith, M., Hasle, N. & Jensen, H. H. 1993. Electrodermal activity in
    anxiety disorders. *Acta Psychiatrica. Scand.* 88: 350–355.
Blazer, D. G., Hughes, D. & George, L. K. 1987. Stressful life events and the onset
    of a generalized anxiety syndrome. *Am. J. Psychiatry* 144: 1178–1183.
Blazer, D. G., Hughes, D., George, L. K. et al. 1991. Generalized anxiety disorder.
    In *Psychiatric Disorders in America: The Epidemiologic Catchment Area
    Study*, eds. L. N. Robins, D. A. Regier, pp. 180–203, Free Press, New York.
Borkovec, T. D. & Inz, J. 1990. The nature of worry in generalized anxiety
    disorder: A predominance of thought activity. *Behav. Res. Ther.* 28: 153–158.
Borkovec, T. D., Lyonfields, J. D. & Wiser, S. L. 1993. An examination of image
    and thought processes in generalized anxiety. *Behav. Res. Ther.* 31: 321–324.
Borkovec, T. D. & Lyonfields, J. D. (In Press). Worry: Thought suppression of
    emotional processing. In *Vigilance and Avoidance*, ed. H. Krohne, Hogrefe

and Huber, Toronto.

Borkovec, T. D., Mathews, A. M., Chambers, A. et al. 1988. The effects of relaxation training with cognitive therapy or nondirective therapy and the role of relaxation-induced anxiety in the treatment of generalized anxiety. *J. Consult. Clin. Psychol.* 58: 883–888.

Borkovec, T. D., Shadick, R. N. & Hopkins, M. 1991. The nature of normal and pathological worry. In *Chronic Anxiety: Generalized Anxiety Disorders and Mixed Anxiety-Depression*, eds. R. M. Rapee, D. H. Barlow, pp. 29–51, Guilford Press, New York.

Borkovec, T. D. & Whisman, M. A. 1996. Psychosocial treatment for generalized anxiety disorder. In *Long-Term Treatment for the Anxiety Disorders*, eds. M. Mavissakalian, R. F. Prien, pp. 201–219, American Psychiatric Press, Washington, DC.

Brawman-Mintzer, O. & Lydiard, R. B. 1996. Generalized anxiety disorder: Issues in epidemiology. *J. Clin. Psychiatry* 57: 3–8.

Brawman-Mintzer, O. & Lydiard, R. B. 1997. Generalized anxiety disorder. In *Psychiatry*, eds. A. Tasman, J. Kay, J. A. Lieberman, Saunders, Philadelphia.

Brawman-Mintzer, O., Lydiard, R. B., Emmanuel, N. et al. 1993. Psychiatric comorbidity in patients with generalized anxiety disorder. *Am. J. Psychiatry* 150: 1216–1218.

Breslau, N. & Davis, G. C. 1985. DSM-III generalized anxiety disorder: An empirical investigation of more stringent criteria. *Psychiatry Res.* 14: 231–238.

Breslau, N., Davis, G. C. & Prabucki, K. 1987. Searching for evidence on the validity of generalized anxiety disorder: Psychopathology in children of anxious mothers. *Psychiatry Res.* 20: 197–285.

Brown, T. A. & Barlow, D. H. 1992. Comorbidity among anxiety disorders: Implications for treatment and DSM-IV. *J. Consult. Clin. Psychol.* 60: 835–844.

Brown, T. A., Barlow, D. H. & Liebowitz, M. R. 1994. The empirical basis of generalized anxiety disorder. *Am. J. Psychiatry* 151: 1272–1280.

Brown, T. A., Martin, M. A. & Barlow, D.H. 1992. Psychometric properties of the Penn State Worry Questionnaire in a clinical anxiety disorders sample. *Behav. Res. Ther.* 30: 33–37.

Brown, T. A., Moras, K., Zinbarg, R. E. et al. 1993a. Diagnostic and symptom distinguishability of generalized anxiety disorder and obsessive-compulsive disorder. *Behav. Ther.* 24: 227–240.

Brown, T. A., O'Leary, T. A. & Barlow, D.H. 1993b. Generalized anxiety disorder. In *Clinical Handbook of Psychological Disorders: A Step-by-Step Treatment Manual*, Second Edition, ed. D. H. Barlow, Guilford Press, New York.

Bruce, M., Scott, N., Shine P. et al. 1992. Anxiogenic effects of caffeine in patients with anxiety disorders. *Arch. Gen. Psychiatry* 49: 867–869.

Butler, G., Cullington, A., Hibbert, G. et al. 1988. Anxiety management for persistent generalized anxiety. *Br. J. Psychiatry* 151: 535–542.

Butler, G., Fennell, M., Robson, P. et al. 1991. Comparison of behavior therapy and cognitive therapy in the treatment of generalized anxiety disorder. *J. Consult. Clin. Psychol.* 59: 167–175.

Cadieux, R. J. 1996. Azapirones: An alternative to benzodiazepines for anxiety. *Am. Fam. Physician* 53: 2349–2353.

Cameron, O. G., Smith, C. B., Lee, M. A. et al. 1990. Adrenergic status in anxiety disorders: Platelet alpha-2-adrenergic receptor binding, blood pressure, pulse, and plasma catecholamines in panic and generalized anxiety disorder patients and in normal subjects. *Biol. Psychiatry* 28: 3–20.

Cameron, O. G., Thyer, B. A., Nesse, R. M. et al. 1986. Symptom profiles of patients with DSM-III anxiety disorders. *Am. J. Psychiatry* 143: 1132–1137.

Catalan, J., Gath, D., Edmonds, G. et al. 1984. The effectives of nonprescribing of anxiolytics in general practice. I. Controlled evaluation of psychiatric and social outcome. *Br. J. Psychiatry* 144: 593–602.

Charney, D. S., Woods, S. W. & Heninger, G.R. 1987. Noradrenergic function in generalized anxiety disorder: Effects of yohimbine in healthy subjects and patients with generalized anxiety disorder. *Psychiatry Res.* 27: 173–182.

Chiaie, R. D., Pancheri, P., Casacchia, M., Stralta, P., Kotzalidis, G. D. & Zibellini, M. 1995. Assessment of the efficacy of buspirone in patients affected by generalized anxiety disorder, shifting to buspirone from prior treatment with lorazepam: A placebo-controlled, double-blind study. *J. Clin. Psychopharmacol.* 15: 12–19.

Clark, D. A., Beck, A. T. & Beck, J. S. 1994. Symptom differences in major depression, dysthymia, panic disorder, and generalized anxiety disorder. *Am. J. Psychiatry* 151: 205–209.

Cloninger, C. R. 1986. A unified biosocial theory of personality and its role in the development of anxiety states. *Psychiatr. Dev.* 3: 167–226.

Cloninger, C. R. 1988. Anxiety and theories of emotions. In *Handbook of Anxiety*, Vol. 2, eds. R. Noyes, M. Roth, G. D. Burrows, pp. 1–29, Elsevier, Amsterdam.

Cloninger, C. R., Martin, R. L., Clayton, P. et al. 1981. A blind follow-up and family study of anxiety neurosis: Preliminary analysis of the St. Louis 500. In *Anxiety: New Research and Changing Concepts*, eds. D. F. Klein, J. Rabkin, pp. 137–148, Raven Press, New York.

Clow, A., Glover, V., Sandler, M. et al. 1988. Increased urinary tribulin output in generalized anxiety disorder. *Psychopharmacology* 95: 378–380.

Craske, M. G., Rapee, R. M., Jackel, L. et al. 1989. Qualitative dimensions of worry in DSM-III-R generalized anxiety disorder subjects and nonanxious controls. *Behav. Res. Ther.* 27: 397–402.

Crowe, R. R., Noyes, R., Pauls, D. L. et al. 1983. A family study of panic disorder. *Arch. Gen. Psychiatry* 40: 1065–1069.

Davies, M. H., Rose, S. & Cross, K. W. 1983. Life events, social interaction and psychiatric symptoms in general practice: A pilot study. *Psychol. Med.* 13: 159–163.

Davis, J. M. 1992. Slow wave sleep and 5-HT2 receptor sensitivity in generalized anxiety disorder: A pilot study with ritanserin. *Psychopharmacology* 108: 387–389.

Derogatis, L. R. 1983. *SCL-90-R Administration, Scoring and Procedures Manual*, Second Edition. Procedures Psychometric Research, Baltimore.

DiNardo, P. A., Moras, K., Barlow, D. H. et al. 1993. Reliability of DSM-III-R anxiety disorder categories using the Anxiety Disorders Interview Schedule-Revised (ADIS-R). *Arch. Gen. Psychiatry* 50: 251–256.

DiNardo, P. A., O'Brien, G. T., Barlow, D. H. et al. 1983. Reliability of DSM-III anxiety disorder categories using a new structured interview. *Arch. Gen. Psychiatry* 40: 1070–1074.

Durham, R. C. & Allan, T. 1993. Psychological treatment of generalized anxiety disorder. *Br. J. Psychiatry* 163: 19–26.

Durham, R. C., Murphy, T., Allan, T., Richard, K., Treliving, L. R. & Fenton, G.

W. 1994. Cognitive therapy, analytic psychotherapy and anxiety management training for generalized anxiety disorder. *Br. J. Psychiatry* 165: 315–323.

Eysenck, H. J. & Eysenck, M. W. 1985. *Personality and Individual Differenes: A Natural Science Approach*, Plenum Press, New York.

Fava, G. A. & Kellner, R. 1991. Prodromal symptoms in affective disorders. *Am. J. Psychiatry* 148: 823–830.

Finlay-Jones, R. & Brown, G. W. 1981. Types of stressful life events and the onset of anxiety and depressive disorders. *Psychol. Med.* 11: 803–815.

Fossey, M. D. & Lydiard, R. B. 1990. Placebo response in patients with anxiety disorders. In *Handbook of Anxiety*, Vol. 4, eds. R. Noyes, M. Roth, G. D. Burrows, pp. 27–56, Elsevier, Amsterdam.

Fossey, M. D., Lydiard, R. B., Ballenger, J. C. et al. 1993. Cerebrospinal fluid thyrotropin-releasing hormone concentrations in patients with anxiety disorders. *J. Neuropsychiatry Clin. Neurosci.* 4: 335–337.

Fossey, M. D., Lydiard, R. B., Ballenger, J. C. et al. 1996. Cerebrospinal fluid corticotropin-releasing factor concentrations in patients with anxiety disorders and normal comparison subjects. *Biol. Psychiatry* 39: 703–707.

Freud, S. 1959. The justification for detaching from neurasthenia a particular syndrome: The anxiety neurosis. In *Collected Papers*, Vol. 1, pp. 76–106, Basic Books, New York.

Fyer, A. J., Mannuzza, S., Martin, L. Y. et al. 1989. Reliability of anxiety assessment. II. Symptom agreement. *Arch. Gen. Psychiatry* 46: 1102–1110.

Ganzini, L., McFarland, B. H. & Cutler, D. 1990. Prevalence of mental disorders after catastrophic financial loss. *J. Nerv. Ment. Dis.* 178: 680–685.

Garvey, M. J., Cook, B. & Noyes, R. 1988. The occurrence of a prodome of generalized anxiety in panic disorders. *Compr. Psychiatry* 29: 445–449.

Garvey, M. J., Noyes, R., Woodman, C. et al. 1993. A biological difference between panic disorder and generalized anxiety disorder. *Biol. Psychiatry* 34: 572–575.

Garvey, M. J., Noyes, R., Woodman, C. et al. 1995. Relationship of generalized anxiety symptoms to urinary 5-hydroxyindoleacetic acid and vanillymandelic acid. *Psychiatry Res.* 57: 1–5.

Gasperini, M., Battaglia, M. & Diaferia, G. 1990. Personality features related to generalized anxiety disorder. *Compr. Psychiatry* 31: 363–368.

Geil, R., TenHorn, G. H., Ormel, J. et al. 1978. Mental illness, neuroticism and life events in a Dutch village sample: A follow-up. *Psychol. Med.* 8: 235–243.

Gelder, M. 1991. Psychological treatment for anxiety disorders: Adjustment disorders with anxious mood, generalized anxiety disorders, panic disorder, agoraphobia, and avoidant personality disorder. In *The Clinical Management of Anxiety Disorders*, eds. W. Coryell, G. Winokur, pp. 10–27, Oxford University Press, New York.

Gray, J. A. 1987. *The Psychology of Fear and Stress*, Second Edition, Cambridge University Press, Cambridge.

Greenblatt, D. J., Shacher, R. I., Diroll, M. et al. 1981. Benzodiazepines: A summary of pharmacokinetic properties. *Br. J. Pharmacol.* 11: 11S–16S.

Greer, S. 1969. The prognosis of anxiety states. In *Studies in Anxiety*, ed. M. D. Lader, pp. 151–157, Royal Medico-Psychological Association, London.

Grillon, C. & Buchsbaum, M. S. 1987. EEG topography of response to visual stimuli in generalized anxiety disorder. *Electoencephalogr. Clin. Neurophysiol.* 66: 337–348.

Hamilton, M. 1959. The assessment of anxiety states by rating. *Br. J. Med. Psychol.* 32: 50–55.

Harris, G. J. & Hoehn-Saric, R. 1995. Functional neuroimaging in biological psychiatry. In *Advances in Biological Psychiatry*, ed. J. Panksepp, pp. 113–160, JAI Press, Greenwich, CT.

Hazlett, R., McLeod, D. R. & Hoehn-Saric, R. 1994. Muscle tension in generalized anxiety disorder: Elevated muscle tonus or agitated movement? *Psychophysiology* 31: 189–195.

Hibbert, G. A. 1984. Ideational components of anxiety: Their origin and content. *Br. J. Psychiatry* 144: 618–624.

Hoehn-Saric, R. 1982. Comparison of generalized anxiety disorder with panic disorder patients. *Psychopharmacol. Bull.* 18: 104–108.

Hoehn-Saric, R., Borkovec, T. D. & Nemiah, J.C. 1995. Generalized anxiety disorder. In *Treatment of Psychiatric Disorders*, Second Edition, ed. G. O. Gabbard, pp. 1537–1567, American Psychiatric Press, Washington, DC.

Hoehn-Saric, R., Hazlett, R. L. & McLeod, D. R. 1993. Generalized anxiety disorder with early and late onset of anxiety symptoms. *Comp. Psychiatry* 34: 291–298.

Hoehn-Saric, R. & Masek, B. 1981. Effects of naloxone on normals and chronically anxious patients. *Biol. Psychiatry* 16: 1041–1050.

Hoehn-Saric, R. & McLeod, D. R. 1993. Somatic manifestations of normal and pathological anxiety. In *Biology of Anxiety Disorders*, eds. R. Hoehn-Saric, D. R. McLeod, pp. 177–222, American Psychiatric Press, Washington, DC.

Hoehn-Saric, R. & McLeod, D. R. 1990. Generalized anxiety disorder in adulthood. In *Handbook of Child and Adult Psychopathology: A Longitudinal Perspective*, eds. M. Hersen, C. L. Last, pp. 247–260, Pergamon Press, New York.

Hoehn-Saric, R., McLeod, D. R., Lee, Y. B. et al. 1991. Cortisol levels in generalized anxiety disorder. *Psychiatry Res.* 38: 313–315.

Hoehn-Saric, R., McLeod, D. R. & Zimmerli, W.D. 1988. Differential effects of alprazolam and imipramine in generalized anxiety disorder: Somatic versus psychic symptoms. *J. Clin. Psychiatry* 49: 293–301.

Hoehn-Saric, R., McLeod, D. R. & Zimmerli, W. D. 1989a. Symptoms and treatment responses of generalized anxiety disorder patients with high versus low levels of cardiovascular complaints. *Am. J. Psychiatry* 146: 854–859.

Hoehn-Saric, R., McLeod, D. R. & Zimmerli, W. D. 1989b. Somatic manifestations in women with generalized anxiety disorder: Psychophysiological responses to psychological stress. *Arch. Gen. Psychiatry* 46: 1113–1119.

Hoehn-Saric, R., McLeod, D. R. & Zimmerli, W. D. 1989b. Somatic manifestations in women with generalized anxiety disorder. *Arch. Gen. Psychiat.* 46: 1113–1119.

Hollister, L. E., Muller-Oerlinghausen, B., Rickels, K. et al. 1993. Clinical uses of benzodiazepines. *J. Clin. Psychopharmacol.* 13 (Suppl. 1): 1S–169S.

Holt, P. E. & Andrews, G. 1989. Hyperventilation and anxiety in panic disorder, social phobia, GAD and normal controls. *Behav. Res. Ther.* 27: 453–460.

Hunt, C. & Singh, M. 1991. Generalized anxiety disorder. *Int. Rev. Psychiatry* 3: 215–229.

Huxley, P. J., Goldberg, D. P., Maguire, G. P. et al. 1979. The prediction of the course of minor psychiatric disorders. *Br. J. Psychiatry* 145: 535–543.

Ifeld, F. W. J. 1979. Persons at high risk for symptoms of anxiety. In *Clinical*

Anxiety/Tension in Primary Medicine, ed. B. Brown, Excerpta Medica, Princeton, NJ.

Inz, J. 1990. *EEG activity in generalized anxiety disorder*. Doctoral dissertation, Penn State University, University Park, PA.

Kahn, R. J., McNair, D. H., Lipman, R. S. et al. 1986. Imipramine and chlordiazepoxide in depressive and anxiety disorders. II. Efficacy in anxious outpatients. *Arch. Gen. Psychiatry* 43: 79–85.

Kales, A., Soldatos, C. R., Bixler, E. O. et al. 1983. Early morning insomnia with rapidly eliminated benzodiazepines. *Science* 220: 95–100.

Kendler, K. S. 1996. Major depression and generalized anxiety disorder: Same genes, (partly) different environments – revisited, *Br. J. Psychiatry* 168: 68–75.

Kendler, K. S., Neale, M. C., Kessler, R. C. et al. 1992a. Generalized anxiety disorder in women: A population-based twin study. *Arch. Gen. Psychiatry* 49: 267–272.

Kendler. K. S., Neale, M. C., Kessler, R. C. et al. 1992b. Childhood parental loss and adult psychopathology in women: A twin study perspective. *Arch. Gen. Psychiatry* 49: 109–116.

Kerr, T. A., Schapira, K., Roth, M. et al. 1970. The relationship between the Maudsley Personality Inventory and the course of affective disorders. *Br. J. Psychiatry* 116: 11–19.

Khan, A., Lee, E., Dager, S. et al. 1986. Platelet MAO-B activity in anxiety and depression. *Biol. Psychiatry* 21: 847–849.

Klein, D. F. 1964. Delineation of two drug responsive anxiety syndromes. *Psychopharmacologia* 5: 397–408.

Klein, D. F. 1981. Anxiety reconceptualized. In *Anxiety: New Research and Changing Concepts*, eds. D. F. Klein, J. G. Rabkin, pp. 235–263, Raven Press, New York.

Klein, D. F. & Fink, M. 1962. Psychiatric reaction patterns to imipramine. *Am. J. Psychiatry* 199: 432–438.

Koenigsberg, H. W., Kaplan, R. D., Gilmore, M. M. et al. 1985. The relationship between syndrome and personality disorder in DSM-III: Experience with 2462 patients. *Am. J. Psychiatry* 142: 207–212.

Kollai, M. & Kollai, B. 1992. Cardiac vagal tone in generalized anxiety disorder. *Br. J. Psychiatry* 151: 831–835.

Kushner, M. G., Shear, K. J. & Beitman, B. O. 1990. The relationship between alcohol problems and the anxiety disorders. *Am. J. Psychiatry* 147: 685–695.

Lader, M. 1994. Treatment of anxiety. *Br. Med. J.* 309: 321–342.

Laria, M. F., Munno, I., Lydiard, R. B. et al. 1996. The influence of stress intrusion on immunodepression in generalized anxiety disorder patients and controls. *Psychosom. Med.* 58: 138–142.

Leenstra, A. S., Ormel, J. & Giel, R. 1995. Positive life change and recovery from depression and anxiety: A three-stage longitudinal study of primary care attenders. *Br. J. Psychiatry* 166: 333–343.

Liebowitz, M. R., Hollander, E., Schneier, F. et al. 1990. Anxiety and depression: Discrete diagnostic entities? *J. Clin. Psychopharmacol.* 10: 615–665.

Lyonfields, J. D., Borkovec, T. D. & Thayer, J. F. 1995. Vagal tone in generalized anxiety disorder and the effects of aversive imagery and worrisome thinking. *Behav. Ther.* 26: 457–466.

Maier, W., Buller, R., Philipp, M. et al. 1988. The Hamilton Anxiety Scale: Reliability, validity, and sensitivity to change in anxiety and depressive disorders. *J. Affect. Dis.* 14: 61–68.

Mancini, C., Van Ameringen, M. & Macmillan, H. 1995. Relationship of childhood sexual and physical abuse to anxiety disorders. *J. Nerv. Ment. Dis.* 183: 309–314.

Mancuso, D. M., Townsend, M. H. & Mercante, D. E. 1993. Long-term follow-up of generalized anxiety disorder. *Comp. Psychiatry* 34: 441–446.

Mann, A. H., Jenkins, R. & Belsey, E. 1981. The twelve-month outcome of patients with neurotic illness in general practice. *Psychol. Med.* 11: 535–550.

Mannuzza, S., Fyer, A. J., Klein, D. F. et al. 1986. Schedule for Affective Disorders and Shizophrenia – Lifetime Anxiety (SADS-LA): Rationale and conceptual development. *J. Psychiatr. Res.* 20: 317–325.

Mannuzza, S., Fyer, A. J., Martin, M. S. et al. 1989. Reliability of anxiety assessment. I: Diagnostic agreement. *Arch. Gen. Psychiatry* 46: 1093–1101.

Marks, I. M. & Lader, M. 1973. Anxiety states (anxiety neurosis): A review. *J. Nerv. Ment. Dis.* 156: 3–18.

Marks, M. 1989. Behavioral psychotherapy for generalized anxiety disorder. *Int. Rev. Psychiatry* 1: 235–244.

Marten, P. A., Brown, T. A., Barlow, D. H. et al. 1993. Evaluation of the ratings comprising the associated symptom criteria of DSM-III-R generalized anxiety disorder. *J. Nerv. Ment. Dis.* 181: 676–682.

Massion, A. O., Warshaw, M. G. & Keller, M. B. 1993. Quality of life and psychiatric morbidity in panic disorder and generalized anxiety disorder. *Am. J. Psychiatry* 150: 600–607.

Mathew, R. J., Ho, B. T., Francis, D. J. et al. 1982. Catecholamines and anxiety. *Acta Psychiatr. Scand.* 65: 142–147.

Mathew, R. J., Ho, B. T. & Kralik, P. 1979. Anxiety and serum prolactin. *Am. J. Psychiatry* 5: 716–718.

Mathew, R. J., Ho, B. T., Taylor, D. L. et al. 1981. Catecholamine and dopamine-B-hydroxylase in anxiety. *J. Psychosom. Res.* 25: 499–504.

Mathew, R. J. & Wilson, W. H. 1990. Behavioral and cerebrovascular effects of caffeine in patients with anxiety disorders. *Acta Psychiatr. Scand.* 82: 17–22.

Mathew, R. J., Wilson, W. H., Blazer, D. G. et al. 1993. Psychiatric disorders in adult children of alcoholics: Data from the Epidemiologic Catchment Area project. *Am. J. Psychiatry* 150: 793–800.

Mauri, M., Sarno, N., Rossi, V. M. et al. 1992. Personality disorders associated with generalized anxiety, panic, and recurrent depressive disorders. *J. Pers. Disord.* 6: 162–167.

Mavissakalian, M. R., Hamann, M. S., Haidar, S. A. et al. 1993. DSM-III personality disorders in generalized anxiety, panic/agoraphobia, and obsessive-compulsive disorders. *Comp. Psychiatry* 34: 243–248.

Mendlewicz, J., Papadimitriou, G. & Wilmotte, J. 1993. Family study of panic disorder: Comparison with generalized anxiety disorder, major depression, and normal subjects. *Psychiatr. Genetics* 3: 73–78.

Meyer, T. J., Miller, M. L., Metzger, R. L. et al. 1990. Development and validation of the Penn State Worry Questionnaire. *Behav. Res. Ther.* 28: 487–495.

Munjack, D. J., Baltazar, P. L., DeQuattro, V. et al. 1989. Generalized anxiety disorders: Some biochemical aspects. *Psychiatry Res.* 32: 35–43.

Munjack, D. J., Brown, R. A. & McDowell, D. E. 1993. Existence of hyperventilation in panic disorder with and without agoraphobia, GAD, and normals: Implications for the cognitive theory of panic. *J. Anxiety Dis.* 7: 37–48.

Munjack, D. J. & Palmer, R. 1988. Thyroid hormones in panic disorder, panic disorder with agoraphobia and generalized anxiety disorder. *J. Clin. Psychiatry* 6: 223–229.

Murphy, J. M., Oliver, D. C., Sobal, A. M. et al. 1986. Diagnosis and outcome: Depression and anxiety in a general population. *Psychol. Med.* 16: 117–126.

Nestadt, G., Romanoski, A. J., Samuels, J. F. et al. 1992. The relationship between personality and DSM-III Axis I disorders in the population: Results from an epidemiological survey. *Am. J. Psychiatry* 149: 1228–1233.

Newman, S. C. & Bland, R. C. 1994. Life events and the 1-year prevalence of major depressive episode, generalized anxiety disorder, and panic disorder in a community sample. *Comp. Psychiatry* 35: 76–82.

Nietzel, M. I., Bernstein, D. A. & Russell, R. L. 1988. Assessment of anxiety and fear. In *Behavioral Assessment: A Practical Handbook*, eds. A. S. Bellack, M. Hersen, Pergamon Press, New York.

Nisita, C., Petracca, A., Akiskal, H. S. et al. 1990. Delimitation of generalized anxiety disorder: Clinical comparisons with panic and major depressive disorder. *Comp. Psychiatry* 31: 409–415.

Noyes, R. 1988a. Revision of the DSM-III classification. In *Handbook of Anxiety*, Vol. II, eds. R. Noyes, M. Roth, G. D. Burrows, pp. 81–107, Elsevier, Amsterdam.

Noyes, R. 1988b. Beta-blocking drugs in anxiety disorders. In *Handbook of Anxiety Disorders*, eds. C. G. Last, M. Hersen, pp. 445–459, Pergamon Press, New York.

Noyes, R., Clancy, J., Hoenk, P. R. et al. 1980. The prognosis of anxiety disorders. *Arch. Gen. Psychiatry* 37: 173–178.

Noyes, R., Clarkson, C., Crowe, R. R. et al. 1987. A family study of generalized anxiety disorder. *Am. J. Psychiatry* 144: 1019–1024.

Noyes, R., Crowe, R. R., Harris, E. L. et al. 1986. Relationship between panic disorder and agoraphobia: A family study. *Arch. Gen. Psychiatry* 43: 227–232.

Noyes, R., Garvey, M. J., Cook, B. L. et al. 1988. Benzodiazepine withdrawal: A review of the evidence. *J. Clin. Psychiatry* 49: 382–389.

Noyes. R., Woodman, C., Garvey, M. J. et al. 1992. Generalized anxiety disorder vs. panic disorder: Distinguishing characteristics and patterns of comorbidity. *J. Nerv. Ment. Dis.* 180: 369–379.

Nyström, S. & Lindegård, B. 1975. Predisposition for mental syndromes: A study comparing predisposition for depression, neurasthenia and anxiety state. *Acta Psychiatr. Scand.* 51: 69–76.

Oakley-Browne, M. A. & Joyce, P. R. 1992. New perspectives for the epidemiology of anxiety disorders. In *Handbook of Anxiety*, Vol. V, eds. G. D. Burrows, M. Roth, R. Noyes, pp. 57–78, Elsevier, Amsterdam.

Onstad, S. I., Torgersen, S. & Kringler, E. 1991. High interrater reliability for the Structured Clinical Interview for DSM-III-R, Axis I (SCID-I). *Acta Psychiatr. Scand.* 84: 167–173.

Öst, L-G. 1987. Description of a coping technique and review of controlled studies. *Behav. Res. Ther.* 25: 397–409.

Otto, M. W., Pollack, M. H., Sachs, G. S. et al. 1993. Discontinuation of benzodiazepine treatment: Efficacy of cognitive-behavioral therapy for patients with panic disorder. *Am. J. Psychiatry* 150: 1485–1490.

Palinkas, L. A., Petterson, J. S., Russell, J. et al. 1993. Community patterns of psychiatric disorders after the Exxon Valdez oil spill. *Am. J. Psychiatry* 150: 1517–1523.

Papadimitrious, G. N., Kerkhofs, M., Kempenaers, C. et al. 1988. EEG sleep studies in patients with generalized anxiety disorder. *Psychiatry Res.* 26: 183–190.

Perry, P. J., Garvey, M. J. & Noyes, R. 1990. Benzodiazepine treatment of generalized anxiety disorder. In *Handbook of Anxiety*, Vol. 4, eds. R. Noyes, M. Roth, G. D. Burrows, pp. 111–124, Elsevier, Amsterdam.

Pomara, N., Stanley, B., Block, R. et al. 1984. Diazepam impairs performance in normal elderly subjects. *Psychopharmacol. Bull.* 20: 37–39.

Power, K. G., Jerrom, D. W., Simpson, R. J. et al. 1991. A controlled comparison of cognitive behavior therapy, diazepam and placebo in the management of generalized anxiety. *Behav. Psychol.* 17: 1–14.

Power, K. G., Simpson, M. B., Swanson, J. et al. 1990b. A controlled comparison of cognitive-behavior therapy, diazepam, and placebo, alone and in combination, for the treatment of generalized anxiety disorder. *J. Anx. Disord.* 4: 269–292.

Power, K. G., Simpson, R. J., Swanson, J. et al. 1990a. Controlled comparison of pharmacological and psychological treatment of generalized anxiety disorder in primary care. *Br. J. Gen. Pract.* 40: 289–294.

Rapee, R. M. 1985. Distinctions between panic disorder and generalized anxiety disorder: Clinical presentation. *Aust. N.Z. J. Psychiatry* 19: 227–232.

Rapee, R. M. 1989. Boundary issues: GAD and somatoform disorders; GAD and psychophysiological disorders. Paper prepared by the generalized anxiety disorder subcommittee for DSM–IV.

Rapee, R. M. 1991a. Generalized anxiety disorder: A review of clinical features and theoretical concepts. *Clin. Psychol. Rev.* 11: 419–440.

Rapee, R. M. 1991b. Psychological factors involved in generalized anxiety. In *Chronic Anxiety: Generalized Anxiety Disorder and Mixed Anxiety–Depression*, eds. R. M. Rapee, D. H. Barlow, pp. 76–94, Guilford Press, New York.

Raskin, M., Peeke, H. V. S., Dickman, W. et al. 1982. Panic and generalized anxiety disorders: Developmental antecedents and precipitants. *Arch. Gen. Psychiatry* 39: 687–689.

Rey, J. M., Plapp, J. M. & Wever, C. 1992. Epidemiology of anxiety disorders of childhood and adolescence. *Handbook of Anxiety*, Vol. 5, eds. G. D. Burrows, M. Roth, R. Noyes, pp. 309–328, Elsevier, Amsterdam.

Reynolds, C. F., Shaw, D. H., Newton, T. F. et al. 1983. EEG sleep in outpatients with generalized anxiety: A preliminary comparison with depressed outpatients. *Psychiatry Res.* 8: 81–89.

Rickels, K., Case, W. G. & Diamond L. 1980. Relapse after short-term drug therapy in neurotic outpatients. *Int. Pharmacopsychiatry* 15: 186–192.

Rickels, K., Case, W. G., Downing, R. et al. 1986. One-year follow-up of anxious subjects treated with diazepam. *J. Clin. Psychopharmacol.* 6: 32–36.

Rickels, K., Downing, R., Schweizer, E. et al. 1993. Antidepressants for the treatment of generalized anxiety disorder. *Arch. Gen. Psychiatry* 50: 884–895.

Rickels, K., Gordon, P. E., Zamostien, B. B. et al. 1970. Hydroxyzine and chlordiazepoxide in anxious neurotic outpatients: A collaborative controlled study. *Compr. Psychiatry* 11: 457–474.

Rickels, K. & Schweizer, E. 1990. The clinical course and long-term management of generalized anxiety disorder. *J. Clin. Psychopharmacol.* 20: 1015–1105.

Rickels, K., Schweizer, E., Case, G. et al. 1990. Long-term therapeutic use of benzodiazepines. II. Effects of gradual discontinuation. *Arch. Gen. Psychiatry*

47: 908–910.

Rickels, K., Wiseman, K., Norstad, N. et al. 1982. Buspirone and diazepam in anxiety: A controlled study. *J. Clin. Psychiatry* 43: 81–86.

Riskind, J. Beck, A. T., Brown, G. et al. 1987b. Taking the measure of anxiety and depression: Validity of the reconstructed Hamilton scales. *J. Nerv. Ment. Dis.* 175: 474–479.

Riskind, J. H., Beck, A. T., Berchick, R. J. et al. 1987a. Reliability of DSM-III diagnoses for major depression and generalized anxiety disorder using the Structured Clinical Interview for DSM-III. *Arch. Gen. Psychiatry* 44: 817–820.

Riskind, J. H., Hohmann, A. A., Beck, A. T. et al. 1991. The relation of generalized anxiety disorder to depression in general and dysthymic disorder in particular. In *Chronic Anxiety: Generalized Anxiety Disorders and Mixed Anxiety-Depression*, eds. R. M. Rapee, D. H. Barlow, pp. 153–171, Guilford Press, New York.

Rocca, P., Ferrero, P., Gualerzi, A. et al. 1991. Peripheral-type benzodiazepine receptors in anxiety disorders. *Acta Psychiatr. Scand.* 84: 537–544.

Rosenbaum, A. H., Schatzberg, A. F., Jost, F. A., III. et al. 1983. Urinary free cortisol levels in anxiety. *Psychosomatics* 24: 835–837.

Roth, M., Gurney, C. & Garside, R. F. 1972. Studies in the classification of affective disorders. I. The relationship between anxiety states and depressive illness. *Br. J. Psychiatry* 121: 147–161.

Sanderson, W. C. & Barlow, D. H. 1990. A description of patients diagnosed with DSM-III-R generalized anxiety disorder. *J. Nerv. Ment. Dis.* 178: 588–591.

Sanderson, W. C. & Wetzler S. 1991. Chronic anxiety and generalized anxiety disorder: Issues in comorbidity. In *Chronic Anxiety: Generalized Anxiety Disorders and Mixed Anxiety-Depression*, eds. R. M. Rapee, D. H. Barlow, pp. 199–135, Guilford Press, New York.

Sartorius, N, Ustun, T.B., Lecrubier, U. & Wittchen, H-U. 1996. Depression comorbid with anxiety: Result from the WHO study on psychological disorders in primary health care. *Br. J. Psychiatry* 168: 38–43.

Schneider, L. S. 1996. Overview of generalized anxiety disorder in the elderly. *J. Clin. Psychiatry* 57 (Suppl. 7): 34–45.

Schneider, L. S., Munjack, D., Severson, J. A. et al. 1987. Platelet [3H] imipramine binding in generalized anxiety disorder, panic disorder, and agoraphobia with panic attacks. *Biol. Psychiatry* 22: 59–66.

Schweizer, E. & Rickels, K. 1991. Pharmacotherapy of generalized anxiety disorder. In *Chronic Anxiety: Generalized Anxiety Disorder and Mixed Anxiety-Depression*, eds. R. M. Rapee, D. H. Barlow, Guilford Press, New York.

Schweizer, E. E., Swenson, C. M., Winokur, A. et al. 1986. The dexamethasone suppression test in generalized anxiety disorder. *Br. J. Psychiatry* 149: 320–322.

Sevy, S., Papadimitrious, G. N., Surmont, D. W. et al. 1989. Noradrenergic function in generalized anxiety disorders, major depressive disorders, and healthy subjects. *Biol. Psychiatry* 25: 141–152.

Shader, R. I. & Greenblatt, D. J. 1983. Some current treatment options for symptoms of anxiety. *J. Clin. Psychiatry* 44: 21–30.

Shapiro, A. K., Stuening, E. L., Shapiro, E. et al. 1983. Diazepam: How much better than placebo? *J. Psychiatr. Res.* 17: 51–73.

Shore, J. H., Vollmer, W. M. & Tatum, E. L. 1989. Community patterns of

post-traumatic stress disorders. *J. Nerv. Ment. Dis.* 177: 681–685.
Shores, M. M., Glabin, T., Cowley, D. S. et al. 1992. The relationship between
    anxiety and depression: A clinical comparison of generalized anxiety
    disorder, dysthymia disorder, panic disorder, and major depressive disorder.
    Comp. Psychiatry 33: 237–244.
Skre, I., Onstad, S., Torgersen, S. et al. 1993. A twin study of DSM-III-R anxiety
    disorders. *Acta Psychiatr. Scand.* 88: 85–92.
Smith, E. M., North, C. S., McCool, R. E. et al. 1990. Acute postdisaster
    psychiatric disorders: Identification of persons at risk. *Am. J. Psychiatry* 147:
    202–206.
Smith, E. M., Robins, L. N., Przybeck, T. R. et al. 1986. Psychosocial
    consequences of a disorder. In *Disaster Stress Studies: New Methods and
    Findings*, ed. J. H. Shore, American Psychiatric Press, Washington, DC.
Snaith, R. T., Baught, F. J., Clayden, A. D. et al. 1982. The Clinical Anxiety Scale:
    An instrument derived from the Hamilton Anxiety Scale. *Br. J. Psychiatry*
    141: 518–523.
Solomon, K. & Hart, R. 1978. Pitfalls and prospects in clinical research on
    antianxiety drugs: Benzodiazepines and placebo – a review. *J. Clin. Psychol.*
    39: 823–833.
Sorby, N. G. D., Reavley, W. & Huber, J. W. 1991. Self help program for anxiety
    in general practice: Controlled trial of an anxiety management booklet. *Br. J.
    Gen. Pract.* 41: 417–420.
Speilberger, C. D. 1972. Anxiety as an emotional state. In *Anxiety: Current Trends
    in Theory and Research*, Vol. I, ed. C. D. Speilberger, pp. 24–49, Academic
    Press, New York.
Starcevic, V., Fallon, S., Uhlenhuth, E. H. 1994. The frequency and severity of
    generalized anxiety symptoms: Toward a less cumbersome
    conceptualization. *J. Nerv. Ment. Dis.* 182: 80–84.
Swinson, R. P., Cox, B. J. & Fergus, K. D. 1993. Diagnostic criteria in generalized
    anxiety disorder treatment studies. *J. Clin. Psychopharmacol.* 13: 455.
Thayer, J. F., Friedman, B. H. & Borkovec, T. D. 1996. Autonomic characteristics
    of generalized anxiety disorder and worry. *Biol. Psychiatry* 39: 255–266.
Thyer, B. A., Parrish, R. T., Curtis, G. C. et al. 1985. Ages of onset of DSM-III
    anxiety disorders. *Comp. Psychiatry* 26: 113–122.
Tiller, J. W. G., Biddle, N., Maguire, K. P. et al. 1988. The dexamethasone
    suppression test and plasma dexamethasone in generalized anxiety disorder.
    Biol. Psychiatry 23: 261–270.
Tollefson, G. D., Montague-Clouse, J. & Tollefson, S. L. 1992. Treatment of
    comorbid generalized anxiety in a recently detoxified alcohol population
    with a selective serotonergic drug (buspirone). *J. Clin. Psychopharmacol.* 12:
    19–26.
Torgersen, S. 1983. Genetic factors in anxiety disorders. *Arch. Gen. Psychiatry* 40:
    1085–1089.
Torgersen, S. 1986. Childhood and family characteristics in panic and generalized
    anxiety disorders. *Am. J. Psychiatry* 143: 630–632.
Tweed, J. L., Schoenbach, J. J., George, L. K. et al. 1989. The effects of childhood
    parental death and divorce on six-month history of anxiety disorders. *Br. J.
    Psychiatry* 154: 823–828.
Tyrer P. 1976. *The Role of Bodily Feelings on Anxiety.* Oxford University Press,
    London.
Tyrer, P. 1986. Classification of anxiety disorders: A critique of DSM-III. *J.*

Affect. Dis. 11: 99–104.

Uhde, T. W., Boulenger, J. P., Roy-Byrne, P. P. et al. 1985. Longitudinal course of panic disorder: Clinical and biological considerations. *Prog. Neuropsychopharmacol. Biol. Psychiatry* 9: 39–51.

Uhlenhuth, E. H., DeWitt, H. H., Balter, M. B. et al. 1988. Risks and benefits of long-term benzodiazepine use. *J. Clin. Psychopharmacol.* 8: 161–167.

Walker, L. G. 1990. The measurement of anxiety. *Postgrad. Med. J.* 66 (Suppl.2): S11–S17.

Weissman, M. M. 1990. Panic and generalized anxiety: Are they separate disorders? *J. Psychiat. Res.* 24: 157–162.

Whitaker, A., Johnson, J., Shaffer, D. et al. 1990. Uncommon troubles in young people: Prevalence estimates of selected psychiatric disorders in a nonreferred adolescent population. *Arch. Gen. Psychiatry* 47: 487–496.

White, J. & Keenan, M. 1992. Stress control: A controlled comparative investigation of large group therapy for generalized anxiety disorder. *Behav. Psychol.* 20: 97–114.

Williams, J. B. W., Gibbon, M., First, M. B. et al. 1992. The Structured Clinical Interview for DSM-III-R (SCID). II. Multisite test-retest reliability. *Arch. Gen. Psychiatry* 49: 630–636.

Wilson, W. H. & Mathew, R. J. 1993. Cerebral blood flow and metabolism in anxiety disorders. In *Biology of Anxiety Disorders*, eds. R. Hoehn-Saric, D. R. McLeod, pp. 1–59 American Psychiatric Press, Washington, DC.

Wittchen, H-U. & von Zerssen, D. 1987. *Verlaufe behandelter und unbehandelter. Depressionen and Angst-storungen. Erine klinish-psychiatrishe and epidemiologische Verlaufsauter-suchung.* Springer, Berlin.

Wittchen, H-U., Zhoa, S., Kessler, R. C. et al. 1994. DSM-III-R generalized anxiety disorder in the National Comorbdity Survey. *Arch. Gen. Psychiatry* 51: 355–364.

Wittchen, H-U., Kessler, R. C., Zhao, S. & Abelson, J. 1995. Reliability and clinical validity of UM-CIDI DSM-III-R. *Gen. Anx. Dis.* 29: 95–110.

Woodman, C. L., Noyes, R., Black, D. et al. 1995. Course and outcome of generalized anxiety disorder and panic disorder. Presented at the *Anxiety Disorders Association of America Annual Meeting*, Pittsburg, PA, April 6–9, 1995.

Woodman, C. L. 1993. The genetics of panic disorder and generalized anxiety disorder. *Ann. Clin. Psychiatry* 5: 231–240.

World Health Organization 1993. *The ICD-10 Classification of Mental and Behavioral Disorders: Diagnostic Criteria for Research.* World Health Organization, Geneva.

Wu, J. C., Buchsbaum, M. S., Hershey, T. G. et al. 1991. PET in generalized anxiety disorder. *Biol. Psychiatry* 29: 1181–1199.

Yonkers, K. A., Warshaw, M. G. & Massion, A. O. 1996. Phenomenology and course of generalized anxiety disorder. *Br. J. Psychiatry* 168: 308–313.

Zwemer, W. & Deffenbacher, J. 1984. Irrational beliefs, anger and anxiety. *J. Counseling Psychol.* 31: 391–393.

3

Panic disorder and agoraphobia

Definition

Panic disorder is characterized by attacks of extreme anxiety accompanied by sympathetic arousal. These attacks resemble the fight or flight response described by Cannon (1929) but occur in the absence of danger. During attacks, patients experience overwhelming fear and have an urge to flee or find help. With repeated attacks, they grow fearful of situations or circumstances from which escape might be difficult (e.g., confined places) or where help might not be available (e.g., when alone or a distance from home) should something catastrophic happen (e.g., heart attack, insanity). Fear and avoidance of such situations is termed agoraphobia.

Panic disorder with or without agoraphobia is the most frequent and severe anxiety disorder encountered in clinical populations. Attacks and alarming symptoms prompt many patients to seek treatment, but their somatic presentation (e.g., palpitations, shortness of breath) often causes the diagnosis to be missed. Untreated, the disorder seriously affects the quality of life and, due to chronicity, exacts heavy social and economic costs (Salvador-Carulla et al., 1995); however, with the development of precise diagnostic criteria and effective treatments, increasing numbers are receiving the help they need.

Da Costa (1871) described an affliction among soldiers of the Union Army that resembled panic. Its most constant features were palpitations, chest pain, and shortness of breath. He believed it represented an abnormal reaction to exertion and gave it the label 'irritable heart'. In 1895, Freud published a description of anxiety neurosis, a disorder he separated from the broader category of neurasthenia that Beard (1869) had popularized. Freud viewed anxiety as the primary manifestation and provided a classical description of panic attacks. He attributed the neurosis to sexual repression of the Victorian era.

The first account of agoraphobia is credited to Westphal (1872). In 1872, he described three men who feared streets and public places (Boyd & Crump, 1991). The term agoraphobia comes from the Greek word 'agora' that means market place. The agoraphobic person does not fear public places per se, but having panic attacks in such settings. Apart from the fact that most agoraphobic persons are women, Westphal's description remains a classic. Agoraphobia was introduced into the current classification by Marks (1970) who distinguished it from social and specific phobias.

Diagnostic criteria

Panic disorder first appeared in the DSM classification in 1980, although criteria had been proposed earlier by Feighner et al. (1972). It was the result of removing a more discrete and sharply defined category from anxiety neurosis (DSM-II), and its essential feature became the panic attack (American Psychiatric Association, 1968). Agoraphobia also first appeared in DSM-III, the result of subdividing phobic neurosis. In the new classification, agoraphobia was viewed as a classically conditioned response to situations in which panic attacks had occurred (Klein, 1981). In ICD-9 agoraphobia was given independent status and seen as a distinctive syndrome of multiple fears, not necessarily arising from panic attacks (World Health Organization, 1978).

The DSM-III criteria called for at least 3 panic attacks in a three week period (American Psychiatric Association, 1980); however, substantial impairment was found in persons having less frequent attacks, indicating that this arbitrary threshold was too high (Klerman et al., 1991). To correct this problem, the frequency criterion was modified, then replaced (American Psychiatric Association, 1987). DSM-IV requires recurrent unexpected panic attacks plus at least 1 month of persistent concern about having additional attacks, worry about the implications or consequences of attacks (e.g., having a heart attack, losing control), or a significant change in behavior related to attacks (e.g., frequent visits to the doctor) (Table 3.1).

DSM-IV includes criteria for panic attacks (Table 3.2) in recognition of the fact that attacks occur in other anxiety and non-anxiety disorders (American Psychiatric Association, 1994). Panic attacks are discrete periods of intense apprehension, fearfulness, or terror often associated with feelings of impending doom. During attacks, symptoms such as shortness of breath, palpitations, chest pain or discomfort, choking or smothering sensations, and fear of dying or losing control are present. The relationship of attacks to situational triggers has diagnostic significance. *Unexpected*

Table 3.1. *DSM-IV criteria for panic attack*

A discrete period of intense fear or discomfort, in which four (or more) of the
following symptoms developed abruptly and reached a peak within 10 minutes:

(1) palpitations, pounding heart, or accelerated heart rate
(2) sweating
(3) trembling or shaking
(4) sensations of shortness of breath or smothering
(5) feeling of choking
(6) chest pain or discomfort
(7) nausea or abdominal distress
(8) feeling dizzy, unsteady, lightheaded, or faint
(9) derealization (feelings of unreality) or depersonalization (being detached
    from oneself)
(10) fear of losing control or going crazy
(11) fear of dying
(12) paresthesias (numbness or tingling sensations)
(13) chills or hot flushes

Table 3.2. *DSM-IV criteria for panic disorder*

A. Both (1) and (2):
   (1) recurrent unexpected panic attacks
   (2) at least one of the attacks has been followed by 1 month (or more) of one
       (or more) of the following:
       (a) persistent concern about having additional attacks
       (b) worry about the implications of the attack or its consequences (e.g.,
           losing control, having a heart attack, 'going crazy')
       (c) a significant change in behavior related to the attacks
B. Absence of agoraphobia
C. The panic attacks are not due to the direct physiological effects of a substance
   (e.g., a drug of abuse, a medication) or a general medical condition (e.g.,
   hyperthyroidism)
D. The panic attacks are not better accounted for by another mental disorder,
   such as social phobia (e.g., occurring on exposure to feared social situations),
   specific phobia (e.g., on exposure to a specific phobic situation),
   obsessive-compulsive disorder (e.g., on exposure to dirt in someone with an
   obsession about contamination), post-traumatic stress disorder (e.g., in
   response to stimuli associated with a severe stressor), or separation anxiety
   disorder (e.g., in response to being away from home or close relatives)

Reprinted with permission from the American Psychiatric Association (1994).

(uncued) attacks occur in panic disorder, whereas *situationally bound* (cued)
attacks occur in other anxiety disorders. In the presence of agoraphobia,
attacks are commonly *situationally predisposed*; i.e., they are likely to occur
in certain situations (e.g., while driving, in a crowded store) but do not
always do so.

Persons with agoraphobia may or may not have a history of panic

Table 3.3. *DSM-IV criteria for agoraphobia without a history of panic disorder*

A. Anxiety about being in places or situations from which escape might be difficult (or embarrassing) or in which help may not be available in the event of having an unexpected or situationally predisposed panic attack or panic-like symptoms. Agoraphobic fears typically involve characteristic clusters of situations that include being outside the home alone, being in a crowd or standing in a line, being on a bridge, and traveling in a bus, train, or automobile
B. The situations are avoided (e.g., travel is restricted) or else are endured with marked distress or with anxiety about having a panic attack or panic-like symptoms, or require the presence of a companion
C. The anxiety or phobic avoidance is not better accounted for by another mental disorder, such as social phobia (e.g., avoidance limited to social situations because of fear of embarrassment), specific phobia (e.g., avoidance limited to a single situation like elevators), obsessive-compulsive disorder (e.g., avoidance of dirt in someone with an obsession about contamination), post-traumatic stress disorder (e.g., avoidance of stimuli associated with a severe stressor), or separation anxiety disorder (e.g., avoidance of leaving home or relatives)
D. Criteria have never been met for panic disorder
E. The disturbance is not due to the direct physiological effects of a substance (e.g., a drug of abuse, a medication) or a general medical condition
F. If an associated general medical condition is present, the fear described in criterion A is clearly in excess of that usually associated with the condition

---

Reprinted with permission from the American Psychiatric Association (1994).

disorder (Table 3.3). Agoraphobia is a fear of places or situations from which escape might be difficult (or embarrassing) or help unavailable in the event of a panic attack or panic symptoms (e.g., fear of collapse or losing control). The fear typically leads to avoidance of a variety of situations such as being alone or away from home, being in crowded places, traveling in an automobile, bus, or airplane, or being on a bridge or elevator. Some persons are able to enter feared situations when accompanied by a trusted companion.

The ICD-10 criteria for panic disorder are very similar but do not specify a threshold beyond recurrent attacks (Table 3.4) (WHO, 1993). The agoraphobia of ICD-10 is an independent disorder with no requirement for panic attacks (Table 3.5).

Reliability and validity

Reliability

Estimates of the diagnostic reliability of panic disorder range from excellent to very poor. Early studies, relying on the Diagnostic Interview

Table 3.4. *ICD-10 criteria for panic disorder (episodic paroxysmal anxiety)*

A. The individual experiences recurrent panic attacks that are not consistently associated with a specific situation or object and that often occur spontaneously (i.e., the episodes are unpredictable). The panic attacks are not associated with marked exertion or with exposure to dangerous or life-threatening situations
B. A panic attack is characterized by all of the following:
  1. it is a discrete episode of intense fear or discomfort
  2. it starts abruptly
  3. it reaches a maximum within a few minutes and lasts at least some minutes
  4. at least four of the symptoms listed below must be present, one of which must be from items a to d:

  autonomic arousal symptoms
  a. palpitations or pounding heart, or accelerated heart rate
  b. sweating
  c. trembling or shaking
  d. dry mouth (not due to medication or dehydration)

  symptoms involving chest and abdomen
  e. difficulty breathing
  f. feeling or choking
  g. chest pain or discomfort
  h. nausea or abdominal distress (e.g., churning in stomach)

  symptoms involving mental state
  i. feeling dizzy, unsteady, faint, or lightheaded
  j. feelings that objects are unreal (derealization), or that the self is distant or 'not really here' (depersonalization)
  k. fear of losing control, 'going crazy,' or passing out
  l. fear of dying

  general symptoms
  m. hot flashes or cold chills
  n. numbness or tingling sensations
C. Panic attacks are not due to a physical disorder, organic mental disorder, or other mental disorders such as schizophrenia and related disorders, mood disorders, or somatoform disorders

---

Reprinted with permission from WHO (1993).

Schedule, found kappa values that were unacceptable (Helzer et al., 1985); however, in settings where the base rate was high (e.g., psychiatric patients) and professional interviewers were used, the results were better. In a sample of anxiety clinic patients, Mannuzza et al. (1989) obtained kappas of 0.76 for panic disorder and 0.81 for panic disorder with agoraphobia, using the Schedule for Affective Disorders and Schizophrenia, Lifetime Anxiety Version. Similarly, DiNardo et al. (1993), using the Anxiety Disorders Interview Schedule, Revised Version, reported a kappa of 0.75 for panic with or without agoraphobia but poor agreement for uncomplicated panic disorder (kappa 0.39) and panic with severe agoraphobia (kappa 0.40).

Table 3.5. *ICD-10 criteria for agoraphobia*

A. There is marked and consistently manifest fear in, or avoidance of, at least two of the following situations:
   1. crowds
   2. public places
   3. traveling alone
   4. traveling away from home
B. At least two symptoms of anxiety in the feared situation must have been present together, on at least one occasion since the onset of the disorder, and one of them must have been an autonomic arousal symptom (i.e., palpitations, sweating, trembling, or dry mouth). The symptoms are the same as those listed under criterion B for panic disorder
C. Significant emotional distress is caused by the avoidance or by the anxiety symptoms, and the individual recognizes that these are excessive or unreasonable
D. Symptoms are restricted to, or predominate in, the feared situations or contemplation of the feared situations
E. Fear or avoidance of situations is not the result of delusions, hallucinations, or other disorders such as organic mental disorder, schizophrenia and related disorders, mood disorders, or obsessive-compulsive disorder, and is not secondary to cultural beliefs

---

Reprinted with permission from WHO (1993).

Also, Williams et al. (1992a), using the Structured Clinical Interview for DSM-III-R, obtained good to excellent agreement among patients who had been prescreened for participation in a treatment study. In a study of psychiatric patients and non-patients, the same investigators obtain kappas of only 0.58 and 0.59 (Williams et al., 1992b). Overall the findings show that, as base rates for panic fall (i.e., outside of anxiety clinics), so do kappa values.

Validity

The classification of panic disorder has been a subject of controversy from the time of its appearance. At issue has been its relationship to generalized anxiety disorder on the one hand and agoraphobia on the other. Generalized anxiety disorder first appeared in DSM-III as a residual category for anxious patients without panic attacks (American Psychiatric Association, 1980). As such, it was poorly defined and could not be diagnosed reliably (DiNardo et al., 1983). In DSM-III-R, distinguishing features (i.e., excessive, uncontrolled worry) were identified and the disorder was given independent status (American Psychiatric Association, 1987). Even with this redefinition, some see generalized anxiety disorder as a poorly-defined heterogeneous category, overlapping with other anxiety and depressive disorders (Breier et al., 1985; Andrews, 1993). Still, studies examining the relationship between panic and generalized anxiety disorder have tended to support the current separation (Chapter 2).

The bringing together of panic and agoraphobia in DSM-III also caused debate. These syndromes coexist in a majority of patients, raising the question of whether they represent a single entity, as in DSM-IV, or separate disorders, as in ICD-10 (American Psychiatric Association, 1994; World Health Organization, 1993). According to the American view, agoraphobia is secondary to repeated unexpected panic attacks (Klein, 1981). It is not a separate disorder but a more severe variant of panic, the primary biological disturbance. According to the European view, panic attacks are a variable feature of many disorders and not an essential feature of agoraphobia (Marks, 1987). Accordingly, agoraphobia is a syndrome of multiple fears that need not include panic attacks or fear of them.

Alhough not conclusive, the evidence favors the unitary concept (reviewed by McNally, 1994). To begin with, most agoraphobic patients report having had panic attacks. In clinical samples, fewer than 10% have never experienced them. The high prevalence of agoraphobia without panic attacks observed in the commuinity appears to have been an artifact of the survey method. When Horwath et al. (1993) reinterviewed persons so diagnosed in the Epidemiologic Catchment Area study, they found only one subject with the disorder. Studies examining initial symptoms have yielded conflicting results. Many patients report unexpected panic attacks followed, within days, by increasing agoraphobia (Uhde et al., 1985; Aronson & Logue, 1987), whereas others report agoraphobia before their first attack (Lelliott et al., 1989). Of course, all of the above data are based on retrospective reports.

Evidence which suggests that agoraphobia is a more severe variant of panic disorder comes from clinical and family studies (Schneier et al., 1991). Noyes et al. (1987b) found that agoraphobic patients had an earlier onset, less frequent remissions, and more severe symptoms; compared to patients with panic disorder, they appeared to have a more severe illness. Data from a family study were interpreted in a similar manner. In that study, Noyes et al. (1986a) found that first degree relatives of agoraphobic probands had an increased risk for both panic disorder and agoraphobia, whereas relatives of panic probands had an increased risk for panic disorder but not agoraphobia. Follow-up and treatment studies point in the same direction. Remissions are more likely to occur in panic disorder, and panic attacks respond more rapidly to medication and at lower dose than do agoraphobic symptoms (Mavissakalian & Perel, 1995; Keller et al., 1994).

The boundary between agoraphobia and social phobia is also important as far as validity is concerned. Social phobia is a disorder of multiple phobias that frequently coexists with agoraphobia (Degonda & Angst, 1993); however, the separation of these disorders is firmly established (reviewed in Chapter 4). Another disorder that frequently coexists with panic is hypochondriasis. An estimated 25–50% of panic patients also have this disturbance (Noyes et al., 1986b; Starcevic et al., 1992). Barsky et al. (1994), however, found primary care patients with panic disorder and hypochondriasis distinguishable on the basis of clinical features.

Measurement

Structured interviews

A series of structured clinical interviews for DSM-IV psychiatric diagnoses are available, and one of them, the Anxiety Disorders Interview Schedule for DSM-IV (ADIS-IV), was developed specifically for anxiety clinic populations (Brown et al., 1994). The ADIS-IV is used to assess anxiety disorders and permits differential diagnosis according to DSM-IV. Screening for other psychiatric disorders is included. The lifetime version contains a diagnostic timeline for determining temporal sequence and course of various disorders plus rating scales (i.e., Hamilton Anxiety Scale) for establishing level of symptoms. The reliability of the instrument has been established (DiNardo et al., 1993). Another structured interview, the Schedule for Affective Disorders and Schizophrenia, Lifetime Anxiety Version, focuses on anxiety disorders and was designed especially for research examining classification (Mannuzza et al., 1986). Other structured interviews include the Composite International Diagnostic Interview, the Diagnostic Interview Schedule, and the Structured Clinical Interview for DSM-IV (reviewed by Page, 1991).

Panic diary

Accurate assessment of panic attacks is important in clinical work and research. Such assessment is difficult because retrospective reporting tends to yield an overestimate (de Beurs et al., 1992). For this reason, a daily self-report of panic attacks or panic diary is an important tool. The diary usually includes the time of day, duration and severity of attacks, as well as whether attacks were unexpected, situationally bound, or situationally predisposed. The Conference on Standardized Assessment of Panic Disorder recommend a monitoring period of 1 month because of their variability (Shear & Maser, 1994). With a diary, several dimensions of anticipatory anxiety can also be rated on linear scales. These include the percentage of the day spent worrying about having a panic attack, the likelihood of experiencing a panic attack in the next week, and the expected severity of attacks, should they occur.

Symptom rating scales

Several instruments are available for measuring the tendency to fear anxiety-related bodily sensations. These include the Anxiety Sensitivity Index, Agoraphobic Cognitions Questionnaire, Body Sensations Questionnaire, Panic Appraisal Inventory, and Panic Belief Questionnaire (reviewed by Shear & Maser, 1994). The Anxiety Sensitivity Index (ASI) contains 16 items that express concern about possible consequences of anxiety (Peterson & Reiss, 1992). These are rated on five-point Likert scales (0 very little to 4 very much). Scores range from 0 to 64 and the mean for normal subjects is 19. The ASI has high internal consistency and satisfactory test-retest reliability.

Patients with panic disorder experience anxiety symptoms that are not necessarily linked to panic or the anticipation of panic. These general anxiety symptoms may be measured by one of a number of commonly used scales, including the Hamilton Anxiety Scale, Sheehan Patient-Rated Anxiety Scale, Beck Anxiety Inventory, and Zung Anxiety Scale (Hamilton, 1959; Zung, 1971; Sheehan, 1983; Beck et al., 1988). The Hamilton Anxiety Scale is a widely used clinician-rated instrument used to measure level of symptoms and change with treatment. The recently developed Beck Anxiety Inventory emphasizes panic symptoms (Beck & Steer, 1990). Instruments for the assessment of panic disorder have been reviewed by Shear & Maser (1994).

Several scales have been developed for the measurement of agoraphobic symptoms. It is important to assess both fear and avoidance because the proportion of each varies among patients. Also, the assessment should emphasize the patient's response to feared situations when unaccompanied. The brief Fear Questionnaire (FQ), developed by Marks & Mathews (1979), is a standardized scale that is used for research and clinical purposes (Arrindell, 1989). Its agoraphobia subscale is made up of five items rated on 9-point linear scales (0 would not avoid it to 8 always avoid it). The FQ has adequate psychometric properties and 82–90% accuracy in classifying social phobics and agoraphobics (Cox et al., 1991). Normative data are available for the general population as well as phobic populations, and the instrument is sensitive to change. A self-report Agoraphobia Scale (AS) was recently developed by Öst (1990). It consists of 20 items covering typical agoraphobic situations that are rated for anxiety/discomfort (0–4) and avoidance (0–2). The AS has adequate psychometric properties and picks up change in treated samples.

Epidemiology

Prevalence

Panic disorder is relatively common in the general population. In studies reviewed by Wittchen & Essau (1993), the lifetime prevalence of panic disorder is about 2%, and for agoraphobia it is roughly 5%. Between 7% and 14% of persons in the general population report having had one or more panic attacks in their lifetime. Rates for attacks and panic disorder from the National Comorbidity Survey are shown in Table 3.6 (Eaton et al., 1994). Persons with attacks not meeting criteria for panic disorder are similar in terms of demographics, suggesting that attacks are part of the panic spectrum (von Korff et al., 1985; Eaton et al., 1994). This spectrum may even include limited-symptom attacks which had a lifetime prevalence of 2.2% in San Antonio (Katerndahl & Realini, 1993). Compared to persons with panic disorder, those with attacks have fewer panic symptoms, fewer attacks, less panic-related worry, lower anxiety sensitivity, and less panic-related avoidance (Telch et al., 1989).

Panic disorder is especially common in primary care where estimates of current prevalence range from 1.4% to 8.0% (Finlay-Jones & Brown, 1981; Katon et al., 1986, 1992; von Korff et al., 1987; Taylor et al., in press). Patients with the disorder typically present with somatic complaints (Katon, 1984). These are most often neurological (e.g., headache, dizziness, 44%), cardiovascular (e.g., chest pain, tachycardia, 33%), and gastrointestinal (e.g., epigastric distress, irritable bowel syndrome, 33%). Persons with panic in the community are high utilizers of medical services (Boyd, 1986). In fact, their utilization exceeds that of any other psychiatric disorder and includes emergency medical services, admissions for physical problems, and specialty services (Klerman et al., 1991); the cost of this high utilization is substantial (Simon et al., 1995).

Panic disorder is prevalent among patients who present with unexplained symptoms (Katon et al., 1992). For example, 33–43% of patients with chest pain and normal coronary arteries have this disorder. Similarly, 13% with unexplained dizziness have panic (Linzer et al., 1990). Somatic presentations of this kind often result in costly and invasive procedures and

Table 3.6. *Prevalence estimates (1 month and lifetime) for panic attacks and disorders in the general population*

	1 Month (%)	Lifetime (%)
Fearful spell	3.8	15.6
Intense fearful spell	3.0	11.3
Panic attack	2.2	7.3
Recurrent panic attacks	1.7	4.2
Panic disorder	1.5	3.5
Agoraphobia without panic disorder	—	5.3

Source: Modified from Eaton et al. (1994). © 1994, American Psychiatric Association. Reprinted with permission.

delay in making the diagnosis (Katon, 1991). In fact, relatively few patients actually receive the treatment they need. One study found that approximately 10% of primary care patients have anxiety symptoms or disorders, including panic, that are not treated (Fifer et al., 1994).

Comorbidity

There is considerable overlap between panic disorder and agoraphobia in the general population; up to half of those with panic report agoraphobia (Eaton et al., 1994). Likewise many, but not all, persons with agoraphobia give a history of panic attacks (Lelliott et al., 1989). In the Epidemiologic Catchment Area study, a sizable proportion were identified who had never had attacks, but, when re-interviewed, these subjects were found to have other (mostly phobic) disorders, not agoraphobia (Horwath et al., 1993). Agoraphobia is also closely associated with social phobia.

Comorbidity is extremely common among persons with panic disorder. The Epidemiologic Catchment Area study found that 91% of persons with panic disorder and 84% of those with agoraphobia had other disorders as well (Robins & Regier, 1991). The comorbidity rates were especially high for other anxiety and depressive disorders, but relatively low for substance use disorders (Merikangas et al., 1996). High odds ratios were reported for phobias (11) and major depressive disorder (25). High rates of comorbidity have been found in clinical populations as well (DiNardo & Barlow, 1990).

Risk factors

Panic disorder is roughly twice as common in women as in men, and agoraphobia shows an even greater female preponderance (Eaton et al.,

1991, 1994). Despite speculation about the importance of role conflict, the greater prevalence in women is unexplained. The prevalence of panic disorder is greatest in persons aged 15–24 years. Although originally considered a disorder of adulthood, there is evidence that it occurs in children and adolescents (Hayward et al., 1989; Moreau & Weissman, 1992; Bernstein et al., 1996). Panic disorder is relatively rare in the elderly (Flint, 1994). In this age group, panic and agoraphobia either persist from earlier in life or arise in association with physical illness. A relationship between education and the disorder was found in the National Comorbidity Survey (NCS) (Eaton et al., 1994). In that study, persons with fewer than 12 years of education were 10 times as likely to have panic disorder as persons with 16 years or more. Although an early onset of the disorder may interfere with education, less education may be an indicator of vulnerability to stressors. Other indices of socioeconomic status, such as occupational class and income, have weaker associations with the disorder.

Family and twin studies

Panic disorder is highly familial (Crowe et al., 1983). Lifetime rates among first degree relatives of patients with panic disorder are shown in Table 3.7. These are considerably higher than rates among relatives of control probands. Among relatives – as in the general population – women are affected twice as often as men. Also, these relatives have higher rates of panic attacks not meeting criteria for panic disorder. For example, Maier et al. (1993a) reported that 17.6% of panic relatives had had attacks compared to 6.9% of control relatives. In addition, there is an increased prevalence of agoraphobia among the relatives of panic probands who also have agoraphobia. For instance, Noyes et al. (1986a) found agoraphobia in 11.6% of the relatives of agoraphobic probands compared to 1.9% of the relatives of panic probands.

Family data have been examined in an effort to determine the relationship between panic and other anxiety, depressive and substance use disorders. The separation of panic and generalized anxiety disorder was supported by studies described earlier (Crowe et al., 1983; Noyes et al., 1986a). Also, the much-debated relationship between panic disorder and major depression has been clarified. In one study, Goldstein et al. (1994) compared relatives of three proband groups: panic only, major depression only, and both panic and major depression. They found elevated rates of panic disorder in relatives of probands with panic disorder with or without major depression, but not in relatives of probands with major depression

Table 3.7. *Prevalence of (lifetime) panic disorder among the relatives of panic disorder and control probands*

	Panic disorder relatives (%)	Control relatives (%)
Crowe et al. (1983)	17.3	1.8
Noyes et al. (1986a)[a]	8.3	4.2
Maier et al. (1993a)	7.7	1.5
Goldstein et al. (1994)	14.2	0.8
Mendlewicz et al. (1993)	13.2	0.9

[a]Agoraphobic probands.

and no panic disorder. Conversely, they found elevated rates of major depression in relatives of probands with major depression with or without panic disorder, but not in relatives of probands with panic disorder and no major depression. These findings are supported by some but not all studies (Coryell et al., 1988; Maier et al., 1993a).

Twin studies indicate that genetic factors are imporatnt in panic disorder. In a small clinical sample, Torgersen (1983) found a concordance of 31% among co-twins of probands with panic disorder or agoraphobia with panic attacks. None of the dizygotic twins was concordant. In another Norwegian study, 42% of monozygotic twins were concordant for panic compared to 17% of dizygotic twins (Skre et al., 1993). An additional study indicated that genetic factors may be important in early separation anxiety (Manicavasgar et al., 1995). More recently, Kendler et al. (1993) completed a twin study based on a large sample from the Virginia Twin Registry. Pairwise concordance was 24% for monozygotic and 11% for dizygotic twins. Using a variety of statistical models, these authors found that family aggregation of panic disorder is due largely to genetic factors; however, they estimated the inherited vulnerability at a modest 30–40%, less than the estimated 65% for manic depressive illness and schizophrenia.

Given the importance of genetic factors, attention has been directed toward possible modes of inheritance (Woodman, 1993). The disorder does not fit a simple Mendelian pattern, so more complex models, involving a single major locus with incomplete penetrance or multifactorial polygenic inheritance, have been considered. A variety of mathematical models have been developed to determine whether transmission patterns can be explained by known genetic mechanisms (Crowe, 1990). Pauls et al. (1980), using a pedigree analysis, found a pattern consistent with monogenic transmission. Crowe et al. (1983) reported that a polygenic model that took gender into account gave an acceptable fit and Vieland et al. (1993) found that, based on a segregation analysis, neither a single dominant nor a single recessive gene could be ruled out.

Advances in molecular genetics have led to the identification of an increasing number of genetic markers that can be used to examine the relationship of a disorder to loci on various chromosomes. In this way the gene or genes responsible for a disorder may be identified. Panic disorder, because there is evidence for genetic transmission, is a candidate for study with linkage markers. Several groups are pursuing studies but, as yet, no linkage has been found. One strategy has been to look for linkage with candidate genes that are involved in neurotransmitter regulation. Studies ruling out linkage to genes for adrenergic receptors, tyrosine hydroxylase, and benzodiazepine receptors have been published (Mutchler et al., 1990; Wang et al., 1992).

Etiology and pathogenesis

Nervous system dysfunction

Global cerebral arousal

It is not clear whether patients with panic disorder are in a persistent state of overarousal or respond excessively to stimuli ignored by others. A measure of hyperarousal is sleep disturbance, and in one survey, two-thirds of the patients complained of moderate to severe sleep difficulty (Stein et al., 1993a). Disturbance of sleep architecture in panic patients consists of increased sleep latency, decreased sleep time, and decreased sleep efficiency, but not the reduced REM latency seen in major depression (Mellman & Uhde, 1989b; Stein et al., 1993; Ferini-Strambi et al, 1996). Thus, sleep studies show that many, but not all, panic patients are hyperaroused.

Brain metabolism is another measure of arousal. A small positron emission tomography (PET) study (Reiman et al., 1984) found no difference in overall cerebral blood flow between panic patients at rest and normal controls; however, in an extended study, the same authors reported abnormally high brain metabolism (Reiman et al., 1986). Still, increased blood flow might have resulted from the imaging procedure itself (Gur et al., 1987). Another group, measuring glucose metabolism, found no elevation in patients (Nordahl et al., 1990). Ambulatory monitoring studies, discussed below, revealed no cardiovascular hyperarousal except when patients were anxious. Judging from sleep studies, panic disorder patients appear mildly hyperaroused but, when they are not anxious, their brain metabolism does not differ from that of normals.

Locus coeruleus and the noradrenergic system

There is good agreement that three brain regions, namely the brain stem, the limbic system, and the prefrontal cortex, are intimately involved in the neurobiology of panic disorder (Gorman et al., 1989); however, investigators differ concerning the extent to which each contributes. Early evidence connecting specific regions to panic attacks was obtained by Redmond (1977). Redmond demonstrated that locus coeruleus activation produced anxious behavior in monkeys, while blocking its activity had a calming effect. The locus coeruleus is the main noradrenergic nucleus with projections to wide areas of the brain, including limbic system and cortex. This nucleus and its connections constitute an 'alarm system' that can be triggered by internal or external stimuli. In persons with panic disorder, this system is thought to be hypersensitive and subject to unprovoked reactions. Klein (1981) hypothesized that certain persons are more sensitive to anxiety-provoking stimuli because of having an innate alarm mechanism with a low threshold. He saw this defective mechanism as the source of separation anxiety and the root of panic disorder.

Pharmacological challenge studies have appeared to confirm Klein's hypothesis. Charney and colleagues (1984) administered yohimbine, an alpha-2-antagonist that increases locus coeruleus activity, to panic disorder patients and normal controls. Panic patients were more sensitive to the drug than non-anxious individuals and developed panic attacks together with elevated plasma MHPG, the main cerebral metabolite of norepinephrine. As predicted from animal studies, clonidine, an alpha-2-agonist that lowers locus coeruleus activity, reduced panic attacks in patients (Hoehn-Saric et al., 1981). Panic patients have also shown a blunted growth hormone response to clonidine (Charney et al., 1992; Brambilla et al., 1995), indicating that they have an alpha-2-noradrenergic receptor dysfunction. Only patients with frequent panic attacks responded excessively to a yohimbine challenge (Charney et al., 1984), and not all studies found the blunted growth hormone response to clonidine (Gann et al., 1995). Platelet alpha-2-receptor function is as an indirect measure of cerebral receptor function but the results of studies have not been conclusive. For instance, Cameron et al. (1990) found lower density binding sites in panic patients, while Charney et al. (1989) found no difference in density but a decrease in affinity.

The central role of the locus coerules in anxiety has been questioned

further by other studies. No differences in cerebrospinal fluid norepinephrine or its metabolites have been found in panic patients and controls
(Eriksson et al., 1991). Also, no increase in MHPG, indicative of locus
coeruleus hyperactivity, has been found during panic attacks induced by
sodium lactate (Carr et al., 1986), carbon dioxide inhalation (Woods et al.,
1988a), caffeine challenge (Boulenger et al., 1984), or exposure to panic-
inducing situations (Woods et al., 1987). Buspirone increases locus coeruleus activity yet acts as an anxiolytic (Sanghera et al., 1982). Moreover,
other factors may alter locus coeruleus function. These include excitation
by corticotropin-releasing factor, acetylcholine, and substance P; and inhibition by opiates, GABA, serotonin, and epinephrine (Charney et al., 1990).
In anxiety disorder patients receiving clonidine, Hoehn-Saric et al. (1981)
observed a reduction in panic attacks and fluctuations in generalized
anxiety despite high overall distress. More recent studies in animals have
confirmed the clinical observations that the locus coeruleus may function
as a gain control for arousal (Aston-Jones et al., 1991) but may not be the
primary locus of anxiety.

Serotonergic raphe nuclei

The fact that selective serotonin reuptake inhibitors suppress panic attacks
suggests that the serotonergic system is important in panic disorder; however, the role that this system plays is not well understood. There is, of
course, strong interdependence between the serotonergic and noradrenergic systems (Asnis et al., 1992). The serotonergic raphe nuclei have a
dampening effect on the locus coeruleus and may prevent the excessive
firing responsible for panic attacks; however, the serotonergic system is
complex, having at least 16 receptors with diverse functions. No differences
in cerebrospinal fluid serotonin or its metabolites have been found between
panic patients and controls (Eriksson et al., 1991). While drugs that increase serotonin at all receptor sites effectively control panic attacks, no
such effects have been demonstrated with drugs that target individual
serotonin receptors. Neither buspirone (Sheehan et al., 1993), a partial
$5HT_{1a}$ agonist, nor ritanserin, a $5HT_2$ antagonist (den Boer & Westenberg,
1990), nor ondansetron, a $5HT_3$ receptor antagonist (Charney et al., 1990),
have outperformed placebo in the suppression of panic attacks.

The results of serotonergic challenges are suggestive but not conclusive.
Tryptophan is the precursor of serotonin. Dietary depletion of tryptophan worsens depression but does not alter panic (Goddard et al.,
1994); intravenous tryptophan does not increase prolactin excessively
(Charney & Heninger, 1986); and 5-hydroxytryptophan, given therapeuti-

cally, is only modestly effective (Kahn et al., 1987). An acute presynaptic increase of serotonin by fenfluramine had an anxiogenic effect in one study (Targum & Marshall, 1989), but not another (Judd et al., 1994). On the other hand, direct stimulation of $5HT_2$ receptors with a partial agonist, mCPP, induced anxiety and attacks in panic patients (Kahn & Moore, 1993). Following a challenge with the selective partial $5HT_{1a}$ agonist, ipsapirone, panic patients had impaired hypothermic as well as ACTH and cortisol responses, indicating subsensitivity of the pre- and postsynaptic $5HT_{1a}$ receptors (Lesch et al., 1992). Platelet serotonin was higher in patients who had increased uptake (Norman et al., 1988) and decreased high-affinity [3H]LSD binding (Norman et al., 1990). This finding points to serotonergic hyperactivity in panic disorder; however, discrepancies between platelet studies make conclusions difficult (Leonard, 1990).

Medullary respiratory centers

Panic attacks are associated with shortness of breath and hyperventilation. In theory, panic attacks might be a consequence of hyperventilation-induced hypocapnia or heightened sensitivity of brain stem chemoreceptors. Hyperventilation may cause symptoms of anxiety, and chronic hyperventilation may cause seemingly spontaneous panic attacks (Margraf et al., 1986). For this reason, some researchers have concluded that panic disorder and the hyperventilation syndrome are synonymous (Lum, 1976). Hyperventilation occurs during panic attacks, but it is not clear whether overbreathing triggers attacks, or more likely, is a consequence of sudden anxiety. Hyperventilation only infrequently induces panic attacks in the laboratory (Gorman et al., 1984). Arterial blood gases in non-panicking patients are not different from those of controls, and experimentally induced hypercarbia or hypocarbia alone are not sufficient to cause panic (Zandbergen, 1992). Zandbergen (1992) concluded that hyperventilation is a consequence, rather than a cause, of panic attacks. Panic disorder patients, however, show abnormal breathing patterns during sleep as indicated by increased irregularity in tidal volume during REM sleep and by an increased rate of microapneas (Stein et al., 1995a). The respiratory stimulant, doxapram, can cause attacks as well as breathing irregularities in panic patients (Abelson et al., 1996). Thus, panic disorder patients may have some constitutional or acquired abnormality in respiratory function.

Sodium lactate infusion and carbon dioxide challenge are believed to cause panic through a buildup of carbon dioxide. In the case of sodium lactate, carbon dioxide is a metabolic end product. This buildup causes central hypercapnia and acidosis which results in panic (Gorman et al., 1984). Another variant of the central acidosis hypotheses was proposed by Carr & Sheehan (1984). According to these authors, sodium lactate, carbon dioxide and hyperventilation all produce systemic alkalosis. This alkalosis results in central ischemia that decreases intracellular pH in ventral medullary chemoreceptors, resulting in panic. These theories have not been proven experimentally.

The most recent theory involving medullary chemoreceptors was proposed by Klein (1993). According to this author, physiological misinterpretation by a suffocation monitor produces sudden respiratory distress followed by hyperventilation, panic, and an urge to flee. The cause of this false suffocation alarm is hypersensitivity of medullary chemoreceptors to carbon dioxide; therefore, acute hyperventilation does not necessarily induce panic attacks. Gorman et al. (1988) observed an association between panic and exaggerated ventilatory response as well as elevated plasma norepinephrine, and concluded that carbon dioxide receptors were oversensitive. The increase in norepinephrine, however, might have been caused by an anxiety-induced increase in muscle activity. Ley (1994) states that there is no empirical evidence to support the proposed neurological 'suffocation alarm' mechanism. Neither Zandbergen (1992) nor Woods et al. (1988a) found evidence for hypersensitive carbon dioxide receptors in panic disorder patients. Also, Hibbert & Pilsbury (1989) found no association between PCO_2 levels and the type of symptoms reported.

Limbic system

The limbic system integrates internal and external inputs into response patterns. This is probably the brain region in which emotions, including anxiety, are generated. Gray (1982) outlined the importance of the septohippocampal system for anxiety. More recent studies have established the importance of the amygdala, particularly in the acquisition of learned anxiety responses (Davis et al., 1994; Phillips & LeDoux, 1992). Chapter 1 on normal anxiety contains more information on this subject. The functions of the hippocampus and amygdala are modified by inputs from noradrenergic and serotonergic nuclei of the brain stem as well as prefrontal cortex. Heightened arousal results in stronger associations between situations and anxiety following exposure. Subsequently, anxiety occurs whenever the situation presents itself, and in extreme instances, this leads to phobic reactions. The suddenness of panic attacks and the development of attacks in individuals who abuse cocaine suggest that limbic kindling may develop in patients (Post et al., 1993); however, the findings from electroencephalographic and structural imaging studies have been normal in such patients (Uhde & Kellner, 1987; Lepola et al., 1990b; de Cristofaro et al., 1993). Roy-Byrne et al. (1986a) found no electroencephalographic abnormalities of the kind seen in patients with temporal lobe epilepsy. Specific electroencephalographic patterns may accompany certain symptoms. For instance, panic patients with depersonalization respond to odor stimulation differently than patients without depersonalization, suggesting activation of temporal regions (Locatelli et al., 1993).

Temporal lobe abnormalities are more frequent in panic disorder patients than one would expect by chance. Several studies have shown a comparatively frequent occurrence of focal paroxysmal discharges and seizures (Weilburg et al., 1995; George & Ballenger, 1992). Interestingly, panic attacks are more frequently associated with morphological or electrophysiological abnormalities in the right than in the left temporal area. Stimulation of the right superior temporal gyrus and parahippocampal region produces overwhelming fear (Penfield & Jasper, 1954), and most partial complex seizures associated with ictal fear originate from the right temporal lobe (Hermann et al., 1992). Ontiveros et al. (1989) and Fontaine et al. (1990) found neuroanatomical abnormalities on magnetic resonance imaging (MRI) scans – mostly involving the right temporal lobe – four times more frequent in panic patients than normal controls. More than half of patients with morphological abnormalities had electroencephalographic abnormalities as well (Dantendorfer et al., 1994).

In panic patients, mean blood flow velocity, measured with transcranial Doppler ultrasound, was greater in the right than in the left middle cerebral artery (Cerisoli et al., 1996). Metabolic asymmetries have also been reported in panic patients using imaging techniques. For example, Reiman et al. (1986) described asymmetry in cerebral blood flow and oxygen metabolism between the right and the left parahippocampal gyrus with higher activity on the right. Nordahl et al. (1990) reported hippocampal asymmetry in glucose metabolism; however, another study using single positron emission computed tomography (SPECT) found decreased cerebral blood flow in both hippocampal regions in panic patients (de Cristofaro et al., 1993). Reiman et al. (1989) also measured cerebral blood flow with PET before and during lactate-induced panic. Panic was associated with significant blood flow increases in the temporal poles bilaterally; insular cortex, claustrum, and lateral putamen; superior colliculus; and left anterior vermis. Others (Drevets et al., 1992) observed similar blood flow changes during jaw clenching, indicating that they might represent artifact. Stewart et al. (1988) examined blood flow changes, using SPECT with 133-xenon inhalation, during lactate-induced panic attacks. Sodium lactate significantly increased flow in controls and patients who did not panic but not in those who panicked. This suggests that hyperventilation prevented an increase in blood flow that might have occurred otherwise.

Frontal lobes

The prefrontal cortex exercises brain executive function. It receives inputs from other parts of the brain, integrates, assesses, plans and decides upon action. This region also influences functions of lower brain regions, including the limbic system and brain stem nuclei. In addition, it modifies perception and response to external stimuli and generates anticipatory anxiety. For instance, isoproterenol, a beta-adrenergic agonist that does not penetrate the blood–brain barrier, induces attacks in panic patients (Nesse et al., 1984). A similar mechanism may be responsible for lactate-induced panic attacks. Thus, procedures that cause panic-like bodily sensations may induce attacks psychologically by triggering an alarm response. Heightened anticipatory anxiety increases the probability that sodium lactate will induce panic (Targum, 1991), while repeated administration of lactate reduces the probability of attacks (Bonn et al., 1971). Similarly, if a patient believes that he can control carbon dioxide administration, his or her panic symptoms may be reduced (Sanderson et al., 1989). Also, repeated exposure to carbon dioxide reduces anxiety in panic patients (van den Hout et al., 1987). The angiogenic effects of yohimbine are also reduced by reassurance (Albus et al., 1992). Thus, prefrontal activity modifies the formation and severity of panic attacks. It is also through prefrontal activity that psychosocial interventions have their effect.

Two cerebral blood flow studies using SPECT found frontal lobe changes in panic patients. One reported significant right–left asymmetry in the inferior frontal cortex (de Cristofaro et al., 1993). The other found bilateral frontal reductions in blood flow among patients who had received yohimbine but not in controls (Woods et al., 1988b). Presently, these results are difficult to interpret. Davidson (1992) demonstrated that increased activity in the right frontal area is associated with increased vulnerability to anxiety and depression, while increased activity in the left hemisphere is associated with decreased vulnerability. Therefore, it is of interest that, in brain imaging and electrophysiological studies of panic patients, the right hemisphere more frequently exhibits pathology.

Other neurotransmitter systems

Cerebrospinal fluid levels of corticotropin-releasing hormone do not appear to be altered in panic patients (Jolkkonen et al., 1993); however, corticotropin-releasing hormone stimulation produces lower ACTH and cortisol responses in these patients, suggesting that they are chronically hypercortisolemic (Roy-Byrne et al., 1986b). While less than one-third of patients were non-suppressors when given the dexamethasone suppression test (Judd et al., 1987), subtle ACTH and cortisol abnormalities were observed over a 24-hour period (Abelson et al., 1996b) when dexamethasone and corticotropin-releasing hormone challenge tests were combined (Schriber et al., 1996). Patients who were dexamethasone non-suppressors had more symptoms of anxiety and social disability after 3 years than suppressors (Coryell et al., 1991). Thus, panic patients may have subtle changes in the hypothalamic–pituitary–adrenal axis, and more pronounced abnormalities may be associated with more severe pathology.

Adenosine has a calming effect in animals (Pelleg & Porter, 1990). Challenges with caffeine, an adenosine antagonist, cause panic disorder patients to respond with anxiety and to panic at lower doses than non-anxious individuals (Boulenger et al., 1984). Injections of caffeine reduced global cerebral blood flow in patients and controls but showed no regional differences (Cameron et al., 1990a).

Panic disorder patients exhibit enhanced sensitivity to the cholecystokinin tetrapeptide (CCK) (Bradwejn et al., 1991). The mechanism of the panicogenic effect of CCK is not known. In animals a functional antagonism between CCK and benzodiazepines has been demonstrated (Bradwejn & de Montigny, 1984). Also, CCK stimulates hypothalamic–pituitary–adrenal function in rats (Kalimaris et al., 1992). In panic patients, lower CCK concentrations have been found in cerebrospinal fluid (Lydiard et al., 1992a).

Reduced cerebrospinal fluid levels of GABA (Rimon et al., 1995) and elevated plasma neuropeptide Y (Boulenger et al., 1996) have also been reported, but no abnormalities in cerebrospinal fluid opioids or somatostatin have been found (Lepola et al., 1990a).

Microstimulation of the thalamus

Recently, Lenz et al. (1995), by electrical microstimulation posterior to the nucleus ventralis caudalis of the thalamus, produced panic-like attacks without changes in heart rate or blood pressure in a patient who had had spontaneous attacks. It appears that panic attacks can form engrams in certain regions of the brain that, when stimulated, induce 'as if' experiences including bodily changes. This may explain why ambulatory monitors often record no changes during panic attacks and why, in spite of mild bodily changes, panic attacks are so frightful.

Physiological dysfunction

Patients with panic disorder show few physiologic abnormalities in the non-anxious state. For instance, there is no cardiovascular hyperactivity among such patients at rest (Hoehn-Saric & McLeod, 1993). Cardiovascular studies have found few differences between relaxed panic patients and controls. On baseline measures, one-third of 19 studies showed increased heart rate and systolic blood pressure in panic patients, and one-quarter showed increased diastolic blood pressure. Skin conductance was elevated in two studies and one reported elevated forehead muscle tension. Highly anxious patients have also exhibited greater chest muscle activity than less anxious patients (Lynch et al., 1991). Several, but not all, studies have found physiological evidence of hyperventilation at baseline. Only one found elevations of stress hormones and this study has been criticized on methodological grounds. Disparate findings may have been due to differences in the severity of panic disorder and experimental design. Frequently, baseline measures for potentially stressful experiments were obtained without allowing time for full relaxation.

We found that, when panic patients were exposed to psychological stressors, this led not to an exaggerated but a more restricted skin conductance response than that seen in non-anxious controls. This and other evidence points to diminished autonomic flexibility of the kind seen in other chronic anxiety disorders (Hoehn-Saric et al., 1991). Also, Yeragani et al. (1990) as well as Klein et al.(1995) reported decreased heart rate variability, indicative of an increase in vagal withdrawal in panic patients. Physiological challenges, such as postural changes, Valsalva maneuver, and treadmill exercise, generally induce stronger cardiovascular responses in panic patients than in controls (Hoehn-Saric & McLeod, 1993). These changes are interpreted as signs of increased autonomic lability but may also be attributed to lower physical fitness. Stein et al. (1994) matched patients and controls for physical fitness and found no difference in vagal tone at rest or during physical challenge. In two studies that measured response to auditory stimuli, slower habituation of skin conductance was observed (Lader et al., 1967; Roth et al., 1990). Thus, panic patients habituate slowly to innocuous stimuli.

The recording of physiological parameters during spontaneous panic attacks is technically difficult; therefore, only limited information is available on naturally occurring attacks. Lader & Mathews (1970) recorded changes in three patients who panicked during recording sessions. Their attacks were associated with sudden increases in heart rate, along with increases in skin conductance, finger pulse volume, and forearm blood flow. The physiological state of these patients normalized within a few minutes. Other studies, including those carried out with ambulatory monitors, have also observed heart rate, blood pressure and respiratory changes during unprovoked attacks (Hoehn-Saric & McLeod, 1993). The most comprehensive study of such attacks was conducted by Woods et al. (1987) who exposed patients to situations in which they frequently panicked. For instance, they took a patient who feared bridges to a bridge. During attacks, they observed increases in heart rate, but blood pressure, plasma MHPG, cortisol, growth hormone, and prolactin remained within the prepanic range. On the other hand, Ko et al. (1983) found that the plasma levels of MHPG were elevated after attacks caused by exposure to phobic situations. Thus, although they are sometimes strong, the physiological changes observed during panic rarely match the subjective experience (Lader & Mathews, 1970). It is assumed that changes during attacks reflect a sudden increase in sympathetic tone, but a reduction in vagal tone has also been postulated (George et al., 1989).

During behavioral interventions, such as systematic exposure to feared situations, increased heart rate accompanies heightened anxiety. As treatment progresses, clinical manifestations and heart rate decrease but not at the same rate. Subjective and behavioral manifestations respond earlier than heart rate, reflecting the desynchrony that has been observed during behavior treatment of simple phobias. In one study (Craske et al., 1987), increased heart rate was associated with a good outcome. Patients who were willing to approach feared situations responded with greater increases in heart rates than did hesitant, non-assertive patients.

Psychological factors

Although hereditary and biological factors have received recent emphasis, environmental factors have traditionally been viewed as important in the development of anxiety disorders. Most models assume a genetically determined, temperamental substrate for personality development that may include traits of timidity, shyness, and avoidance of risk-taking (Parker, 1988; Biederman et al., 1990). Developmental factors, including relationships with parents and parental attitudes, may interact with temperamental factors to foster traits of emotional dependence, immaturity, and neuroticism, and these may in turn increase vulnerability to adult anxiety (Roth et al., 1972; Arrindell et al., 1989). Stressful life events, if perceived as threatening, may play a role in the onset of an anxiety disorder (Finlay-

Jones & Brown, 1981; Andrews, 1988). Likewise, factors such as social class and social support may hasten or retard the development of pathological anxiety. Finally, coping style, both cognitive and behavioral, may have a bearing on who develops anxiety and who does not.

Temperament

Recent work has focused on temperamental differences that might form a basis of vulnerability to panic and, perhaps, other anxiety disorders. Temperament refers to stable response patterns that are evident early in life and that influence later personality development. One such temperamental category, known as behavioral inhibition, is characterized by a consistent tendency to display fear and withdraw from unfamiliar settings, people or objects. Kagan and colleagues (1989) report that behavioral inhibition occurs in about 15% of infants and children. Characteristic behaviors, that can be identified in the laboratory at an early age, persist in school-age children (Rosenbaum et al., 1994). The physiological correlates of behavioral inhibition point to lower threshold for arousal and sympathetic inhibition that are consistent with hypothesized neurophysiologic mechanisms in anxiety disorders.

A series of studies have linked this temperamental pattern to risk for anxiety disorders. For instance, Rosenbaum et al. (1988) found behavioral inhibition in 70–85% of the children of parents with panic disorder compared to 15% in children of non-anxious parents. Also, behaviorally inhibited children showed increased rates of anxiety disorders compared to normal controls (Beiderman et al., 1990). When these children were reassessed after 3 years, even more anxiety disorders had emerged (Beiderman et al., 1993). Finally, when the parents of behaviorally inhibited children were examined, they were found to have higher rates of both childhood and adult anxiety disorders (Rosenbaum et al., 1992). These results suggest that early behavioral inhibition may be involved in the later development of panic and other anxiety disorders.

Childhood environment

The role of early environment in the etiology of panic disorder with or without agoraphobia has been the subject of theorizing and empirical investigation. Hypotheses concerning factors important in the later development of the disorder arose from attachment theory. According to this theory, the human infant is endowed with a behavioral system that ensures closeness to a caretaker, thereby increasing its chance of survival (Bowlby,

1969). If the caretaker is not sensitive and responsive to the child, separation anxiety or fearfulness in the face of threatened loss of that person may arise. Based on extensive study of childhood attachment, Bowlby (1973) hypothesized that this anxiety plays an important role in panic and agoraphobia. Klein (1981) elaborated on this theme and, along with Gittleman & Klein (1984), reported high rates of childhood separation anxiety and school phobia among patients with agoraphobia.

Several studies show that adult agoraphobics have more often experienced childhood separation anxiety than non-patient controls (reviewed by de Ruiter & van Ijzendoorn, 1992). One study showed a higher rate of such anxiety among panic patients with agoraphobia than those without (Deltito et al., 1986); however, these studies did not show a difference between panic patients and neurotic controls in the frequency of this childhood disturbance, which suggests that separation anxiety is a nonspecific factor in adult psychopathology. Also, the relatively low frequency (23% across studies) suggests that it has limited importance (de Ruiter & van Ijzendoorn, 1992).

Adverse events and circumstances in childhood are associated with the development of panic disorder but it is not clear how specific or important such factors are. One potentially important event is separation from a parent by death or divorce. Early studies rather consistently found that patients with panic and agoraphobia had been separated from a parent more often than controls (reviewed by Tweed et al., 1989; Brown & Harris, 1993). More recent studies have demonstrated the same thing in non-clinical populations. In two of them, 28–32% of persons with panic disorder reported that their parents had been separated or divorced compared to 13–16% of persons with generalized anxiety disorder (Tweed et al., 1989; Brown & Harris, 1993). Also, two studies showed associations between parental death and both panic disorder and agoraphobia (Tweed et al., 1989; Kendler et al., 1992). In these studies, separation from the mother was a stronger predictor of panic than separation from the father.

The issues of how important early parental separation is to the subsequent development of anxiety or depressive disorders was examined by Brown & Harris (1993). They assessed the impact of parental loss within the context of the overall childhood environment. Using an index of childhood adversity, they found that parental loss added little to the prediction of an anxiety disorder once early adversity had been taken into account. According to them, overall environment is the critical factor and loss of a parent is important only because it increases the likelihood of negative early experience. The elements of such adversity included physical and sexual abuse, parental indifference or neglect, as well as separation from a parent by death or divorce, and roughly half of persons with panic and agoraphobia experience such early events or circumstances (Brown & Harris, 1993; Stein et al., 1995b).

Research on parenting style has relied upon self-report questionnaires, asking agoraphobics to retrospectively assess the caregiving they received. The dimensions of affection and protection have been of particular interest based on Bowlby's theory. De Ruiter and van Ijzendoorn (1992) found that, across studies they reviewed, agoraphobics rated their parents lower on affection and higher on overprotection than did normal controls (Parker, 1979; Arrindell et al., 1989). They concluded that agoraphobic patients view their parents as having been highly unaffectionate but only moderately overprotective. Three studies compared agoraphobics to social phobics. In these, agoraphobics recalled more parental affection and less overprotection than did the social phobics. The findings from comparisons between agoraphobics and normals support the hypothesized role of early separation anxiety in agoraphobia, but findings from the agoraphobic-social phobic comparison do not (de Ruiter & van Ijzendoorn, 1992).

Life events

Major life events appear important in precipitating panic disorder (Mathews et al., 1981; Barlow, 1988). Research has shown that anxiety disorders are more often preceded by threatening events, whereas depressive disorders more often follow losses (Finlay-Jones & Brown, 1981). With respect to panic and agoraphobia, events involving the threat of separation and interpersonal conflict have been implicated (Goldstein & Chambless, 1978; Klein, 1981). Controlled studies have found major life events associated with the onset in a majority of patients (Pollard et al., 1989). For example, Faravelli & Pallanti (1989) found that 64% of panic patients experienced negative events in the year prior to onset compared to 35% of normal controls. Importantly, they found independent events (i.e., not influenced by the development of the disorder) frequent among those with panic disorder.

The life events that precede panic and agoraphobia appear to be nonspecific and their overall importance in the etiology is unclear (Roy-Byrne et al., 1986c; Rapee et al., 1990). Events involving separation and interpersonal conflict are frequent, but other types of events are reported as well (Pollard et al., 1989). In fact, some patients report an onset associated with biological factors such as substance use. For example, some patients who have a panic attack during marijuana intoxication subsequently experience recurrent attacks not related to the drug (Roy-Byrne & Uhde, 1988). According to Brown et al. (1993), who studied a population of high-risk inner city women, negative life events and circumstances in adulthood may have limited importance. When they took childhood adversity into account, they found the relationship of panic and agoraphobia to *adult* adversity to be weak.

Personality

Studies have consistently demonstrated high levels of personality pathology in patients with panic disorder and agoraphobia. Although subject to varied interpretation, the findings generally point toward a personality predisposition to the disorder. This conclusion is tentative because traits have usually been assessed in symptomatic individuals whose personality functioning may be influenced by their morbid state. The reported prevalence of personality disorders has ranged in most studies from 27% to 58% (reviewed by Brooks et al., 1989; Mavissakalian, 1990). Disorders from the anxious cluster have been reported with the greatest frequency and avoidant, dependent, histrionic and borderline personality disorders have been found most consistently. Studies using dimensional measures have found increased harm avoidance, anxiety sensitivity, and neuroticism (Saviotti et al., 1991; Hoffart, 1995). Some studies, but not all, have shown greater personality disturbance among agoraphobic than panic patients. For instance, Reich et al. (1987) observed dependent personality disorder more frequently among patients with agoraphobia than those with panic disorder.

Investigators have used several approaches in examining the relationship between abnormal personality and panic disorder. In two epidemiological studies, the traits of persons who later developed anxiety disorders were compared to those who did not (Nyström & Lindegård (1975). Their results were similar. Angst & Vollrath (1991) found that military inductees, who later developed panic or generalized anxiety disorder, had more nervousness, depressiveness, inhibition, low frustration tolerance, and neuroticism than those who did not. Another approach involved examination of remitted or recovered patients. Here, successfully treated patients were found to have avoidant traits as well as greater anxiety sensitivity and harm avoidance than healthy controls (Saviotti et al., 1991; Mavissakalian & Hamann, 1992). This evidence suggests that a personality substrate for panic and agoraphobia exists, although the influence of prodromal or residual anxiety symptoms cannot be ruled out.

The personality disturbance associated with panic may, to some degree, be a non-specific consequence of the disorder. Comparisons between patients with panic and other disorders, such as major depressive and obsessive-compulsive disorder, have in most instances shown similar personality features (Reich & Troughton, 1988; Mavissakalian et al., 1990; Sciuto et al., 1991; Skodol et al., 1995). Also, some personality traits change with treatment (Mavissakalian & Hamann, 1987). For example, when Noyes et al. (1991a) assessed personality in a large group of patients before treatment and again 3 years later, they found substantial improvement in the same traits – dependent, avoidant, and histrionic – that had distinguished patients from normal controls originally. To some extent, such change may reflect a lifting of morale associated with treatment, but some improvement in personality functioning may be a direct result of treatment.

Cognitive dysfunction

Observation of cognitive disturbances during panic attacks (i.e., fear of dying, going crazy or doing something uncontrolled) led to their inclusion in the DSM criteria. Such disturbances also led to theories about the role of cognitive factors in the pathogenesis of panic disorder. Beck et al. (1974) and Hibbert (1984) noted that patients view their panic symptoms as extremely dangerous. For example, palpitations may be viewed as a sign of impending catastrophe (e.g., heart attack). Goldstein & Chambless (1978) suggested that this fear of fear might be the result of interoceptive conditioning. Clark (1986), on the other hand, proposed that panic attacks may result from catastrophic misinterpretation of bodily sensations. Self-monitoring studies have confirmed that cognitions of this kind accompany attacks (Westling & Öst, 1993). These theories have been influential and have led to the development of effective therapies, but still require proof (McNally, 1994). Most, but not all, attacks are accompanied by catastrophic cognitions, but it is not clear whether they give rise to, or result from, panic.

Still another cognitive formulation emphasizes anxiety sensitivity or an enduring tendency to fear anxiety symptoms (Reiss & McNally, 1985). Persons with high anxiety sensitivity are believed to panic because of the potential for harm that symptoms represent. Studies show that patients with panic disorder have high anxiety sensitivity, as measured by the Anxiety Sensitivity Index, and that this distinguishes them from patients with generalized anxiety disorder (McNally, 1992). Anxiety sensitivity may develop in the absence of panic, may predict who will develop attacks under challenge conditions (e.g., lactate infusion), and may constitute a risk factor for the development of panic disorder (McNally, 1994).

Predictability and controllability are cognitive factors that may also be important in the occurrence of panic attacks (McNally, 1994). There is evidence that heightened expectation may increase the likelihood of having a panic attack. Also, a sense of control or lack of it may be important (Barlow, 1988). When panic patients who believed they had control over the amount of carbon dioxide they were inhaling were compared with those who believed they had no control, the rate of panic was lower in those who had an illusion of control (Sanderson et al., 1989). Patients often report that they are more prone to panic in situations involving less control (e.g., riding in, compared to driving, an automobile).

Clinical picture

Clinical characteristics

Panic attacks

The essential feature of panic disorder is recurrent, discrete, anxiety or panic attacks. Such attacks are characterized by unexpected, extreme anxiety or fear, accompanied by a variety of alarming, autonomically-mediated symptoms (Aronson & Logue, 1988). The latter result from excitation of the sympathetic nervous system and include palpitations or racing heart, chest tightness or pain, and shortness of breath. Hyperventilation that accompanies this autonomic surge may contribute additional symptoms, most commonly dizziness and paraesthesias (Bass et al., 1987). Other somatic symptoms such as nausea, an urge to defecate, blurred vision, and extreme weakness may result from parasympathetic activation. Typically, symptoms begin suddenly and crescendo rapidly, reaching a peak within 10 minutes. Attacks usually last 10–30 minutes, rarely as long as an hour. They leave a patient fatigued or drained (Starcevic, 1991).

Anxiety or panic attacks are variable in their frequency, intensity, and what provokes them. Some patients report many attacks per day while others experience one or two a year. They range in intensity from mild to extreme. Mild attacks, not meeting DSM-IV criteria, are referred to as limited-symptom attacks. Many attacks, especially early in the illness, are unexpected (uncued), but others are provoked by a variety of physiological or emotional stimuli (Roy-Byrne & Uhde, 1988). Some patients, for example, find that physical exertion will trigger attacks, and therefore, avoid it. Others report that anger or excitement (e.g., sexual arousal) may provoke attacks yet states of relaxation may do so as well. Also, a variety of substances may give rise to attacks. For example, caffeine not only increases anxiety symptoms but may cause attacks (Charney et al., 1985). Many patients become aware of this and restrict their use of the substance. Alcohol may cause attacks 6–12 hours after ingestion.

Anticipatory anxiety

In addition to attacks, patients experience anticipatory anxiety. Anticipatory anxiety is characterized by worry about the possibility of future attacks and/or their consequences. With repeated panics patients become preoccupied with what might be done to forestall attacks or to terminate them should they occur. They report a feeling of uneasiness or foreboding as well as a sense of vulnerability and loss of control. They also experience general anxiety symptoms, including impaired concentration, irritability, and impatience. In addition, many find they have little stamina and wear out easily. Their uneasiness is accompanied by restlessness, inability to relax, muscle tension, and difficulty falling or staying asleep. During the day many are bothered by imbalance, blurred vision, trouble swallowing, abdominal distress, etc., symptoms that add to their apprehension and preoccupation with how they feel.

Behavioral manifestations

Although acutely anxious patients may show outward physiological or behavioral signs, most chronically anxious patients do not appear distressed except during attacks. Then, they may appear pale and diaphoretic. They may also look frightened, distractible and emotionally labile. Many are tremulous, restless, and may terminate an activity or leave a situation abruptly. In the emergency room, where patients often present, they may be hyperventilating. During severe attacks, transient increases in heart rate and blood pressure may be recorded. Chronically anxious patients sometimes appear worried, drawn or fatigued, but overall lack of outward sign contributes to skepticism on the part of others.

Cognitive symptoms

Panic attacks are often accompanied by catastrophic misinterpretation of the danger they represent (Beck et al., 1974; Hibbert, 1984). Typically patients fear dying, going crazy or collapsing. There is an immediacy and conviction about such possibilities; in the midst of strong attacks patients believe that something catastrophic is, at that moment, happening (Argyle, 1988). In response to palpitations, chest pain, and shortness of breath they may believe they are having a heart attack. With dizziness and depersonalization patients may feel they are going crazy, and lightheadedness, weakness and flushing may be interpreted as imminent collapse. Some attacks are triggered by anxious thoughts or the anticipation of a phobic situation (Argyle, 1988); however, as an attack intensifies, thoughts become more narrowly focused, more intrusive, more credible and harder to exclude from awareness (Hibbert, 1984). Some patients even visualize scenes of a feared event taking place.

Agoraphobia

Persons with agoraphobia are characteristically fearful of crowded or confined places (e.g., stores, restaurants, theaters), traveling distances from home (e.g., car, bus, airplane), or being alone or away from safe persons (Marks, 1987). As a result of their fears, they avoid such situations and restrict their activities, sometimes to a severe degree (e.g., become housebound). Agoraphobic persons often experience panic attacks in the feared situations, but these attacks are unpredictable (situationally predisposed), occurring at one time but not the next (Mathews et al., 1981). Some patients find that they can enter phobic situations with relative comfort in the company of a trusted person, such as a spouse or friend, when they could not otherwise (Foa et al., 1984). Others enter phobic situations when they are not crowded or sit near an exit (e.g., church, theater). When at home, their minds are filled with fearful anticipation of future encounters and how these might be avoided.

Hypochondriasis and depersonalization

Many patients with panic disorder experience hypochondriasis (Noyes et al., 1986b; Barsky et al., 1994). Hypochondriacal patients are preoccupied with the fear of developing or having serious physical disease despite evidence to the contrary (American Psychiatric Association, 1994). The unrealistic anticipation of danger that accompanies attacks persists and causes patients to seek unnecessary medical care and reassurance which has little effect. Starcevic et al. (1992) reported that half of the panic patients they examined had hypochondriacal fears and beliefs. Such beliefs are more common in patients with heightened anxiety sensitivity (i.e., unrealistic fear of bodily sensations) and agoraphobic symptoms (Otto et al., 1992a; Starcevic et al., 1992).

Other patients report depersonalization. This is an altered awareness of the self characterized by a feeling of strangeness or unreality. Patients often experience this alarming symptom complex during attacks or periods of severe anxiety (Roth, 1960). It is accompanied by a sense of detachment, loss of emotion, altered perception, and self-scrutiny that are difficult to describe. The disturbance may be a response to heightened arousal such as that normal persons experience in the face of life-threatening danger (Noyes et al., 1977). It is associated with more severe panic disorder and agorphobia (Cassano et al., 1989).

Panic variants

Some patients are awakened from sleep by attacks. These appear to be spontaneous physiological events that occur without perceptual or cognitive antecedent. They have been reported in 40–69% and a few patients claim predominant or even exclusive sleep attacks (Mellman & Uhde, 1989a; Labbati et al., 1994). Electroencephalographic studies show that these attacks occur during stage 2 or 3 sleep and are not associated with dreams or night terrors that arise from other stages (Mellman & Uhde, 1989b). Patients who experience sleep attacks often report other attacks induced by relaxation or sleep deprivation. They also have a longer duration of illness, more comorbidity, and more frequent anxiety disorders in childhood, which suggests that they have a more severe illness (Mellman & Uhde, 1989a, b; Labbati et al., 1994).

Some patients who otherwise have typical panic attacks report no anxiety associated with them. Beitman et al. (1987) found that nearly a third of cardiology patients with panic disorder experienced no fear with attacks. These patients were similar to those with typical attacks except for less severe anxiety and fewer phobic symptoms (Kushner & Beitman, 1990). Patients of this kind may be incapable of expressing emotions (i.e., alexithymic). Studies establishing a linkage between this subgroup and panic disorder, including family, follow-up, and challenge studies have been done (Beitman et al., 1991; Kushner et al., 1992). According to Kushner & Beitman (1990), a substantial minority of panic patients in medical populations have non-fear panic.

Pattern of morbidity

Anxiety disorders, especially panic, are associated with significant impairment in quality of life (Salvador-Carulla et al., 1995). For instance, the impairment in functioning in patients with untreated anxiety studied by Fifer et al. (1994) was similar to that observed in patients with chronic physical diseases such as diabetes and congestive heart failure. The consequences of panic disorder in the community are summarized in Table 3.8.

Table 3.8. *Morbidity associated with panic disorder, major depressive disorder, and no mental disorder in the general population*

	Panic disorder	Major depression	No disorder	p*
General health ratings				
Physical (% fair/poor)	35	29	24	0.01
Emotional (% fair/poor)	38	39	16	0.01
Psychiatric problems				
Alcohol abuse (% ever)	27	18	11	0.01
Drug abuse (% ever)	18	14	4	0.01
Attempted suicide (% ever)	20	15	2	0.01
Marital functioning				
Getting along (% not well)	12	14	2	0.01
Confided in partner (% seldom/never)	19	13	7	0.05
Told worries (% seldom/never)	27	19	17	NS
Financial dependency				
Welfare or disability (% currently)	2	16	12	0.01

*p values for persons with panic disorder vs. no mental disorder. *Source*: Modified from Markowitz et al. (1989). Copyright 1989, American Medical Association. Reprinted with permission.

They include subjective feelings of poor physical and emotional health, alcohol and drug abuse, increased likelihood of suicide attempts, impaired social and marital functioning, and financial dependency (Markowitz et al., 1989). As the table shows, persons with panic disorder reported impairment comparable to, or exceeding, that reported by persons with major depression. Comorbidity with major depression, agoraphobia, and substance abuse does not explain such findings. Also, persons with panic attacks not meeting criteria for panic disorder had significant morbidity (Klerman et al., 1991). Similar impairment in quality of life has been found in clinical populations (Massion et al., 1993). Patients who are employed lose more work days, and a substantial minority are unemployed on account of their condition (Seigel et al., 1990). Thus, the social costs of panic disorder are high (Leon et al., 1995).

Natural history

Onset

The onset of panic disorder peaks in the early adult years (Thyer et al., 1985; von Korff et al., 1985). Half of patients presenting for treatment experienced anxiety disorders during childhood (Pollack et al., 1996). The disorder often begins suddenly with an unexpected attack, although some patients report gradually increasing anxiety symptoms beforehand. Prodromal generalized anxiety, phobic, and hypochondriacal symptoms have all been reported, but whether agoraphobic symptoms sometimes predate initial attacks remains controversial (Klein, 1981; Fava et al., 1988; Lelliott et al., 1989; Faravelli et al., 1992). Similar *residual* symptoms have been observed in patients who no longer have attacks (Katon et al., 1987). Both prodromal and residual symptoms may be manifestations of a vulnerability to the disorder.

The onset is commonly associated with precipitating events or circumstances. These are often emotionally disturbing events such as the death of a loved one, divorce, financial loss, etc., but physical illness and events associated with hormonal change occur as well (Faravelli & Pallanti, 1989; Pollard et al., 1989). Panic disorder may begin after childbirth, and one survey of childbearing women found that 11% had had their first panic attack postpartum (Sholomskas et al., 1993). Likewise, precipitation of the disorder by oral contraceptives (i.e., progesterone and estrogen) and estrogen replacement has been reported (Deci et al., 1992; Dembert et al., 1994). Occasionally the onset occurs at puberty or the menopause in women (Hayward et al., 1992; Swales & Sheikh, 1992).

Many women report premenstrual increases in anxiety symptoms and panic frequency. Although such changes have been difficult to document by prospective monitoring, at least one study showed an increase in the rate of attacks during the late luteal phase (Kaspi et al., 1994). Changes in panic symptoms with pregnancy and postpartum have been reviewed by Shear & Mammen (1995). Some patients experience improvement late in the first trimester although the influence of pregnancy appears variable (Villeponteaux et al., 1992; Cohen et al., 1994a; Northcott & Stein, 1994). More consistent is postpartum worsening that may occur in one- to two-thirds of women but is less likely in those receiving pharmacotherapy (Cohen et al., 1994b; Northcott & Stein, 1994).

Symptoms of panic disorder show considerable variation over time. A diurnal pattern has been observed with greatest attack frequency in late morning and early afternoon (Geraci & Uhde, 1992; Kenardy et al., 1992). Also, patients with the disorder report marked day-to-day and week-to-week fluctuations in symptoms. Many feel, on arising, that they will have a bad day and that attacks are likely to occur. In addition, agoraphobic patients will sometimes panic in phobic situations but other times will not. The reasons for such variability are not understood. One retrospective study identified seasonal variation in symptom intensity with a peak in winter months and a lesser peak in summer (Marriott et al., 1994).

Course and outcome

Epidemiological studies indicate that panic disorder, like anxiety disorders in general, is either chronic or recurrent (Wittchen, 1988). Cross-sectional studies have found low, 1-year recovery rates (Oakley-Browne et al., 1989). Even among new cases, longitudinal investigations have demonstrated long-standing prodromes which suggest that such cases may arise from and return to a pool of persons with subthreshold symptoms (Murphy et al., 1989). In reviewing community studies, Angst & Vollrath (1991) found recovery rates that ranged between 12% and 25% for anxiety disorders (panic disorder and generalized anxiety disorder). After many years, most subjects still had residual symptoms and about half had social and work impairment.

Similar conclusions have come from studies of clinical samples. Most early studies, reviewed by Greer (1969), Marks & Lader (1973), and Roy-Byrne & Cowley (1995) involved psychiatric patients, among whom 41–59% were found to be recovered or much improved. Recent studies have tended to support this impression (reviewed by Noyes, 1992; Katschnig & Amering, 1994). Among panic patients followed-up after 3 years, Noyes et al. (1990) reported that two-thirds had absent or mild symptoms and one-third were free of panic attacks. Also, Katschnig et al. (1991) found that after 2–6 years 39% were free of panic attacks (i.e., past year) and 60% had absent or mild phobic avoidance. In these studies relatively few patients were completely free of symptoms despite continuing medication. Consistent with this impression of chronicity, Keller et al. (1994) observed high rates of relapse among patients who had remitted.

A review of clinical studies shows that the nature of the patient sample influences outcome. For instance, patients from general medical practice appear to do better than those from psychiatric practice (Wheeler et al., 1950; Noyes et al., 1980; Ormel et al., 1993). Among psychiatric patients, outpatients do better than inpatients (Krieg et al., 1987). Also, Keller & Baker (1992) noted that patients studied recently have had a better outcome and concluded that the course has improved with modern treatments. Supporting their view, a number of recent studies have described naturalistically treated patients as doing especially well (Nagy et al., 1989; Noyes et al., 1989a). For example, Mavissakalian & Michelson (1986) reported that two-thirds of a series of agoraphobic patients treated with imipramine and exposure had recovered 2 years later.

Panic patients who have responded to cognitive behavioral therapy appear to have a favorable outcome for 5 or more years after treatment.

Those who receive interoceptive exposure have, perhaps, the best long-term course (McNally, 1994). Agoraphobic patients who responded to behavioral therapy have also maintained their improvement. In a review of studies, O'Sullivan & Marks (1991) found that 76% of patients were much improved 1–9 years after treatment. The average improvement of target symptoms was roughly 50% for all patients. Nevertheless, they noted that residual symptoms and impairment were typical, and that 15–25% had one or more depressive episodes during the follow-up period. Longer follow-ups showed that many patients had seen a doctor about psychological symptoms or taken medication (Beck et al., 1992).

Several investigators have followed patients treated with medication (reviewed by Noyes, 1992). To begin with, they showed that relapse is frequent following the discontinuation of effective medication. Rebound and withdrawal phenomena make the assessment of change following discontinuation of benzodiazepines especially difficult (Noyes et al., 1991b). Many, if not most, patients remain on medication over long periods (Nagy et al., 1989; Noyes et al., 1990). One study showed significant adverse effects of long-term tricyclic antidepressants, the most notable being weight gain (Noyes et al., 1989b). Despite these problems, drug-treated patients have had a good overall outcome (Nagy et al., 1989; Noyes et al., 1989a, 1990). There is preliminary evidence that some patients benefit from medication beyond the time of its actual administration (Mavissakalian & Perel, 1992).

Predictors of outcome

Predictors of outcome in panic disorder were reviewed by Noyes (1992). Among demographic variables, female gender and low socioeconomic status appear weakly associated with poor prognosis. With respect to clinical features, more severe initial symptoms are associated with worse outcome and greater agoraphobia is predictive of more severe symptoms at follow-up. Also, longer duration is associated with poorer outcome.

A recent prospective study examined potential predictors in some detail. Noyes et al. (1990) followed up 89 subjects with panic disorder 3 years after they had participated in a drug treatment study. They found that some baseline measures were more predictive of symptoms and others more predictive of social adjustment, but that demographic variables were relatively unimportant on either count. Subjects of lower social class and less extensive social networks had less favorable social adjustment at outcome. Also, most measures of symptom severity at baseline were predictive of symptom severity, symptom-related disability, and social adjustment at outcome. Strongest correlations were observed between abnormal personality traits, level of anxiety symptoms and duration of illness at baseline and level of anxiety symptoms and social adjustment at follow-up.

This study also found a relationship between comorbidity and the outcome (Noyes et al., 1990). Panic subtypes (uncomplicated, limited phobic avoidance, and extensive phobic avoidance) were predictive of greater symptom severity and worse social adjustment. Similarly, Keller et al. (1994) reported a 0.37 probability of remission for panic disorder compared to a 0.16 probability for panic with agoraphobia. Comorbid personality disorders also predict unfavorable outcome. Noyes et al. (1990) found personality-disordered panic subjects to have more severe symptoms and social adjustment 3 years later. Other investigators have reported similar findings and have noted that personality disorders predict poor response to treatment (Reich, 1988; Pollack et al., 1990).

Complications

Mood and substance use disorders are the most frequent and important coexisting disturbances in patients with panic (Noyes, 1990). Coexisting anxiety disorders may also have a significant impact, especially social phobia (Stein et al., 1989). Whether coexisting disturbances represent complications or independent disorders has been the subject of debate (Maser & Cloninger, 1990). Proponents of the concept of secondary depression note that such depression follows the onset of a primary illness and differs from primary depression in important ways (Winokur, 1990). Regardless of what the relationship may be, it is clear that comorbid depression and alcoholism influence the course and outcome of panic disorder and have serious additional consequences of their own.

Major depression

Major depression occurs in a substantial proportion of patients with panic disorder. According to the ECA study, the risk of major depression in persons with panic disorder is more than 10 times that of persons with no disorder (Boyd et al., 1984; Eaton et al., 1991; Merikangas et al., 1996). Between 30% and 70% of panic patients have experienced at least one episode of major depression (Lesser, 1990). The frequency appears to vary with the population studied and the duration of illness; the longer a patient has been ill the more likely he or she is to have experienced depression. There may be an over-representation of patients with depression in clinical samples because the mood disturbance often leads to treatment seeking (Woodruff et al., 1972).

Patients with coexisting depression appear to have more severe panic disorder. Lesser et al. (1988) found that patients with depression had more severe symptoms, and Breier et al. (1984) found more frequent attacks in depressed compared with non-depressed patients. Likewise, Noyes et al. (1990) found that patients with major depression had more severe anxiety symptoms, more frequent panic attacks, greater phobic avoidance and more symptom-related disability. Consistent with the greater severity, patients with coexisting depression appear to have a less favorable course and outcome. Noyes et al. (1990) observed that patients with current or past major depression had more severe symptoms and symptom-related disability at follow-up than did subjects without major depression. Also, they were more likely to experience episodes of depression during the follow-up interval than were those who had no history of depression.

The impact of major depression upon panic symptoms and their response to treatment remains uncertain. More severe anxiety symptoms are likely to develop during an episode of depression (Noyes et al., 1990). Whether the coexistence of depression influences treatment response has been the subject of debate (Marks & O'Sullivan, 1989). Some investigators have found patients with major depression less responsive to drug and behavior therapy but others have not (Lesser, 1990). Many patients with coexisting depression respond to antianxiety drugs (Lesser et al., 1988).

Alcohol use disorders

Community surveys show that the risk for alcohol dependence more than doubles in the presence of panic disorder (Helzer & Pryzbeck, 1988; Kessler et al., 1997). Surveys of clinical populations have consistently found that a significant proportion of anxious patients also suffer from alcohol or sedative drug abuse (Cowley, 1992). Quitkin et al. (1972) called attention to the co-occurrence of these conditions by reporting a series of ten patients with phobic anxiety complicated by drug dependence. They viewed the use of sedative drugs and alcohol as misguided attempts at self-medication and noted that, when drug abuse became the primary focus of attention, the underlying anxiety disorder was often overlooked (Kushner et al., 1996). Emphasizing the importance of treating the primary disturbance, these authors followed their patients for up to 3 years and observed that those on imipramine avoided return to drug abuse whereas those not treated relapsed.

Studies of alcohol dependence in patients with anxiety disorders have been reviewed by Kushner et al. (1990), and George et al. (1990). Prevalence estimates range from 7% to 28% for lifetime alcohol abuse or dependence in patients with panic disorder (Otto et al., 1992b). The risk of alcohol disorders in these patients exceeds that in the general population. Studies have also shown a high prevalence of anxiety disorders among alcoholics. Studies of panic disorder among alcoholic inpatients have yielded lifetime estimates of 2–21% (Cowley, 1992). Among men with panic, the rate of alcoholism ranged from 5% to 8%, higher than that in the general population (Schuckit, 1986). Among patients with anxiety disorders, alcoholism occurs predominantly in men, reflecting their greater overall susceptibility to alcohol disorders (Woodruff et al., 1972).

When they coexist, an anxiety disorder usually comes before but may follow an alcohol disorder (George et al., 1990; Kushner et al., 1990; Kessler et al., 1997). The relationship between such disorders appears to be complex (Kushner et al., 1990). For example, even though many patients use alcohol to relieve anxiety symptoms, many also report more severe anxiety with heavy drinking (Smail et al., 1984). Of course, alcohol withdrawal causes anxiety symptoms, and stressors associated with heavy drinking may increase them as well. Family studies have shown an increased risk of alcohol disorders among relatives of panic probands which suggests that these disorders have a shared vulnerability (Noyes et al., 1986a; Maier et al., 1993b).

Mortality

Another consequence of panic disorder is increased mortality. Among panic disorder patients, Coryell et al. (1982) found a death rate that exceeded that of the general population. They located 113 former inpatients with panic disorder an average of 35 years after admission and found that, according to age and sex-specific population figures, patients with panic had significant excess mortality due to unnatural causes. Suicide was responsible for 20% of deaths, a rate comparable to the 16% observed in a unipolar depression comparison group. This rate was also as high as the 15% typical of patients with primary depression followed for long periods (Guze & Robins, 1976).

A high rate of suicide has been a consistent finding in follow-up studies of panic disorder (Allgulander & Lavori, 1991). In reviewing them, Noyes (1991) noted that, with one exception, more than 15% of deaths had been suicides. In addition, a recent study showed that coexisting anxiety may contribute to suicide in patients with depressive disorders (Fawcett et al.,

1990). The features most strongly predictive of suicide in the 32 of 954 depressed patients who killed themselves over a 10-year period included panic attacks, psychic anxiety, global insomnia, diminished concentration, and alcohol abuse.

ECA data also pointed to an increased risk of suicide in panic disorder. They showed that 20% of persons with panic disorder had attempted suicide compared to 6% in persons with other disorders and 1% of those with no disorder (Weissman et al., 1989). According to these figures, the risk of suicide associated with panic disorder was comparable to that with major depression. They also showed that, while coexisting disorders increased the risk, the likelihood of an attempt in uncomplicated panic subjects was high (Johnson et al., 1990). Of course, because attempters and completers represent separate populations, attempts may not yield information about completed suicides. Also, low rates of suicide have been reported in some clinical populations (Friedman et al., 1992).

Serious suicidal behavior is associated with greater severity and comorbidity among panic patients (Lepine et al., 1993; Appleby, 1994). For instance, Noyes et al. (1991c) followed up 81 patients after 7 years and found that five had made serious suicide attempts and three more had completed suicide. They found that subjects who had made serious attempts were younger and had had an earlier onset of illness than subjects who had not made attempts. More of the serious attempters had personality disorders and coexisting major depression. At the time of initial assessment, the serious attempters had more severe symptoms and more often reported disturbed early environments. Thus, severity and chronicity may be non-specific correlates of suicide among persons with panic and other psychiatric illnesses.

There is also evidence of increased mortality due to natural causes in panic disorder. Coryell et al. (1982) found the risk for cardiovascular death among men twice that for men in the general population. This, and more recent evidence, is reviewed in Chapter 7.

Differential diagnosis

Anxiety disorders due to general medical conditions

There are a variety of medical conditions that may cause panic attacks and others that may produce panic-like symptoms. In either case it is important to rule out such conditions, especially when symptoms are of recent origin. A careful history, physical examination, and laboratory screening should be completed, but more extensive evaluation is not usually warranted unless features atypical for panic disorder are present or signs and symptoms of a medical condition known to produce anxiety are elicited. Table 7.6 lists physical conditions that are commonly associated with anxiety (Goldberg, 1992). Some are associated with panic-like episodes and others with actual panic attacks.

Perhaps the most common cardiac conditions associated with recurrent attacks are angina pectoris and arrhythmias. Angina is characterized by episodes of chest pain, dyspnea, and palpitations and is precipitated by exercise or emotional stress. The diagnosis may depend on coronary angiography when symptoms are atypical. A high proportion of patients with chest pain and normal coronary arteries have panic disorder (Katon et al., 1988). Cardiac arrhythmias, such as paroxysmal supraventricular tachycardia, may cause palpitations, chest discomfort, dyspnea, and faintness (Lessmeier et al., 1997). The diagnosis of an arrhythmia may be made by identifying the abnormal rhythm through transtelephonic event monitoring.

A variety of endocrine abnormalities may be associated with anxiety. Although some patients have a history of thyroid problems, laboratory tests do not show a relationship between panic disorder and thyroid disease (Stein & Uhde, 1988). Routine thyroid testing of patients therefore, is not recommended. Hypoglycemia may be associated with symptoms that resemble anxiety attacks (Dietch, 1981). A low blood glucose level is accompanied by sweating, weakness, hunger, tremor, and headache and may be confirmed by measurement of blood glucose levels during an acute episode. Reactive hypoglycemia is identified by an oral glucose tolerance test but should be reserved for patients with postprandial attacks, attacks accompanied by hunger, or those who have had gastric surgery.

Patients with panic disorder are frequently suspected of having pheochromocytoma, a rare catecholamine-secreting tumor of the adrenal gland. Patients with this tumor experience paroxysmal attacks accompanied by blood pressure elevation that are less intense than panic attacks (Starkman et al., 1985). Also, somatic symptoms predominate and phobic avoidance rarely occurs. Routine screening of panic patients for elevated urinary catecholamines is not recommended (Raj & Sheehan, 1987). Hypoparathyroidism is another endocrine disturbance sometimes associated with anxiety. Symptoms include muscle cramps and paresthesias of the hands, feet, and mouth. Carpopedal spasm is a diagnostic sign. Useful diagnostic tests include serum calcium and phosphorous levels.

Partial complex seizures are sometimes difficult to distinguish from panic disorder (Handal et al., 1995). Fear or anxiety may occur as part of the aura or seizure itself. Seizures are distinguished by alterations in consciousness, semi-purposeful movements, and the occurrence of other types of seizures. When such atypical features suggest a seizure disorder, an electroencephalogram, using nasopharyngeal leads or continuous monitoring, may confirm the diagnosis. Anxiety may also accompany postconcussion syndrome (Goldberg, 1992). This syndrome occurs in an estimated 20% of persons with less serious head injuries and consists of sleep difficulty, irritability, lightheadedness, poor concentration, and headaches in addition to anxiety.

Substance-induced anxiety disorders

A variety of drugs may, during intoxication or withdrawal, cause anxiety including panic attacks. A listing of common drugs is shown in Table 7.7. Cocaine may induce panic attacks and even precipitate panic disorder (Aronson & Craig, 1986). Similarly, marijuana intoxication may cause panic, and patients occasionally report that their first attack was provoked by this drug. Alcohol withdrawal is a frequent cause of anxiety symptoms including panic (Schuckit et al., 1990). Abstinence symptoms include anxiety, tremulousness, insomnia, and autonomic arousal producing diaphoresis, flushing, nausea, and tachycardia. Symptoms resulting from abrupt discontinuation of benzodiazepines and other central nervous system sedatives are similar (Noyes et al., 1988). Drugs with short half-lives (e.g., alprazolam, lorazepam) cause earlier and more severe symptoms. Discontinuation of narcotic analgesics also produces a withdrawal syndrome with anxiety.

A variety of other drugs may cause anxiety including panic attacks. In susceptible individuals caffeine may precipitate attacks (Boulenger et al., 1984). Also, caffeine discontinuation may cause anxiety. Nicotine withdrawal has been associated with the onset of panic attacks as well as depression (Hughes et al., 1991). Other drugs that can produce anxiety include alpha adrenergic stimulants such as ephedrine, pseudoephedrine, phenylpropranolamine, and phenylephrine (Goldberg, 1992). Bronchodilators, such as isoproterenal, epinephrine, albuteral, isoetharine, and metaproterenal, may cause anxiety, restlessness, tremor, insomnia. Theophylline may also cause tachycardia, nervousness, and anxiety states.

Psychiatric disorders

Panic attacks may be an associated feature of other anxiety disorders. In these disorders attacks are not unexpected, as in panic, but are either situationally bound or situationally predisposed (American Psychiatric Association, 1994). Thus, in social phobia, attacks are cued by social situations, in obsessive-compulsive disorder by the object of an obsession (e.g., dirt, contamination), in posttraumatic stress disorder by recall or reminder of a stressor, and in specific phobia by exposure to a feared object or situation (e.g., heights, storms). Also, the focus of anxiety distinguishes patients with agoraphobia from other phobic disorders. Agoraphobic persons fear being unable to escape from public situations or obtain help in the event of an attack. In contrast, social phobics fear humiliation or embarrassment and specific phobics fear physical injury resulting from exposure to potentially dangerous situations.

Panic disorder with agoraphobia may be difficult to distinguish from specific phobia when the latter involves situations that are commonly feared by agoraphobics (e.g., driving, flying, closed places). Typically, panic disorder begins with unexpected panic attacks and fear subsequently develops in multiple situations where attacks are likely occur. Specific phobias, on the other hand, typically develop in one or more situations without the occurrence of panic (American Psychiatric Association, 1994). An individual who experiences a panic attack while driving and subsequently avoids driving might have either; however, the person who has panic disorder with agoraphobia is apt to experience attacks in other situations, likely to develop fear of other confining circumstances, likely to fear panic in these situations, and likely to be apprehensive about future attacks whether planning to drive or not. The specific phobic does not have unexpected attacks or fear other confining situations. Also, he or she does not fear having attacks but fears being injured (e.g., motor vehicle accident).

Similarly, panic disorder with agoraphobia may be difficult to distinguish from social phobia (Mannuzza et al., 1990). Persons with both may fear and avoid social situations (e.g., public speaking, eating in restaurants). If an individual experiences a panic attack while speaking in public and then avoids public performance situations due to fear of humiliating panic, he or she may have social phobia. On the other hand, if attacks occur in other situations, and these are avoided out of fear that help might not be available in the event of incapacitation (i.e., panic attack), then agoraphobia may be the appropriate diagnosis. The social phobic fears public scrutiny and is often more comfortable when alone; the agoraphobic often fears being alone and may have panic attacks under such circumstances. A number of demographic and illness characteristics distinguish patients with these phobias (Mannuzza et al., 1990).

When symptoms of major depressive disorder and panic disorder coexist, it is important to determine which disorder is primary. As has been noted, many patients with panic disorder develop major depression and about 20% of individuals with primary major depression experience panic attacks (Coryell et al., 1988). Thus, panic and major depression frequently co-occur, and if the criteria for both disorders are met, both should be diagnosed, but if recurrent attacks are not accompanied by fear of additional attacks, associated concerns, or behavioral change, then a diagnosis of panic disorder should not be made (American Psychiatric Association, 1994). Although not mentioned in the DSM-IV criteria, the temporal relationship between these disorders is important. If panic attacks are limited to an episode of major depression, then depression is the primary disorder (Coryell et al., 1988). If panic attacks had their onset prior to an episode of depression, then panic is the primary disorder. The distinction has treatment and prognostic implications (Coryell et al., 1992).

Individuals with alcohol and substance use disorders commonly report panic attacks. These individuals may or may not warrant a separate anxiety disorder diagnosis. The relationship between use of the substance and anxiety symptoms is not always clear (Kushner et al., 1990). Many patients use alcohol and marijuana in an effort to control symptoms, but others experience attacks as part of alcohol withdrawal. If panic attacks occurred before the onset of heavy drinking and persist after the substance is withdrawn, then an additional diagnosis of panic disorder may be warranted (Schuckit et al., 1990). If attacks are associated with periods of intoxication or withdrawal, a diagnosis of substance-induced anxiety disorder may be appropriate (Chapter 7).

Treatment

Medical management

Effective treatment of panic disorder depends upon establishing and communicating the diagnosis. Initially, many patients are convinced that they are physically ill and resist the idea that their problem may be psychiatric (Katon, 1991). Other patients reject the diagnosis of panic disorder because, for them, it implies weakness or responsibility for symptoms. Of course, examination and reassurance are important first steps when patients exhibit acute symptoms. These measures not only rule out more serious disease, but have an important anxiety-relieving function of their own. In the face of persisting symptoms, education becomes important, and the discussion of diagnosis and prognosis forms a basis for understanding and accepting the disorder. Books written for patients may be helpful, including those by Sheehan (1983), Marks (1978) and Ross (1994). Emotional support is important and may come from meeting and sharing experiences with patients who have similar disorders. Anxiety support groups that provide opportunities for this kind of sharing exist in many communities (Saylor et al., 1990).

Effective treatments are available for panic disorder and agoraphobia (reviewed in Wolfe & Maser, 1994). They include proven pharmacological and psychological therapies, and both should be available to patients. Too often practitioners doubt their skill in administering one or the other or referral patterns favor one approach over the other. Treatment selection should be based on evidence of efficacy. Although psychotherapy is widely believed to be effective and case reports of benefit exist, controlled studies have not been done (Shear et al., 1993). A psychotherapeutic approach to panic disorder has been developed and a manual for panic-focused psychodynamic therapy is available (Milrod et al., 1997; Shear & Weiner, 1997). In choosing an approach, the severity of a patient's illness and coexisting disorders, especially major depressive disorder and alcohol or drug dependence, should be taken into account. Also, the patient's past treatment, including his or her response to it and preference for various modes, should be considered.

Pharmacological treatment

Both pharmacological and psychological treatments are effective but, because there are relatively few studies involving comparisons, not very much is known about which approach is superior for which patients (Wolfe & Maser, 1994). Some psychiatrists believe that medication is important for more severely ill patients, but data supporting this view are sparse (Roy-Byrne, 1992). Drug therapies, despite their ease of administration and apparent cost effectiveness, have several drawbacks. First, side-effects make some drugs difficult to tolerate, causing many patients to discontinue them (Noyes et al., 1989b). Also, the risk of dependence (i.e., benzodiazepines) and of adverse health consequences (i.e., monoamine oxidase inhibitors) diminish the benefit/risk ratio (Noyes et al., 1988). Second, relapse frequently occurs when effective drugs are discontinued, especially the benzodiazepines (Ballenger et al., 1993; Mavissakalian et al., 1993).

There are four main classes of drugs with demonstrated efficacy. These include the tricyclic antidepressants, serotonin uptake inhibitors, mono-amine oxidase inhibitors, and high potency benzodiazepines. All have certain advantages and disadvantages, but equal if not superior efficacy, tolerability, and safety make the serotonin uptake inhibitors (SSRIs) the current drugs of choice.

Regardless of what drug is administered, the treatment of panic and agoraphobia has three phases (Ballenger, 1994). The goal of the acute phase (6–8 weeks) is control of panic attacks. The stabilization or continuation phase (2–6 months) seeks to sustain and extend the initial response and reduce phobic avoidance. In the maintenance phase (6–12 months), the goal is reduction in impairment and the restoration of functioning. Some comment on the method of achieving these goals will be made after reviewing specific treatments.

Tricyclic antidepressants

Effective pharmacological treatment for panic disorder was first reported by Klein (1964). He observed that imipramine blocked panic attacks in agoraphobic patients, but confirmation was delayed for nearly two decades (Sheehan et al., 1980). There have since been a number of controlled trials, and in all of them, imipramine has proven superior to placebo (Ballenger, 1994). In most, the response to imipramine appeared robust. For example, Zitrin et al. (1983) reported that 47% of patients showed marked response (combined with behavior therapy) and 29% showed a moderate response. In contrast, 20% had a marked response to placebo and 45% a moderate response; however, the improvement with imipramine was often not seen until the second week and did not become maximal for 6–10 weeks.

Imipramine is not only capable of controlling panic attacks but of reducing agoraphobic symptoms as well; however, a higher blood level may be required. Mavissakalian & Perel (1995) observed an optimal thera-peutic response for phobias in a range of 110 to 140 ng/ml. The dose required to achieve this level is variable and for some patients may necessi-tate 150–300 mg per day. Although an effective drug, imipramine's side-effects have led a quarter to a third of patients to drop out of various trials (Marks & O'Sullivan, 1989). In addition to anticholinergic side-effects, about 20% experience an overstimulatory response and discontinue the drug before it has had a chance to work. Among those who benefit, weight gain is a common and distressing problem that often leads to discontinu-ation (Noyes et al., 1989b).

Other tricyclic antidepressants have been shown to be effective as well. In controlled trials, clomipramine has proven superior to placebo (Modigh et al., 1992; Wolfe & Maser, 1994). Clomipramine blocks the uptake of serotonin as well as norepinephrine. In contrast to imipramine, this drug appears to have antipanic effects at low doses (e.g., 50 mg daily). A recent controlled trial also showed desipramine more effective than placebo as well (Lydiard et al., 1992b). Clinical experience indicates that other tricyclic antidepressants are also effective, and in the case of nortriptyline, may have fewer side-effects. There is no evidence that electroconvulsive therapy is useful (Fink, 1990).

Serotonin uptake inhibitors

In addition to clomipramine, research has shown that SSRIs are effective in panic and agoraphobia. Controlled trials have been completed for fluoxetine, fluvoxamine, paroxetine, sertraline, and venlafaxine, all but one showing the SSRI superior to placebo (de Beurs et al., 1995; Oehrberg et al., 1995; reviewed by Boyer, 1995). An antipanic response was not observed for 2–3 weeks but was usually strong. For example, Black et al. (1993) reported that 90% of patients were at least moderately improved after 8 weeks of fluvoxamine (230 mg daily). In most studies, SSRIs were well tolerated; however, fluoxetine appeared to cause an overstimulatory response including agitation, restlessness, jitteriness, and insomnia that for many patients was intolerable. In several studies serotonin uptake inhibitors proved more effective than other drugs (den Boer & Westenberg, 1988; Modigh et al., 1992; Bakish et al., 1996) and, based upon a meta analysis, Boyer (1995) concluded that SSRIs may be superior to imipramine and alprazolam.

Monoamine oxidase inhibitors

Sargant & Dally (1962) were the first to report that patients with phobic anxiety respond to monoamine oxidase inhibitors. Early investigators noted that, like the tricyclic antidepressants, these drugs reduce panic attacks but have less effect on anticipatory anxiety. Phenelzine is the monoamine oxidase inhibitor that has been used in most controlled trials (Noyes et al., 1986c). In the largest of these, Sheehan et al. (1980) found phenelzine in a dose of 45–90 mg daily at least as effective than imipramine.

The major drawback to these drugs is the risk of hypertensive crises. They inhibit enzymes that deactivate dietary tyramine, so ingestion of foods containing this substance (e.g., aged cheese, red wine) result in its accumulation and, through release of norepinephrine, increased blood pressure. Patients who use monoamine oxidase inhibitors (MAOIs) must follow a low tyramine diet and run the risk of potentially fatal (though rare) crises. This together with side-effects that include postural hypotension, insomnia, weight gain, and sexual dysfunction have caused these drugs to be reserved for treatment-refractory cases. Recently, reversible and selective MAOIs have been developed that are less likely to affect the metabolism of tyramine or cause blood pressure elevations. Although not available in the USA, reversible MAO inhibitors, moclobemide and brofaromine, have been administered to panic patients in controlled trials (Bakish et al., in press). In one of them, clinically significant improvement was observed in over 70% of patients (van Vliet et al., 1993).

High potency benzodiazepines

Although the benzodiazepines had been widely prescribed for two decades, they were at first believed to be ineffective for panic disorder. When Sheehan (1987) reported that alprazolam might be beneficial, this led to a large multicenter controlled trial (Ballenger et al., 1988). At a mean dose of nearly 6 mg daily, 82% of patients were at least moderately improved compared to 43% on placebo. Improvement was observed in phobic avoidance as well as panic attacks. In a subsequent trial, a fixed dose of 2 mg daily produced improvement that was only slightly less than that from 6 mg daily (Lydiard et al., 1992b). In these trials, improvement was observed in the first week.

Other benzodiazepines have been shown in controlled trials to be equally effective. For example, clonazepam appears to have equivalent antipanic effect, and because of its longer elimination half-life, may have certain clinical advantages (Tesar et al., 1987). In a recent multicenter trial, Noyes et al. (1996) showed that low potency benzodiazepines, such as diazepam, are as effective as high potency drugs. With roughly equivalent doses (i.e., mean of 40 mg diazepam and 4 mg alprazolam) panic patients responded in comparable fashion. Comparisons with imipramine in large scale trials have shown alprazolam to be equally effective (Cross National Collaborative Panic Study, 1992).

Although benzodiazepines produce a rapid therapeutic response and are well tolerated (i.e., dropout rates under 10%), concern about their dependence potential has caused continuing debate. Discontinuation studies have shown that a high proportion of patients experience rebound anxiety and withdrawal symptoms (Pecknold et al., 1988). Also, most relapse. For example, Noyes et al. (1991b) reported that the majority of patients who had responded to alprazolam or diazepam for 8 months relapsed when they rapidly tapered and discontinued their drugs. Anxiety symptoms that were worse than those at baseline and new symptoms were experienced by a substantial minority of patients taking these drugs. A slow taper over 2–3 months reduces this kind of distress, and both pharmacological and psychological treatments during benzodiazepine discontinuation may reduce it still further (Roy-Byrne et al., 1993).

Many long-term benzodiazepine users (i.e., 1 year or more) experience withdrawal symptoms when their drugs are stopped (Noyes et al., 1988; Roy-Byrne & Hommer, 1988). Despite this indication of physical dependence, there is little clinical evidence that tolerance to the therapeutic effects develops or that psychological dependence (i.e., craving, dose escalation, drug-seeking behavior) is widespread. Tolerance to the therapeutic effects may occur in persons who have abused substances, and administration should usually be avoided in such patients (American Psychiatric Association, 1990). The treatment of anxiety in alcohol dependent patients has been reviewed by Nunes et al. (1995). Otherwise, patients may take benzodiazepines in relative safety over long periods (Ballenger et al., 1993).

Drug administration

Patients tend to have misconceptions and fears about medication and about how it will affect them. They need to understand that, although often effective, the benefits of medication are limited. Drugs do not cure anxiety disorders, and symptoms often return when they are stopped. Patients should understand that psychological dependence is unlikely if they follow instructions, and that side-effects, including sedation, tend to be dose-related and subside with continued use. They should understand that antianxiety drugs belong to several classes and that finding one that works best may involve trying first one and then another. Many patients with panic disorder are sensitive to medications and fearful of their effects, so they should be assured that the physician is readily available by telephone. Drugs, especially the antidepressants, should be initiated with small doses (e.g., 25–50 mg fluvoxamine, 10–25 mg imipramine) and increased every 3 or 4 days as tolerated. Patients have a greater sense of control if put in charge of the rate of increase.

Rapid control of symptoms may be accomplished with a benzodiazepine. An antidepressant may also be started, and in several weeks, when its effects are established, the benzodiazepine may be tapered and discontinued (Ballenger, 1994). Clonazepam is preferred by many patients because it can be taken less often (i.e., twice or even once daily), causes less interdose rebound (i.e., symptoms as a dose is wearing off), and has fewer problems with discontinuation (Tesar, 1990). One of the SSRIs other than fluoxetine is the drug of choice for most patients. Sexual dysfunction occurs in about half of patients but may respond to dose adjustment, drug holidays, or counteractive drugs (e.g., cyproheptadine, yohimibine). An overstimulatory response to any of the antidepressants may subside if the dose is kept low initially and a benzodiazepine is used to counteract symptoms (Pohl et al., 1988). Management of antidepressant side-effects has been reviewed by McElroy et al. (1995). When an adequate trial of an antidepressant (e.g., 6–8 weeks of 30–60 mg paroxetine, 150–300 mg imipramine) has shown it to be ineffective, a drug from another class should be tried. When a second drug is ineffective, the physician should review the diagnosis and consider one of several strategies that have been developed for treatment-resistant patients (Rosenbaum, 1992; Pollack et al., 1994; Tiffon et al., 1994). In severe, intractable cases, psychosurgery may be considered (Waziri, 1990).

Psychological treatment

Highly effective psychological treatments for panic and agoraphobia are now available (reviewed by Barlow & Lehman, 1996). These include exposure in vivo for agoraphobia and cognitive behavioral therapy for panic disorder. It is worth noting that this disorder is relatively responsive to non-specific factors (Shear et al., 1994). Treatment studies have shown that 30–50% of patients respond to placebo (Mavissakalian, 1987, 1988; Fossey & Lydiard, 1990). Those with milder symptoms and less prior treatment are most responsive to placebo (Woodman et al., 1994). Factors that contribute to this response include patient education and enhancement of morale, important ingredients in most therapies (Frank, 1973).

Exposure in vivo for agoraphobia

In their first controlled trial of behavior therapy in agoraphobia, Gelder & Marks (1966) employed imaginal systematic desensitization. Subsequent research, reviewed by McNally (1994) and by Chambless & Gillis (1993), has established that exposure is most effective in vivo (i.e., real life rather than imagination). It is the treatment of choice for patients with agoraphobia. In their review of studies, Jansson & Öst (1982) reported that 60–70% of patients who completed treatment showed clinically significant improvement. Subsequent reviewers have agreed. For example, Jacobson et al. (1988) reported an average clinically significant improvement rate of 58% across studies. They also reported a recovery rate of 27% but noted that most patients had residual symptoms following treatment.

Originally exposure was conducted by therapists who accompanied agoraphobic patients into phobic situations. Subsequent research has shown that treatment is effective if carried out by patients alone under the direction and supervision of a therapist (Williams & Zane, 1989). Indeed, its simplest form consists of instructions to an agoraphobic patient to challenge him or herself in phobic situations together with the rationale for doing so. Many patients are able to follow such instructions, especially if given manuals that provide guidance (Andrews et al., 1994). Simple instructions of this kind are effective and should be given to most patients at least initially. Other attempts to improve the effectiveness of exposure have included adding cognitive procedures, breathing re-training, involving spouses, and adding medication.

Exposure therapy usually begins by establishing a hierarchy of phobic situations starting with the least anxiety-provoking. Patients are instructed to place themselves in this situation repeatedly until it is no longer distressing, then move to the next situation, and so on. According to Andrews et al. (1994), there are several ingredients in successful exposure. First, the more exposure exercises represent real situations avoided by patients the better. Second, the more frequently and the longer patients expose themselves the better the result. Third, exposure that continues until anxiety has subsided yields best results. Also, according to this author, exposure that brings about cognitive change may have a better chance of sustained results.

Cognitive behavioral therapy

Several cognitive behavioral approaches have been developed for panic disorder (Chambless & Gillis, 1993; McNally, 1994). One of these seeks to provide patients with coping skills with which to control anxiety and thereby, prevent attacks. Techniques such as applied relaxation and breathing re-training fall into this category (Bonn et al., 1984; Öst, 1987). A second approach calls for interoceptive exposure or exposure to bodily sensations that are triggers of panic (Barlow, 1988). A third approach relies upon correcting the catastrophic misinterpretation of bodily sensations (Clark, 1986). In controlled trials, these techniques or combinations of them have yielded impressive results with 70% or more of patients becoming panic free (Beck et al., 1992; Telch et al., 1993; Clark et al., in press). Also, where long-term follow-ups have been completed, treatment gains appear to have been sustained.

The cognitive behavioral techniques referred to above are described in detail in clinician guides and patient manuals (Andrews et al., 1994). They rely upon patient education, active patient participation and persistence with homework assignments. According to self-efficacy theory, this participation is in itself an important ingredient. Exposure to interceptive cues, for example, involves deliberately invoking certain feared sensations, such as palpitations or shortness of breath until doing so no longer elicits the feared response (Barlow et al., 1989). In order to produce palpitations or dyspnea a patient might run in place or hyperventilate. Breathing retraining involves instructing patients to breath in a slow, measured fashion and to employ such breathing at the first sign of, or in a situation where they anticipate, panic. By controlling hyperventilation and the symptoms associated with it (e.g., lightheadedness, paresthesias), they may interrupt the spiraling anxiety of attacks.

References

Abelson, J. L., Nesse, R. M., Weg, J. G. et al. 1996a. Respiratory psychophysiology and anxiety: Cognitive intervention in the doxapram model of panic. *Psychosom. Med.* 58: 302–313.

Abelson, J. L., Curtis, G. C. & Cameron, O. G. 1996b. Hypothalamic–pituitary–adrenal axis activity in panic disorder: Effects on 24–hour secretion of adrenocorticotropin and cortisol. *J. Psychiatry Res.* 30: 79–93.

Albus, M., Zahn, T. P. & Breier, A. 1992. Anxiogenic properties of yohimbine. II. Influences of experimental set and setting. *Eur. Arch. Psychiatry Clin. Neurosci.* 241: 345–351.

Allgulander, C. 1994. Suicide and mortality patterns in anxiety neurosis and depressive neurosis. *Arch. Gen. Psychiatry* 51: 708–712.

Allgulander, C. & Lavori, P. W. 1991. Excess mortality among 3302 patients with 'pure' anxiety neurosis. *Arch. Gen. Psychiatry* 48: 599–602.

American Psychiatric Association 1968. *Diagnostic and Statistical Manual of Mental Disorders*, Second Edition, American Psychiatric Association, Washington, DC.

American Psychiatric Association. 1980. *Diagnostic and Statistical Manual of Mental Disorders*, Third Edition, American Psychiatric Association, Washington, DC.

American Psychiatric Association. 1987. *Diagnostic and Statistical Manual of Mental Disorders*, Third Edition, Revised, American Psychiatric Association, Washington, DC.

American Psychiatric Association. 1994. *Diagnostic and Statistical Manual of Mental Disorders*, Fourth Edition, American Psychiatric Association, Washington, DC.

American Psychiatric Association. 1990. Benzodiazepine Dependency, Toxicity, and Abuse: A Task Force Report of the American Psychiatric Association, American Psychiatric Association, Washington, DC.

Andrews, G. 1988. Stressful life events and anxiety. In *Handbook of Anxiety*, Vol. 2, eds. R. Noyes, M. Roth, G. D. Burrows, pp. 163–173, Elsevier, Amsterdam.

Andrews, G. 1993. Panic and generalized anxiety disorders. *Curr. Opin. Psychiatry* 6: 191–194.

Andrews, G., Crino, R., Hunt, C. et al. 1994. *The Treatment of Anxiety Disorders: Clinician's Guide and Patient Manuals.* Cambridge University Press, Cambridge.

Angst, J. & Vollrath, M. 1991. The natural history of anxiety disorders. *Acta Psychiatr. Scand.* 84: 446–452.

Appleby, L. 1994. Panic and suicidal behaviour. *Br. J. Psychiatry* 164: 719–721.
Argyle, N. 1988. The nature of cognitions in panic disorder. *Behav. Res. Ther.* 26: 261–264.
Aronson, T. A. & Craig, T. J. 1986. Cocaine precipitation of panic disorder. *Am. J. Psychiatry* 143: 643–645.
Aronson, T. A. & Logue, C. M. 1987. On the longitudinal course of panic disorder: Developmental history and predictors of phobic complications. *Compr. Psychiatry* 28: 344–355.
Aronson, T. A. & Logue, C. M. 1988. Phenomenology of panic attacks: A descriptive study of panic disorder patients' self-reports. *J. Clin. Psychiatry* 49: 8–13.
Arrindell, W. A. 1989. The Fear Questionnaire. *Br. J. Psychiatry* 154: 724–726.
Arrindell, W. A., Kwee, M. G. T., Methorst, G. J. et al. 1989. Perceived parental rearing styles of agoraphobic and socially phobic inpatients. *Br. J. Psychiatry* 155: 526–535.
Asnis, G. M., Wetzler, S., Sanderson, W. C. et al. 1992. Functional interrelationship of serotonin and norepinephrine: Cortisol response to MCPP and DMI in patients with panic disorder, patients with depression, and normal control subjects. *Psychiatry Res.* 43: 65–76.
Aston-Jones, G., Shipley, M. T., Chouvet, G. et al. 1991. Afferent regulation of locus coeruleus neurons: Anatomy, physiology and pharmacology. In *Progress in Brain Research*, eds. C. D. Barnes, O. Pompeiano, pp. 47–75, Elsevier, New York.
Bakish, D., Filteau, M. J., Charbonneau, Y. et al. 1993. A double-blind, placebo-controlled trial comparing fluvoxamine and imipramine in the treatment of panic disorder with or without agoraphobia. Presented at the CINP Regional Workshop. *Current Therapeutical Approaches in Panic and Other Anxiety Disorders.* Nov. 20–22, Monte Carlo.
Bakish, D., Hooper, C. L. & Filteau, M. J. 1996. A double-blind, placebo-controlled trial comparing fluvoxamine and imipramine in the treatment of panic disorder with and without agoraphobia. *Psychopharmacol. Bull.* 32: 135–141.
Bakish, D., Saxena, B. M., Bowen, R. et al. 1993. Reversible monoamine oxidase inhibitors in panic disorder. *Clin. Neuropharmacol.* 16 (Suppl. 2): 577–582.
Ballenger, J. C. 1994. Overview of the pharmacotherapy of panic disorder. In *Treatment of Panic Disorder*, eds. B. E. Wolfe, J. D. Maser, pp. 59–72, American Psychiatric Press, Washington, DC.
Ballenger, J. C., Burrows, G. D., DuPont, R. L. Jr. et al. 1988. Alprazolam in panic disorder and agoraphobia: Results from a multicenter trial. I. Efficacy in short-term treatment. *Arch. Gen. Psychiatry* 45: 413–422.
Ballenger, J. C., Pecknold, J., Rickels, K. et al. 1993. Medication discontinuation in panic disorder. *J. Clin. Psychiatry* 54 (Suppl. 10): 15–21.
Barlow, D. H. 1988. *Anxiety and Its Disorders.* Guilford Press, New York.
Barlow, D. H., Craske, M. G., Cerny, J. A. et al. 1989. Behavioral treatment of panic disorder. *Behav. Ther.* 20: 261–282.
Barlow, D. H. & Lehman, C. L. 1996. Advances in the psychosocial treatment of anxiety disorders: Implications for national health care. *Arch. Gen. Psychiatry* 53: 727–736.
Barsky, A. J., Barnett, M. C. & Cleary, P. D. 1994. Hypochondriasis and panic disorder: Boundary and overlap. *Arch. Gen. Psychiatry* 51: 918–925.
Bass, C., Kartsounis, L. & Lelliott, P. 1987. Hyperventilation and its relation to

anxiety and panic. *Integrative Psychiatry* 5: 274–291.

Beard, G. M. 1869. Neurasthenia or nervous exhaustion. *Boston Med. Surg. J.* 3: 217–221.

Beck, A. T., Apstein, N., Brown, G. et al.: 1988. An inventory for measuring clinical anxiety: Psychometric properties. *J. Cons. Clin. Psychol.* 56: 893–897.

Beck, A. T., Laude, R. & Bohnert, M. 1974. Ideational components of anxiety neurosis. *Arch. Gen. Psychiatry* 31: 319–325.

Beck, A. T., Sokol, L., Clark, D. A. et al. 1992. A crossover study of focused cognitive therapy for panic disorder. *Am. J. Psychiatry* 149: 778–783.

Beck, A. T. & Steer, R. A. 1990. *Beck Anxiety Inventory Manual*, Psychological Corporation, Harcourt-Brace-Javanovich, San Antonio.

Beitman, B. D., Basha, I. & Flaker, G. 1987. Non-fearful panic disorder: Panic attacks without fear. *Behav. Res. Ther.* 25: 487–492.

Beitman, B. D., Kushner, M. G., Basha, I. et al. 1991. Follow-up status of patients with angiographically normal coronary arteries and panic disorder. *JAMA* 265: 1545–1549.

Bernstein, G. A., Borchardt, C. M. & Perwien, A. R. 1996. Anxiety disorders in children and adolescents: A review of the past 10 years. *J. Am. Acad. Child and Adolesc. Psychiatry* 35: 1110–1119.

Biederman, J., Rosenbaum, J. F., Bolduc-Murphy, E. A. et al. 1993. A 3-year follow-up of children with and without behavioral inhibition. *J. Am. Acad. Child Adolesc. Psychiatry* 32: 814–921.

Biederman, J., Rosenbaum, J. F., Hirshfeld, D. R. et al. 1990. Psychiatric correlates of behavioral inhibition in young children of parents with and without psychiatric disorders. *Arch. Gen. Psychiatry* 47: 21–26.

Black, D. W., Wesner, R. & Bowers, W. 1993. A comparison of fluvoxamine, cognitive therapy and placebo in the treatment of panic disorder. *Arch. Gen. Psychiatry* 50: 44–50.

Bonn, J. A., Harrison, J. & Rees, W. L. 1971. Lactate induced anxiety: Therapeutic implications. *Br. J. Psychiatry* 119: 468–471.

Bonn, J. A., Readhead, C. P. & Timmons, B. H. 1984. Enhanced adaptive behavioural response in agoraphobic patients pretreated with breathing retraining. *Lancet* 2: 665–669.

Boulenger, J. P., Jerabec, I., Jolicoeur, F. B. et al. 1996. Elevated plasma levels of neuropeptide Y in patients with panic disorder. *Am. J. Psychiatry* 153: 114–116.

Boulenger, J. P., Uhde, T. W., Wolff, E. A. et al. 1984. Increased sensitivity to caffeine in patients with panic disorders: Preliminary evidence. *Arch. Gen. Psychiatry* 41: 1067–1071.

Bowlby, J. 1969. *Attachment and Loss*, Vol. 1, *Attachment*. (2nd Revised Edition, 1982.) Basic Books, New York.

Bowlby, J. 1973. *Attachment and Loss*, Vol. 2, *Separation: Anxiety and Anger*. Basic Books, New York.

Boyd, J. H. 1986. Use of mental health services for the treatment of panic disorder. *Am. J. Psychiatry* 143: 1569–1574.

Boyd, J. H., Burke, J. D., Gruenberg, E. et al. 1984. Exclusion criteria of DSM-III: A study of co-occurrence of hierarchy-free syndromes. *Arch. Gen. Psychiatry* 41: 983.

Boyd, J. H. & Crump, T. 1991. Westphal's agoraphobia. *J. Anx. Dis.* 5: 77–86.

Boyer, W. 1995. Serotonin uptake inhibitors are superior to imipramine and alprazolam in alleviating panic attacks: A meta-analysis. *Int. Clin.*

Psychopharmacol. 10: 45–49.

Bradwejn, J. & de Montigny, C. 1984. Benzodiazepines antagonize cholecystokinin-induced activation of rat hippocampal neurones. *Nature* 312: 363–364.

Bradwejn, J., Koszycki, D. & Shriqui, C. 1991. Enhanced sensitivity to cholecystokinin tetrapeptide in panic disorder. *Arch. Gen. Psychiatry* 48: 603–610.

Brambilla, F., Perna, G., Garberi, A. et al. 1995. Alpha-2 adrenergic receptor sensitivity in panic disorder: I. GH response to GHRH and clonidine stimulation in panic disorder. *Psychoendocrinolgy* 220: 1–9.

Breier, A., Charney, D. S. & Heninger, G. R. 1984. Major depression in patients with agoraphobia and panic disorder. *Arch. Gen. Psychiatry* 41: 1129–1135.

Breier, A., Charney, D. S. & Heninger, G. R. 1985. The diagnostic validity of anxiety disorders and their relationships to depressive illness. *Am. J. Psychiatry* 142: 787–797.

Brooks, R. B., Baltazar, P. L. & Munjack, D. J. 1989. Co-occurrence of personality disorders with panic disorder, social phobia, and generalized anxiety disorder: A review of the literature. *J. Anx. Dis.* 3: 59–85.

Brown, G. W. & Harris, T. O. 1993. Aetiology of anxiety and depressive disorders in an inner-city population. 1. Early adversity. *Psychol. Med.* 23: 143–154.

Brown, G. W., Harris, T. O. & Eales, M. J. 1993. Aetiology of anxiety and depressive disorders in an inner-city population. 2. Comorbidity and adversity. *Psychol. Med.* 23: 155–165.

Brown, T. A., DiNardo, P. A. & Barlow, D. H. 1994. *Anxiety Disorders Interview Schedule for DSM-IV (ADIS-IV)*, Graywinds, Albany, NY.

Cameron, O. G., Modell, J. G. & Hariharan, M. 1990a. Caffeine and human cerebral blood flow: A positron emission tomography study. *Life Sciences* 47: 1141–1146.

Cameron, O. G., Smith, C. B., Lee, M. A. et al. 1990b. Adrenergic status in anxiety disorders: Platelet alpha-2-adrenergic receptor binding, blood pressure, pulse, and plasma catecholamines in panic and generalized anxiety disorder patients and in normal subjects. *Biol. Psychiatry* 28: 3–20.

Cannon, W. B. 1929. *Bodily Changes in Pain, Hunger, Fear and Rage*, Appleton, New York.

Carr, D. B. & Sheehan, D. V. 1984. Panic anxiety: A new biological model. *J. Clin. Psychiatry* 45: 323–330.

Carr, D. B., Sheehan, D. V., Surman, O. S. et al. 1986. Neuroendocrine correlates of lactate-induced anxiety and their response to chronic alprazolam therapy. *Am. J. Psychiatry* 143: 483–494.

Cassano, G. B., Petracca, A., Perugi, G. et al. 1989. Derealization and panic attacks: A clinical evaluation on 150 patients with panic disorder/agoraphobia. *Compr. Psychiatry* 30: 5–12.

Cerisoli, M., Amore, M., Campanile, S. et al. 1996. Evaluating CBF velocity changes with transcranial Doppler ultrasound. *Am. J. Psychiatry* 153: 477.

Chambless, D. L. & Gillis, M. M. 1993. Cognitive therapy of anxiety disorders. *J. Consult. Clin. Psychol.* 61: 248–260.

Charney, D. S. & Heninger, G. R. 1986. Serotonin function in panic disorders. *Arch. Gen. Psychiatry* 43: 1059–1065.

Charney, D. S., Heninger, G. R. & Breier, A. 1984. Noradrenergic function in panic anxiety. *Arch. Gen. Psychiatry* 41: 751–763.

Charney, D. S., Heninger, G. R. & Jatlow, P. I. 1985. Increased anxiogenic effects of caffeine in panic disorders. *Arch. Gen. Psychiatry* 42: 233–243.

Charney, D. S., Innis, R. B., Duman, R. S. et al. 1989. Platelet alpha-2-receptor binding and adenylate cyclase activity in panic disorder. *Psychopharmacology* 98: 102–107.

Charney, D. S., Krystal, J. J., Southwick, S. M. et al. 1990. Serotonin function in panic and generalized anxiety disorders. *Psychiatr. Ann.* 20: 593–602.

Charney, D. S., Woods, S. W., Krystal, J. H. et al. 1992. Noradrenergic neuronal dysregulation in panic disorder: The effects of intravenous yohimbine and clonidine in panic disorder patients. *Acta Psychiatr. Scand.* 86: 273–282.

Clark, D. M. 1986. A cognitive approach to panic. *Behav. Res. Ther.* 24: 461–470.

Clark, D. M., Salkovskis, P. M., Hackmann, A. et al. In Press. A comparison of cognitive therapy, applied relaxation and imipramine in the treatment of panic disorder. *Br. J. Psychiatry.*

Cohen, L. S., Sickel, D. A., Dimmock, J. A. et al. 1994a. Impact of pregnancy on panic disorder: A case series. *J. Clin. Psychiatry* 55: 284–288.

Cohen, L. S., Sickel, D. A., Dimmock, J. A. et al. 1994b. Postpartum course in women with preexisting panic disorder. *J. Clin. Psychiatry* 55: 289–292.

Coryell, W., Endicott, J., Andreasen, N. C. et al. 1988. Depression and panic attacks: The significance of overlap as reflected in follow-up and family study data. *Am. J. Psychiatry* 145: 293–300.

Coryell, W., Endicott, J. & Winokur, G. 1992. Anxiety syndromes as epiphenomena of primary major depression: Outcome and familial psychopathology. *Am. J. Psychiatry* 149: 100–107.

Coryell, W., Noyes, R. & Clancy, J. 1982. Excess mortality in panic disorder: A comparison with primary unipolar depression. *Arch. Gen. Psychiatry* 39: 701–703.

Coryell, W., Noyes, R. & Reich, J. 1991. The prognostic significance of HPA-axis disturbance in panic disorder: A three-year follow-up. *Biol. Psychiatry* 29: 96–102.

Cowley, D. S. 1992. Alcohol abuse, substance abuse, and panic disorder. *Am. J. Med.* 92 (Suppl. 1A): 415–485.

Cox, B. J., Swinson, R. P. & Shaw, B. F. 1991. Value of the Fear Questionnaire in differentiating agoraphobia and social phobia. *Br. J. Psychiatry* 159: 842–845.

Craske, M. G., Sanderson, W. C. & Barlow, D. H. 1987. How do desynchronous response systems relate to the treatment of agoraphobia: A follow-up evaluation. *Behav. Res. Ther.* 25: 117–122.

Cross National Collaborative Panic Study, Second Phase Investigators. 1992. Drug treatment of panic disorder: Comparative efficacy of alprazolam, imipramine, and placebo. *Br. J. Psychiatry* 160: 191–202.

Crowe, R. R. 1990. Panic disorder: Genetic considerations. *J. Psychiatr. Res.* 24 (Suppl. 2): 129–134.

Crowe, R. R., Noyes, R., Pauls, D. L. et al. 1983. A family study of panic disorder. *Arch. Gen. Psychiatry* 40: 1065–1069.

Da Costa, J. M. 1871. On irritable heart: A functional form of cardiac disorder and its consequences. *Am. J. Med. Sci.* 61: 14–52.

Dantendorfer, K., Amering, M., Berger, P. et al. 1994. High frequency of MRI brain abnormalities in panic disorder. *Psychopharmacol. Bull.* 30: 97.

Davidson, R. J. 1992. Emotion and affective style: Hemispheric substrates. *Psychol. Sci.* 3: 39–43.

Davis, M., Rainnie, D. & Cassell, M. 1994. Neurotransmission in the rat amygdala related to fear and anxiety. *TINS* 17: 208–214.

de Beurs, E., Lange A. & van Dyck, R. 1992. Self-monitoring of panic attacks and retrospective estimates of panic: Discordant findings. *Behav. Res. Ther.* 30: 411–413.

de Beurs, E., van Balkom, A. J. L. M., Lange, A. et al. 1995. Treatment of panic disorder with agoraphobia: Comparison of fluvoxamine, placebo, and psychological panic management combined with exposure and exposure in vivo alone. *Am. J. Psychiatry* 152: 683–691.

de Cristofaro, M. T. R., Sessarego, A., Pupi, A. et al. 1993. Brain perfusion abnormalities in drug-naive, lactate-sensitive panic patients: A SPECT study. *Biol. Psychiatry* 33: 505–512.

de Ruiter, C. & van Ijzendoorn, M. H. 1992. Agoraphobia and anxious-ambivalent attachment: An intergrated review. *J. Anx. Dis.* 6: 365–381.

Deci, P. A., Lydiard, B. & Santos, A. B. 1992. Oral contraceptives and panic disorder. *J. Clin. Psychiatry* 53: 163–165.

Degonda, M. & Angst, J. 1993. The Zurich Study XX. Social phobia and agoraphobia. *Eur. Arch. Psychiatry Clin. Neurosci.* 243: 95–102.

Deltito, J. A., Perugi, G., Maremmani, I. et al. 1986. The importance of separation anxiety in the differentiation of panic disorder from agoraphobia. *Psychiatr. Dev.* 3: 227–236.

Dembert, M. L., Dinneen, M. P. & Opsahl, M. S. 1994. Estrogen-induced panic disorder. *Am. J. Psychiatry* 151: 1246.

den Boer, J.A. & Westenberg, H. G. M. 1988. Effect of serotonin and noradrenaline uptake inhibitors in panic disorder: A double-blind comparative study with fluvoxamine and maprotiline. *Int. Clin. Psychopharmacol.* 3: 59–74.

den Boer, J. A. & Westenberg, H. G. M. 1990. Serotonin function in panic disorder: A double blind placebo controlled study with fluvoxamine and ritanserin. *Psychopharmacology* 102: 85–94.

Dietch, J. T. 1981. Diagnosis of organic anxiety disorders. *Psychosomatics* 22: 661–669.

DiNardo, P. A. & Barlow, D. H. 1990. Syndrome and symptom co-occurrence in the anxiety disorders. In *Comorbidity of Mood and Anxiety Disorders*, eds. J. D. Maser, C. R. Cloninger, pp. 205–230, American Psychiatric Press, Washington, DC.

DiNardo, P. A., Moras, K., Barlow, D. H. et al. 1993. Reliability of the DSM-III-R anxiety disorder categories using the Anxiety Disorders Interview Schedule-Revised (ADIS-R). *Arch. Gen. Psychiatry* 50: 251–256.

DiNardo, P. A., O'Brien, G. T., Barlow, D. H. et al. 1983. Reliability of DSM-III anxiety disorder categories using a new structured interview. *Arch. Gen. Psychiatry* 40: 1070–1074.

Drevets, W. C., Videen, T. O., MacLeod, T. O. et al. 1992. PET images of blood flow changes during anxiety: Correction. *Science* 256: 1696.

Eaton, W. W., Dryman, A. & Weissman, M. M. 1991. Panic and phobia. In *Psychiatric Disorders in America: The Epidemologic Catchment Area Study*, eds. L. N. Robins, D. A. Regier, pp. 155–179, The Free Press, New York.

Eaton, W. W., Kessler, R. C., Wittchen, H-U. et al. 1994. Panic and panic disorder in the United States. *Am. J. Psychiatry* 151: 413–420.

Eriksson, E., Westberg, P., Alling, C. et al. 1991. Cerbrospinal fluid levels of monoamine metabolites in panic. *Psychiatry Res.* 36: 243–251.

Faravelli, C. & Pallanti, S. 1989. Recent life events and panic disorder. *Am. J.*

Psychiatry 146: 622–626.

Faravelli, C., Pallanti, S., Biondi, F. et al. 1992. Onset of panic disorder. *Am. J. Psychiatry* 149: 827–828.

Fava, G. A., Grandi, S. & Canestrari, R. 1988. Prodromal symptoms in panic disorder with agoraphobia. *Am. J. Psychiatry* 145: 1564–1567.

Fawcett, J., Scheftner, W. A., Fogg, L. et al. 1990. Time-reated predictors of suicide in major affective disorder. *Am. J. Psychiatry* 147: 1189–1194.

Feighner, J. P., Robins, E., Guze, S. B. et al. 1972. Diagnostic criteria for use in psychiatric research. *Arch. Gen. Psychiatry* 26: 57–63.

Ferini-Strambi, L., Bellodi, L., Oldani, A. et al. 1996. Cyclic alternating pattern of sleep encephalogram in patients with panic disorder. *Biol. Psychiatry* 440: 225–227.

Fifer, S. K., Mathias, S. D., Patrick, D. L. et al. 1994. Untreated anxiety among adult primary care patients in a health maintenance organization. *Arch. Gen. Psychiatry* 51: 740–750.

Fink, M. 1990. Electroconvulsive treatment of anxiety disorders. In *Handbook of Anxiety*, Vol. 4, eds. R. Noyes, M. Roth, G. D. Burrows, pp. 511–518, Elsevier, Amsterdam.

Finlay-Jones, R. & Brown, G.W. 1981. Types of stressful life events and the onset of anxiety and depressive disorders. *Psychol. Med.* 11: 803–815.

Flint, A. J. 1994. Epidemiology and comorbidity of anxiety disorders in the elderly. *Am. J. Psychiatry* 151: 640–649.

Foa, E. G., Sleketee, G. & Young, M. C. 1984. Agoraphobia: Phenomenological aspects, associated characteristics, and theoretical considerations. *Clin. Psychol. Rev.* 4: 431–457.

Fontaine, R., Breton, G., Dery, R. et al. 1990. Temporal lobe abnormalities in panic disorder: An MRI study. *Biol. Psychiatry* 27: 304–310.

Fossey, M. O. & Lydiard, R. B. 1990. Placebo response in patients with anxiety disorders. In *Handbook of Anxiety*, Vol. 4, eds. R. Noyes, M. Roth, G. D. Burrows, pp. 27–56, Elsevier, Amsterdam.

Frank, J. D. 1973. *Persuasion and Healing*. Johns Hopkins University Press, Baltimore, MD.

Freud, S. 1962. On the grounds for detaching a particular syndrome from neurasthenia under the description 'anxiety neurosis.' In *Standard Edition of the Complete Psychological Work of Sigmund Freud*, Vol. 3, p. 90, Hogarth Press, London.

Friedman, S., Jones, J. C., Chernen, L. et al. 1992. Suicidal ideation and suicide attempts among patinets with panic disorder: A survey of two outpatient clinics. *Am. J. Psychiatry* 149: 680–685.

Gann, H., Riemann, D., Stoll, S. et al. 1995. Growth-hormone response to clonidine in panic disorder patients in comparison to patients with major depression and healthy controls. *Pharmacopsychiatry* 28: 80–83.

Gelder, M. G. & Marks, I. M. 1966. Severe agoraphobia: A controlled prospective trial of behaviour therapy. *Br. J. Psychiatry* 112: 309–319.

George, D. T., Nutt, D. J., Dwyer, B. A. et al. 1990. Alcoholism and panic disorder: Is the comorbidity more than coincidence? *Acta Psychiatr. Scand.* 81: 97–107.

George, D. T., Nutt, D. J., Waxman, R. P. et al. 1989. Panic response to lactate administration in alcoholic and nonalcoholic patients with panic disorder. *Am. J. Psychiatry* 149: 1161–1165.

George, M. S. & Ballenger, J. C. 1992. The neuroanatomy of panic disorder: The emerging role of the right parahippocampal region. *J. Anx. Dis.* 6: 181–188.

Geraci, M. F. & Uhde, T. W. 1992. Diurnal rhythms and symptom severity in panic disorder: A preliminary study of 24-hour changes in panic attacks, generalized anxiety, and avoidance behaviour. *Br. J. Psychiatry* 161: 512–516.

Gittelman, R. & Klein, D. F. 1984. Relationship between separation anxiety and agoraphobic disorders. *Psychopathology* 17 (Suppl.1): 56–65.

Goddard, A. W., Sholomskas, D. E., Walton, K. E. et al. 1994. Effects of tryptophan depletion in panic disorder. *Biol. Psychiatry* 36: 775–777.

Goldberg, R. J. 1992. Medical aspects of panic disorder. *Rhode Island Med.* 75: 265–270.

Goldstein, A. J. & Chambless, D. L. 1978. A reanalysis of agoraphobia. *Behav. Ther.* 9: 47–59.

Goldstein, R. B., Weissman, M. M., Adams, P. B. et al. 1994. Psychiatric disorders in relatives of probands with panic disorder and major depression. *Arch. Gen. Psychiatry* 51: 383–394.

Gorman, J. M., Askanazi, J., Liebowitz, M. R. et al. 1984. Response to hyperventilation in a group of patients with panic disorder. *Am. J. Psychiatry* 141: 857–861.

Gorman, J. M., Fyer, M. R., Goetz, R. et al. 1988. Ventilatory physiology of patients with panic disorder. *Arch. Gen. Psychiatry* 45: 31–39.

Gorman, J. M., Liebowitz, M. R., Fyer, A. J. et al. 1989. A neuroanatomical hypothesis for panic disorder. *Am. J. Psychiatry* 146: 148–161.

Gray, J. A. 1982. *The Neuropsychology of Anxiety*, Oxford University Press, New York.

Greer, S. 1969. The prognosis of anxiety states. In *Studies of Anxiety*, ed. M. Lader, pp. 151–57, Royal Medico-Psychological Association, London.

Gur, R. C., Gur, R. E., Resnick, S. M. et al. 1987. The effect of anxiety on cortical blood flow and metabolism. *J. Cerebr. Blood Flow and Metab.* 7: 173–177.

Guze, S. B. & Robins, E. 1976. Suicide in primary affective disorder. *Br. J. Psychiatry* 117: 437–448.

Hamilton, M. 1959. The assessment of anxiety states by rating. *Br. J. Med. Psychol.* 32: 50–55.

Handal, N. M., Masand, P. & Weilburg, J. B. 1995. Panic disorder and complex partial seizures: A truly complex relationship. *Psychosomatics* 36: 498–502.

Hayward, C., Killen, J. D., Hammer, L. D. et al. 1992. Pubertal stage and panic attack history in sixth and seventh-grade girls. *Am. J. Psychiatry* 149: 1239–1243.

Hayward, C., Killen, J. D. & Taylor, C. B. 1989. Panic attacks in young adolescents. *Am. J. Psychiatry* 146: 1061–1062.

Helzer, J. E. & Pryzbeck, T. R. 1988. The co-occurrence of alcoholism with other psychiatric disorders in the general population and its impact on treatment. *J. Stud. Alcohol* 49: 219–224.

Helzer, J. E., Robins, L. N., McEvoy, L. T. et al. 1985. A comparison of clinical and Diagnostic Interview Schedule diagnoses: Physician reexamination of lay-interviewed cases in the general population. *Arch. Gen. Psychiatry* 42: 657–666.

Hermann, B. P., Wyler, A. R., Blumer, D. et al. 1992. Icatal fear: Lateralizing significance and implications for understanding the neurobiology of pathological fear states. *Neuropsychiatr. Neuropsychol. Behav. Neurol.* 5: 205–210.

Hibbert, G. A. 1984. Ideational components of anxiety: Their origin and content. *Br. J. Psychiatry* 144: 618–624.

Hibbert, G. A. & Pilsbury, D. 1989. Hyperventilation: Is it a cause of panic attacks? *Br. J. Psychiatry* 155: 805–809.

Hoehn-Saric, R. & McLeod, D. R. 1993. Somatic manifestations of normal and pathological anxiety. In *Biology of Anxiety Disorders*, eds. R. Hoehn-Saric, D. R. McLeod, pp. 177–222. American Psychiatric Press, Washington, DC.

Hoehn-Saric, R., McLeod, D. R. & Zimmerli, W. D. 1991. Psychophysiological response patterns in panic disorder. *Acta Psychiatr. Scand.* 83: 4–11.

Hoehn-Saric, R., Merchant, A. F., Keyser, M. L. et al. 1981. Effects of clonidine on anxiety disorders. *Arch. Gen. Psychiatry* 38: 1278–1282.

Hoffart, A. 1995. Psychoanalytical personality types and agoraphobia. *J. Nerv. Ment. Dis.* 183: 139–144.

Horwath, E., Lish, J. D., Johnson, J. et al. 1993. Agoraphobia without panic: Clinical reappraisal of an epidemiologic finding. *Am. J. Psychiatry* 150: 1496–1501.

Hughes, J. R., Gust, S. W., Skoog, K. et al. 1991. Symptoms of tobacco withdrawal. *Arch. Gen. Psychiatry* 48: 52–59.

Jacobson, N. S., Wilson, L. & Tupper, C. 1988. The clinical significance of treatment gains resulting from exposure-based interventions for agoraphobia: A re-analysis of outcome data. *Behav. Ther.* 19: 539–554.

Jansson, L. & Öst, L-G. 1982. Behavioral treatments for agoraphobia: An evaluative review. *Clin. Psychol. Rev.* 2: 311–336.

Johnson, J., Weissman, M. M. & Klerman, G. 1990. Panic disorder, comorbidity and suicide attempts. *Arch. Gen. Psychiatry* 47: 805–808.

Jolkkonen, J., Lepola, U., Bissette, G. et al. 1993. CSF corticotropin-releasing factor is not affected in panic disorder. *Biol. Psychiatry* 33: 136–138.

Judd, F. K., Apostolopoulos, M., Burrows, G. D. et al. 1994. Serotonergic function in panic disorder: Endocrine responses to D-fenfluramine. *Prog. Neuro-Psychopharm. Biol. Psychiatry* 18: 329–337.

Judd, F. K., Norman, T. R., Burrows, G. D. et al. 1987. The dexamethasone suppression test in panic disorder. *Pharmacopsychiatry* 20: 99–101.

Kagan, J., Reznick, J. S. & Gibbons, J. 1989. Inhibited and uninhibited types of children. *Child Dev.* 60: 838–845.

Kahn, R. S. & Moore, C. 1993. Serotonin in the pathogenesis of anxiety. In *Biology of Anxiety Disorders*, eds. R. Hoehn-Saric, D. R. McLeod pp. 61–102, American Psychiatric Press, Washington, DC.

Kahn, R. S., Westenberg, H. G. M., Verhoeven, W. M. A. et al. 1987. Effect of serotonin precursor and uptake inhibitor in anxiety disorders; a double-blind comparison of 5-hydroxytryptophan, clomipramine and placebo. *Int. Clin. Psychopharmacol.* 2: 33–45.

Kalimaris, T. C., Johnson, E. O., Calogero, A. E. et al. 1992. Cholecystokinin-octapeptide stimulates hypothalamic–pituitary–adrenal function in rats: Role of corticotropin-releasing hormone. *Endocrinology* 130: 1764–1774.

Kaspi, S. P., Otto, M. W., Pollack, M. H. et al. 1994. Premenstrual exacerbation of symptoms in women with panic disorder. *J. Anx. Dis.* 8: 131–138.

Katerndahl, D. A. & Realini, J. P. 1993. Lifetime prevalence of panic states. *Am. J. Psychiatry* 150: 246–249.

Katon, W. J. 1984. Panic disorder and somatization: Review of 55 cases. *Am. J. Med.* 77: 101–106.

Katon, W. J. 1991. *Panic Disorder in the Medical Setting*. American Psychiatric

Press, Washington, DC.

Katon, W. J., Hall, M. L., Russo, J. et al. 1988. Chest pain: Relationship of psychiatric illness to coronary arteriography results. *Am. J. Med.* 84: 1–9.

Katon W. J., Vitaliano, P. P., Anderson, K. et al. 1987. Panic disorder: Residual symptoms after the acute attacks abate. *Compr. Psychiatry* 28: 151–158.

Katon, W. J., Vitaliano, P. P., Russo, J. et al. 1986. Panic disorder: Epidemiology in primary care. *J. Fam. Practice* 23: 233–239.

Katon, W. J., Von Korff, M. & Lin, E. 1992. Panic disorder: Relationship to high utilization. *Am. J. Med.* 92: 75–115.

Katschnig, H. & Amering, M. 1994. The long-term course of panic disorder. In *Treatment of Panic Disorder*, pp. 73–82, American Psychiatric Press, Washington, DC.

Katschnig, H., Stolk, J. M., Klerman, G. L. et al. 1991. Discontinuation and long-term follow-up of participants in a clinical drug trial for panic disorder. *Biol. Psychiatry* 1: 657–660.

Keller, M. B. & Baker, L. A. 1992. The clinical course of panic disorder and depression. *J. Clin. Psychiatry* 53 (Suppl. 3): 5–8.

Keller, M. B., Yonkers, K. A., Warshaw, M. G. et al. 1994. Remission and relapse in subjects with panic disorder and panic with agoraphobia: A prospective short-term naturalistic follow-up. *J. Nerv. Ment. Dis.* 182: 290–296.

Kenardy, J., Fried, L., Kraemer, H. C. & Taylor, C. B.: 1992. Psychological precursors of panic attacks. *Br. J. Psychiatry* 160: 668–673.

Kendler, K. S., Neale, M. C., Kessler, R. C. et al. 1992. Childhood parental loss and adult psychopathology in women. *Arch. Gen. Psychiatry* 49: 109–116.

Kendler, K. S., Neale, M. C., Kessler, R. C. et al. 1993. Panic disorder in women: A population-based twin study. *Psychol. Med.* 23: 397–406.

Kessler, R. C., Crum, R. M., Warner, L. A. et al. 1997. Lifetime co-occurrence of DSM-III-R alcohol abuse and dependence with other psychiatric disorders in the National Comorbidity Survey. *Arch. Gen. Psychiatry* 54: 313–321.

Klein, D. F. 1964. Delineation of two drug-responsive anxiety syndromes. *Psychopharmacologia* 5: 397–408.

Klein, D. F. 1981. Anxiety reconceptualized. In *Anxiety: New Research and Changing Concepts*, eds. D. F. Klein, J. G. Rabkin, pp. 235–263, Raven Press, New York.

Klein, D. F. 1993. False suffocation alarms, spontaneous panics, and related conditions. *Arch. Gen. Psychiatry* 50: 306–317.

Klein, D. F. & Fink, M. 1962. Psychiatric reaction patterns to imipramine. *Am. J. Psychiatry* 119: 432–438.

Klein, E., Cnaani, E., Harel, T. et al. 1995. Altered heart rate variability in panic disorder patients. *Biol. Psychiatry* 37: 18–24.

Klerman, G. L., Weissman, M. M., Ouellette, R. et al.1991. Panic attacks in the community. Social morbidity and health care utilization. *JAMA* 265: 742–746.

Ko, G. N., Elsworth, J. D., Ruth, R. H. et al. 1983. Panic-induced elevation of plasma MHPG levels in phobic-anxious patients. *Arch. Gen. Psychiatry* 40: 425–450.

Krieg, J. C., Bronischt, T., Wittchen, H. U. et al. 1987. Anxiety disorders: A long-term prospective and retrospective follow-up study of former inpatients suffering from an anxiety neurosis or phobia. *Acta Psychiatr. Scand.* 76: 36–47.

Kushner, M. G. & Beitman, B. D. 1990. Panic attacks without fear: An overview.

Behav. Res. Ther. 28: 469–479.

Kushner, M. G., Mackenzie, T. B., Fisdon, J. et al. 1996. The effects of alcohol consumption on laboratory-induced panic and state anxiety. *Arch. Gen. Psychiatry* 53: 264–270.

Kushner, M. G., Shera, K. J. & Beitman, B. D. 1990. The relation between alcohol problems and the anxiety disorders. *Am. J. Psychiatry* 147: 685–695.

Kushner, M. G., Thomas, A. M., Bartels, K. M. et al. 1992. Panic disorder history in the families of patients with angiographically normal coronary arteries. *Am. J. Psychiatry* 149: 1563–1567.

Labbati, L. A., Pollack, M. H., Otto, M. W. et al. 1994. Sleep panic attacks: An association with childhood anxiety and adult psychopathology. *Biol. Psychiatry* 36: 57–60.

Lader, M. H., Gelder, M. G. & Marks, I. M. 1967. Palmar skin conductance measures as predictors of response to desensitization. *J. Psychosom. Res.* 11: 283–290.

Lader, M. H. & Mathews, A. 1970. Physiological changes during spontaneous panic attacks. *J. Psychosom. Res.* 14: 377–382.

Lelliott, P., Marks, I. M., McNamee, G. et al. 1989. Onset of panic disorder with agoraphobia: Toward an integrated model. *Arch. Gen. Psychiatry* 46: 1000–1004.

Lenz, F. A., Gracely, R. H., Romanoski, A. J. et al. 1995. Stimulation in the human somatosensory thalamus can reproduce both the affective and sensory dimensions of previously experienced pain. *Nature Med.* 1: 910–913.

Leon, A. C., Portera, L. & Weissman, M. M. 1995. The social costs of anxiety disorders. *Br. J. Psychiatry* 166: 19–22.

Leonard, B. E. 1990. Changes in biogeneric amine neurotransmitters in panic disorder. *Stress Med.* 6: 269–276.

Lepine, J. P., Chignon, J. M. & Teherni, M. 1993. Suicide attempts in patients with panic disorder. *Arch. Gen. Psychiatry* 50: 144–149.

Lepola, U., Jolkkonen, J., Pitkanen, A. et al. 1990a. Cerebrospinal fluid monoamine metabolites and neuropeptides in patients with panic disorder. *Ann. Med.* 22: 237–239.

Lepola, U., Nousiainen, U., Puranen, M. et al. 1990b. EEG and CT findings in patients with panic disorder. *Biol. Psychiatry* 28: 721–727.

Lesch, K. P., Wiesmann, M., Hoh, A. et al. 1992. 5-HT receptor-effector system responsivity in panic disorder. *Psychopharmacology* 106: 111–117.

Lesser, I. M. 1990. Panic disorder and depression: Co-occurrence and treatment. In *Clinical Aspects of Panic Disorder*, pp. 181–191, Wiley-Liss, New York.

Lesser, I. M., Rubin, R. T., Pecknold, J. C. et al. 1988. Secondary depression in panic disorder and agoraphobia. I: Frequency, severity, and response to treatment. *Arch. Gen. Psychiatry* 45: 437–443.

Lessmeier, T. J., Gamperling, D., Johnson-Liddon, J. et al. 1997. Unrecognized paroxysmal supraventricular tachycardia: Potential for misdiagnosis as panic disorder. *Arch. Intern. Med.* 157: 537–543.

Ley, R. 1994. The 'suffocation alarm' theory of panic attacks: A critical commentary. *J. Behav. Ther. Exp. Psychiatry* 25: 269–273.

Lindesay, J. 1991. Phobic disorders in the elderly. *Br. J. Psychiatry* 159: 531–541.

Linzer, M., Felder, A., Hackel, A. et al. 1990. Psychiatric syncope: A new look at an old disease. *Psychosomatics* 31: 181–188.

Locatelli, M., Bellodi, L., Perna, G. et al. 1993. EEG power modifications in panic disorder during a temporolimbic activation task: Relationship with temporal lobe clinical symptomatology. *J. Neuropsychiatry* 5: 409–414.

Lum, L. C. 1976. The syndrome of habitual chronic hyperventilation. In *Modern Trends in Psychosomatic Medicine*, ed. O. Hill, pp. 196–230. Butterworths, London.

Lydiard, R. B., Ballenger, J. C., Laraia, M. T. et al. 1992a. CSF cholecystokinin concentrations in patients with panic disorder and in normal comparison subjects. *Am. J. Psychiatry* 149: 691–693.

Lydiard, R. B., Lesser, I. M., Ballenger, J. C. et al. 1992b. A fixed-dose study of alprazolam 2 mg, alprazolam 6 mg, and placebo in panic disorder. *J. Clin. Psychopharmacol.* 12: 96–103.

Lynch, P., Bakal, D. A., Whitelaw, W. et al. 1991. Chest muscle activity and panic anxiety: A preliminary investigation. *Psychosom. Med.* 53: 80–89.

Maier, W., Lichtermann, D., Meyer, A. et al. 1993a. A controlled family study in panic disorder. *J. Psychiatric Res.* 27 (Suppl. 1): 79–87.

Maier, W., Minges, J. & Lichtermann, D. 1993b. Alcoholism and panic disorder: Co-occurrence and co-transmission in families. *Eur. Arch. Psychiatry Clin. Neurosci.* 243: 205–211.

Manicavasagar, S. D., O'Connell, J. & Morris-Yates, D. 1995. Genetic factors in early separation anxiety: Implications for the genesis of adult anxiety disorders. *Acta Psychiatr. Scand.* 92: 17–24.

Mannuzza, S., Fyer, A., Klein, D. et al. 1986. Schedule for Affective Disorders and Schizophrenia-Lifetime Anxiety (SADS-LA): Rationale and conceptual development. *J. Psychiatr. Res.* 20: 317–325.

Mannuzza, S., Fyer, A. J., Liebowitz M. R. et al. 1990. Delineating the boundaries of social phobia: Its relationship to panic disorder and agoraphobia. *J. Anx. Dis.* 4: 41–59.

Mannuzza, S., Fyer, A. J., Martin, L. Y. et al. 1989. Reliability of anxiety assessment: I. Diagnostic agreement. *Arch. Gen. Psychiatry* 46: 1093–1101.

Margraf, J., Ehlers, A. & Roth, W. T. 1986. Biological models of panic disorder and agoraphobia: A review. *Behav. Res. Ther.* 24: 553–567.

Markowitz, J. S., Weissman, M. M., Ouellette, R. et al. 1989. Quality of life in panic disorder. *Arch. Gen. Psychiatry* 46: 984–992.

Marks, I. M. 1970. The classification of phobic disorders. *Br. J. Psychiatry* 116: 377–386.

Marks, I. M. 1978. *Living with Fear*. McGraw-Hill, New York.

Marks, I. M. 1987. *Fears, Phobias and Rituals*. Oxford University Press, New York.

Marks, I. M., Lader, M. 1973. Anxiety states (anxiety neurosis): A review. *J. Nerv. Ment. Dis.* 156: 3–18.

Marks, I. M. & Mathews, A. M. 1979. Brief standard self-rating for phobic patients. *Behav. Res. Ther.* 17: 263–267.

Marks, I. M. & O'Sullivan, G. 1989. Anti-anxiety drug and psychological treatment effects in agoraphobia/panic and obsessive-compulsive disorders. In *Psychopharmacology of Anxiety*, pp. 196–242, Oxford University Press, New York.

Marriott, P. F., Greenwood, K. M. & Armstrong, S. M. 1994. Seasonality in panic disorder. *J. Affect. Dis.* 31: 75–80.

Maser, J. D. & Cloninger, C. R. 1990. *Comorbidity of Mood and Anxiety Disorders*. American Psychiatric Press, Washington, DC.

Massion, A. O., Warshaw, M. G. & Keller, M. B. 1993. Quality of life and psychiatric morbidity in panic disorder and generalized anxiety disorder. *Am.*

J. Psychiatry 150: 600–607.

Mathews, A. M., Gelder, M. G. & Johnston, D. W. 1981. *Agoraphobia: Nature and Treatment.* Guilford Press, New York.

Mavissakalian, M. 1987. The placebo effect in agoraphobia. *J. Nerv. Ment. Dis.* 175: 95–99.

Mavissakalian, M. 1988. The placebo effect in agoraphobia. *J. Nerv. Ment. Dis.* 176: 446–448.

Mavissakalian, M. 1990. The relationship between panic disorder/agoraphobia and personality disorders. *Psychiatr. Clin. North Am.* 13: 661–684.

Mavissakalian, M. & Hamann, M. S. 1987. DSM-III personality disorder in agoraphobia: II. Changes with treatment. *Compr. Psychiatry* 28: 356–361.

Mavissakalian, M. & Hamann, M. S. 1992. DSM-III personality characteristics of panic disorder with agoraphobia in stable remission. *Compr. Psychiatry* 33: 305–309.

Mavissakalian, M., Hamann, S. & Jones, B. 1990. A comparison of DSM-III personality disorders in panic/agoraphobia and obsessive-compulsive disorder. *Compr. Psychiatry* 31: 238–244.

Mavissakalian, M. & Michelson, L. 1986. Two year follow-up of exposure and imipramine treatment of agoraphobia. *Am. J. Psychiatry* 143: 1106–1112.

Mavissakalian, M. & Perel, J. M. 1992. Clinical experiments in maintenance and discontinuation of imipramine therapy in panic disorder with agoraphobia. *Arch. Gen. Psychiatry* 49: 318–323.

Mavissakalian, M. R. & Perel, J. M. 1995. Imipramine treatment of panic disorder with agoraphobia: Dose ranging and plasma level-response relationships. *Am. J. Psychiatry* 152: 673–682.

Mavissakalian, M. R., Perel, J. M. & deGroot, C. 1993. Imipramine treatment of panic disorder with agoraphobia: The second time around. *J. Psychiatr. Res.* 27: 61–68.

McElroy, S. L., Keck, P. E. & Friedman, L. M. 1995. Minimizing and managing antidepressant side effects. *J. Clin. Psychiatry* 56: 49–55.

McNally, R. J. 1992. Anxiety sensitivity distinguishes panic disorder from generalized anxiety disorder. *J. Nerv. Ment. Dis.* 180: 737–738.

McNally, R. J. 1994. *Panic Disorder: A Critical Analysis,* pp. 173–177, Guilford Press, New York.

Mellman, T. A. & Uhde, T. W. 1989a. Sleep panic attacks: New clinical findings and theoretical implications. *Am. J. Psychiatry* 146: 1204–1207.

Mellman, T. A. & Uhde, T. W. 1989b. Electroencephalographic sleep in panic disorder: A focus on sleep-related panic attacks. *Arch. Gen. Psychiatry* 46: 178–184.

Mendlewicz, J., Papadimitriou, G. & Wilmotte, J. 1993. Family study of panic disorder: Comparison of generalized anxiety disorder, major depression, and normal subjects. *Psychiatr. Genet.* 3: 73–78.

Merikangas, K. R., Angst, J., Eaton, W. et al. 1996. Comorbidity and boundaries of affective disorders with anxiety disorders and substance misuse: Results of an international task force. *Br. J. Psychiatry* 168: 58–67.

Milrod, B., Busch, F., Cooper, A. et al. 1997. *Manual of Panic-Focused Psychodynamic Psychotherapy.* American Psychiatric Press, Washington, DC.

Modigh, K., Westberg, P. & Eriksson, E. 1992. Superiority of clomipramine over imipramine in the treatment of panic disorder: A placebo-controlled trial. *J. Clin. Psychopharmacol.* 12: 251–261.

Moreau, D. & Weissman, M. M. 1992. Panic disorder in children and adolescents: A review. *Am. J. Psychiatry* 149: 1306–1314.

Murphy, J. M., Sobol, A. M., Olivier, D. C. et al. 1989. Prodromes of depression and anxiety. The Stirling County Study. *Br. J. Psychiatry* 155: 490–495.

Mutchler, K., Crowe, R. R., Noyes, R. Jr. et al. 1990. Exclusion of the tyrosine hydroxylase gene in 14 panic disorder pedigrees. *Am. J. Psychiatry* 147: 1367–1369.

Nagy, L. M., Krystal, J. H., Woods, S. W. et al. 1989. Clinical and medication outcome after short-term alprazolam and behavioral group treatment in panic disorder: 2.5-year naturalistic follow-up study. *Arch. Gen. Psychiatry* 46: 993–999.

Nesse, R. M., Cameron, O. G., Curtis, G. C. et al. 1984. Adrenergic function in patients with panic anxiety. *Arch. Gen .Psychiatry* 41: 771–776.

Nordahl, T. E., Semple, W. E., Gross, M. et al. 1990. Cerebral glucose metabolic differences in patients with panic disorder. *Neuropsychopharmacology* 3: 261–272.

Norman, T. R., Gregory, M. S., Judd, F. K. et al. 1988. Platelet serotonin uptake in panic disorder: Comparison with normal controls and the effect of treatment. *Aust. NZ J. Psychiatry* 22: 390–395.

Norman, T. R., Judd, F. K., Staikos, V. et al. 1990. High-affinity platelet [3H]LSD binding is decreased in panic disorder. *J. Affect. Dis.* 19: 119–123.

Northcott, C. J. & Stein, M. B. 1994. Panic disorder in pregnancy. *J. Clin. Psychiatry* 55: 539–542.

Noyes, R. 1991. Suicide in panic disorder: A review. *J. Affect. Dis.* 22: 1–11.

Noyes, R. 1992. Outcome of panic disorder as influenced by illness variables and coexisting syndromes. In *Handbook of Anxiety*, Vol. 5, eds. G. D. Burrows, R. Noyes, M. Roth, pp. 137–160, Elsevier, Amsterdam.

Noyes, R., Burrows, G. D., Reich, J. H. et al. 1996. Diazepam versus alprazolam for treatment of panic disorder. *J. Clin. Psychiatry.* 57: 349–355.

Noyes, R., Chaudhry, D. R. & Domingo, D. V. 1986c. Pharmacologic treatment of phobic disorders. *J. Clin. Psychiatry* 47: 445–452.

Noyes, R., Christiansen, J., Clancy, J. et al. 1991c. Predictors of serious suicide attempts among patients with panic disorder. *Compr. Psychiatry* 32: 261–267.

Noyes, R., Clancy, J., Garvey, M. J. et al. 1987b. Is agoraphobia a variant of panic disorder or a separate illness? *J. Anx. Dis.* 1: 3–13.

Noyes, R., Clancy, J., Hoenk, P. R. et al. 1980. The prognosis of anxiety neurosis. *Arch. Gen. Psychiatry* 37: 173–178.

Noyes, R., Clancy, J., Woodman, C. et al. 1993. Environmental factors related to the outcome of panic disorder: A seven-year follow-up study. *J. Nerv. Ment. Dis.* 181: 529–538.

Noyes, R., Crowe, R. R., Harris, E. L. et al. 1986a. Relationship between panic disorder and agoraphobia: A family study. *Arch. Gen. Psychiatry* 43: 227–232.

Noyes, R., Garvey, M. J., Cook, B. et al. 1991b. Controlled discontinuation of benzodiazepine treatment for patients with panic disorder. *Am. J. Psychiatry* 148: 517–523.

Noyes, R., Garvey, M. J. & Cook, B. L. 1989a. Follow-up study of patients with panic disorder and agoraphobia with panic attacks treated with tricyclic antidepressants. *J. Affect. Dis.* 16: 249–257.

Noyes, R., Garvey, M. J., Cook, B. L. et al. 1988. Benzodiazepine withdrawal: A review of the evidence. *J. Clin. Psychiatry* 49: 382–389.

Noyes, R., Garvey, M. J., Cook, B. L. et al. 1989b. Problems with tricyclic antidepressant use in patients with panic disorder or agoraphobia: Results of a naturalistic follow-up study. *J. Clin. Psychiatry* 50: 163–169.

Noyes, R., Hoenk, P. R., Kuperman, S. et al. 1977. Depersonalization in accident victims and psychiatric patients. *J. Nerv. Ment. Dis.* 164: 401–407.

Noyes, R., Reich, J., Christiansen, J. et al. 1990. Outcome of panic disorder: Relationship to diagnostic subtypes and comorbidity. *Arch. Gen. Psychiatry* 47: 809–818.

Noyes, R., Reich, J., Clancy, J. et al. 1986b. Reduction in hypochondriasis with treatment of panic disorder. *Br. J. Psychiatry* 149: 631–635.

Noyes, R., Reich, J. H., Suelzer, M. et al. 1991a. Personality traits associated with panic disorder: Change associated with treatment. *Compr. Psychiatry* 32: 283–294.

Noyes, R., Woodman, C., Garvey, M. J. et al. 1992a. Generalized anxiety disorder vs. panic disorder: Distinguishing characteristics and patterns of comorbidity. *J. Nerv. Ment. Dis.* 180: 369–379.

Nunes, E. J., McGrath, P. J. & Quitkin, F. M. 1995. Treating anxiety in patients with alcoholism. *J. Clin. Psychiatry* 56: 3–9.

Nyströem, S. & Lindegard, B. 1975. Predisposition for mental syndromes: A study comapring predisposition for depression, neurasthenia, and anxiety state. *Acta Psychiatr. Scand.* 51: 69–76.

Oakley-Browne, M. A., Joyce, P. R., Wells, J. E. et al. 1989. Christchurch Psychiatric Epidemiology Study, part II: Six month and other period prevalences for specific psychiatric disorders. *Aust. NZ J. Psychiatry* 23: 327–340.

Oehrberg, S., Christiansen, P. E. & Behnke, K. et al. 1995. Paroxetine in the treatment of panic disorder: A randomized, double-blind, placebo-controlled study. *Br. J. Psychiatry* 167: 374–379.

Ontiveros, A., Fontaine, R., Breton, G. et al. 1989. Correlation of severity of panic disorder and neuroanatomical changes on magnetic resonance imaging. *J. Neuropsychiatry* 1: 404–408.

Ormel, J., Oldehinkel, T. & Brilman, E. 1993. Outcome of depression and anxiety in primary care. *Arch. Gen. Psychiatry* 50: 759–766.

Öst, L-G. 1990. The Agoraphobia Scale: An evaluation of its reliability and validity. *Behav. Res. Ther.* 28: 323–329.

Öst, L-G. 1987. Applied relaxation: Description of a coping technique and review of controlled studies. *Behav. Res. Ther.* 25: 397–409.

O'Sullivan, G. & Marks, I. M. 1991. Long-term outcome of phobic and obsessive-compulsive disorders after treatment. In *Handbook of Anxiety*, Vol. 4, eds. R. Noyes, G. D. Burrows, M. Roth, pp. 87–108, Elsevier, Amsterdam.

Otto, M. W., Pollack, M. H., Sachs, G. S. et al. 1992a. Hypochondriacal concerns, anxiety sensitivity, and panic disorder. *J. Anx. Dis.* 6: 93–104.

Otto, M. W., Pollack, M. H., Sacks, G. S. et al. 1992b. Alcohol dependence in panic disorder patients. *J. Psychiatr. Res.* 26: 29–38.

Page, A. C. 1991. An assessment of structured diagnostic interviews for adult anxiety disorders. *Int. Rev. Psychiatry* 3: 265–278.

Parker, G. 1979. Reported parental characteristics of agoraphobics and social phobics. *Br. J. Psychiatry* 135: 555–560.

Parker, G. 1988. Developmental factors in anxiety. In *Handbook of Anxiety*, Vol. 2, eds. R. Noyes, M. Roth, G. D. Burrows, pp. 147–162, Elsevier, Amsterdam.

Pauls, D. L., Bucher, K. D., Crowe, R. R. et al. 1980. A genetic study of panic disorder pedigrees. *Am. J. Hum. Genet.* 32: 639–644.

Pecknold, J. C., Swinson, R. P., Kuch, K. et al. 1988. Alprazolam in panic disorder and agoraphobia: Results from a multicenter trial. III. Discontinuation effects. *Arch. Gen. Psychiatry* 45: 429–436.

Pelleg, A. & Porter, R. S. 1990. The pharmacology of adenosine. *Pharmacotherapy* 10: 157–174.

Penfield, W. & Jasper, H. 1954. *Epilepsy and the Functional Anatomy of the Human Brain*. Little Brown, Boston.

Peterson, R. A. & Reiss, S. 1992. *Manual for the Anxiety Sensitivity Index*, Second Edition, International Diagnostic Services, Inc., Worthington, OH.

Phillips, R. G. & LeDoux, J. E. 1992. Differential contribution of amygdala and hippocampus to cued and contextual fear conditioning. *Behav. Neurosci.* 106: 274–285.

Pohl, R, Yeragani, V. K., Balon, R. et al. 1988. The jitteriness syndrome in panic disorder patients treated with antidepressants. *J. Clin. Psychiatry* 49: 100–104.

Pollack, M. H., Otto, M. N., Rosenbaum, J. F. et al. 1990. Longitudinal course of panic disorder: Findings from the Massachusetts General Hospital naturalistic study. *J. Clin. Psychiatry* 51 (Suppl. A): 12–16.

Pollack, M. H., Otto, M. W., Kaspi, S. P. et al. 1994. Cognitive behavior therapy for treatment-refractory panic disorder. *J. Clin. Psychiatry* 55: 200–205.

Pollack, M. H., Otto, M. W., Sabatino, S. et al. 1996. Relationship of childhood anxiety to adult panic disorder: Correlates and influence on course. *Am. J. Psychiatry* 153: 376–381.

Pollard, C. A., Pollard, H. J. & Corn, K. J. 1989. Panic onset and major life events in the lives of agoraphobics: A test of contiguity. *J. Abn. Psychol.* 8: 318–321.

Post, R. M., Weiss, S. R. B., Uhde, T. W. et al. 1993. Implications of cocaine kindling, induction of the proto-oncogene c-fos, and contingent tolerance. In *Biology of Anxiety Disorders*, eds. R. Hoehn-Saric, D. R. McLeod, pp. 121–175, American Psychiatric Press, Washington, DC.

Quitkin, F. J., Rifkin, A., Kaplan, J. et al. 1972. Phobic anxiety syndrome complicated by drug dependence and addiction: A treatable form of drug abuse. *Arch. Gen. Psychiatry* 27: 159–162.

Raj, A. & Sheehan, D. V. 1987. Medical evaluation of panic attacks. *J. Clin. Psychiatry* 48: 309–313.

Rapee, R. M., Litwin, E. M. & Baslow, D. H. 1990. Impact of life events on subjects with panic disorder and on comparison subjects. *Am. J. Psychiatry* 147: 640–644.

Redmond, D. E., Jr. 1977. Alterations in the function of the nucleus locus coeruleus: A possible model for studies of anxiety. In *Animal Models in Psychiatry*, eds. I. Hanin, E. Usdin, pp. 293–305, Pergamon Press, Oxford, New York.

Reich, J. H. 1988. DSM-III personality disorders and the outcome of treated panic disorder. *Am. J Psychiatry* 145: 1149–1152.

Reich, J. H., Noyes, R. & Troughton, E. 1987. Dependent personality disorder associated with phobic avoidance in patients with panic disorder. *Am. J. Psychiatry* 144: 323–326.

Reich, J. H. & Troughton, E. 1988. Comparison of DSM-III personality disordersin recovered depressed and panic disorder patients. *J. Nerv. Ment. Dis.* 176: 300–304.

Reiman, E. M., Raichle, M. E., Butler, F. K. et al. 1984. A focal brain abnormality in panic disorder, a severe form of anxiety. *Nature* 310: 683–685.

Reiman, E. M., Raichle, M. E., Robins, E. et al. 1986. The application of positron emmission tomography to the study of panic disorder. *Am. J. Psychiatry* 143: 469–477.

Reiman, E. M., Raichle, M. E., Robins, E. et al. 1989. Neuroanatomical correlates of a lactate-induced anxiety attack. *Arch. Gen. Psychiatry* 46: 493–499.

Reiss, S. & McNally, R. J. 1985. Expectancy model of fear. In *Theoretical Issues in Behavior Therapy*, eds. S. Reiss, R. R. Bootzin, pp. 107–21, Academic Press, San Diego, CA.

Rimon, R., Lepola, U., Jakkonen, J. et al. 1995. Cerebrospinal fluid gamma-aminobutyric acid in patients with panic disorder. *Biol. Psychiatry* 38: 737–741.

Robins, L. N. & Regier, D. A. 1991. *Psychiatric Disorders in America*. Free Press, New York.

Rosenbaum, J. F. 1992. Evaluation and management of the treatment-resistant anxiety disorder patient. *Bull. Menninger Clin.* 56 (Suppl. 2A): A50–A60.

Rosenbaum, J. F., Biederman, J. & Bolduc, E. A. 1992. Comorbidity of parental anxiety disorders as risk for childhood-onset anxiety in inhibited children. *Am. J. Psychiatry* 149: 475–481.

Rosenbaum, J. F., Biederman, J., Gersten, M. et al. 1988. Behavioral inhibition in children of parents with panic disorder and agoraphobia: A controlled study. *Arch. Gen. Psychiatry* 45: 463–470.

Rosenbaum, J. F., Biederman, J. & Pollock, R. A. 1994. The etiology of social phobia. *J. Clin. Psychiatry* 55 (Suppl. 6): 10–16.

Ross, J. 1994. *Triumph Over Fear*. Bantam books, New York.

Roth, M. 1960. The phobic anxiety-depersonalization syndrome and some general aetiological problems in psychiatry. *J. Neuropsychiatry* 1: 293–306.

Roth, M., Gurney, C. & Garside, R. F. 1972. Studies in the classification of affective disorders. The relationship between anxiety states and depressive illness. *Br. J. Psychiatry* 121: 147–161.

Roth, W. T., Ehlers, A., Taylor, C. B. et al. 1990. Skin conductance habituation in panic disorder patients. *Biol. Psychiatry* 27: 1231–1243.

Roy-Byrne, P. P. 1992. Integrated treatment of panic disorder. *Am. J. Med.* 92 (Suppl. 1A): 495–545.

Roy-Byrne, P. P. & Cowley, D. S. 1995. Course and outcome in panic disorder: A review of recent follow-up studies. *Anxiety* 1: 151–160.

Roy-Byrne, P. P., Geraci, M. & Uhde, T. N. 1986c. Life events and the onset of panic disorder. *Am. J. Psychiatry* 143: 1424–1427.

Roy-Byrne, P. P. & Hommer, D. 1988. Benzodiazepine withdrawal: Overview and implications for the treatment of anxiety. *Am. J. Med.* 84: 1041–1052.

Roy-Byrne, P. P., Sullivan, M. D., Cowley, D. S. et al. 1993. Adjunctive treatment of benzodiazepine discontinuation syndromes: A review. *J. Psychiatr. Res.* 27 (Suppl. 1): 143–153.

Roy-Byrne, P. P. & Uhde, T. W. 1988. Exogenous factors in panic disorder: Clinical and research implications. *J. Clin. Psychiatry* 49: 56–61.

Roy-Byrne, P. P., Uhde, T. W. & Post, R. M. 1986a. Effects of one night's sleep deprivation on mood and behavior in panic disorder. *Arch. Gen. Psychiatry* 43: 895–899.

Roy-Byrne, P. P., Uhde, T. W., Post, R. M. et al. 1986b. The corticotropin-releasing hormone stimulation test in patients with panic disorder. *Am. J. Psychiatry* 143: 896–899.

Salvador-Carulla, L., Segui, J., Fernandez-Cano, P. et al. 1995. Costs and offset effect in panic disorders. *Br. J. Psychiatry* 166 (Suppl. 27): 23–28.

Sanderson, W. C., Rapee, R. M. & Barlow, D. H. 1989. The influence of an illusion of control on panic attacks induced via inhalation of 5.5% carbon dioxide-enriched air. *Arch. Gen. Psychiatry* 46: 157–162.

Sanghera, M. K., McMillen, B. A. & German, D. C. 1982. Buspirone, a non-benzodiazepine anxiolytic, increases locus coerulrus noradrenergic neuronal activity. *Eur. J. Pharmacol.* 86: 107–110.

Sargent, N. & Dally, P. J. 1962. Treatment of anxiety states by antidepressive drugs. *Br. Med. J.* 1: 6–9.

Saviotti, F. M., Grandi, S., Savron, G. et al. 1991. Chracterological traits of recovered patients with panic disorder and agoraphobia. *J. Affect. Dis.* 23: 113–117.

Saylor, K. E., DuPont, R. L. & Brouillard, M. 1990. Self-help treatment of anxiety disorders. In *Handbook of Anxiety*, Vol. 4, eds. R. Noyes, M. Roth, G. D. Burrows, pp. 483–496, Elsevier, Amsterdam.

Schneier, F. R., Fyer, A. J., Martin, L. Y. et al. 1991. A comparison of phobic subtypes within panic disorder. *J. Anx. Dis.* 5: 65–75.

Schriber, W., Lauer, C. J., Krumrey, K. et al. 1996. Disregulation of the hypothalamic–pituitary–adrenocortical system in panic disorder. *Neuropsychopharmacology* 15: 7–15.

Schuckit, M. A. 1986. Genetic and clinical implications of alcoholism and affective disorder. *Am. J. Psychiatry* 143: 140–147.

Schuckit, M. A., Irwin, M. & Brown, S. A. 1990. The history of anxiety symptoms among 171 primary alcoholics. *J. Stud. Alcohol* 51: 34–41.

Sciuto, G., Diaforia, G., Battaglia, M. et al. 1991. DSM-III-R personality disorders in panic and obsessive-compulsive disorder: A comparison study. *Compr. Psychiatry* 32: 450–457.

Shear, M. K., Cooper, A. M., Klerman, G. L. et al. 1993. A psychodynamic model of panic disorder. *Am. J. Psychiatry* 150: 859–866.

Shear, M. K. & Mammen, O. 1995. Anxiety disorders in pregnant and postpartum women. *Psychopharm. Bull.* 31: 693–703.

Shear, M. K. & Maser, J. D. 1994. Standardized assessment for panic disorder research: A conference report. *Arch. Gen. Psychiatry* 51: 346–354.

Shear, M. K., Pilkonis, P. A., Cloitre, M. et al. 1994. Cognitive behavioral treatment compared with nonprescriptive treatment of panic disorder. *Arch. Gen. Psychiatry* 51: 395–401.

Shear, M. K. & Weiner, K. 1997. Psychotherapy for panic disorder. *J. Clin. Psychiatry* 58: 38–43.

Sheehan, D. V. 1983. *The Anxiety Disease*, pp. 126–128, Charles Scribner and Sons, New York.

Sheehan, D. V. 1987. Benzodiazepines in panic disorder and agoraphobia. *J. Affect. Dis.* 13: 169–181.

Sheehan, D. V., Ballenger, J. & Jacobsen, G. 1980. Treatment of endogenous anxiety with phobic, hysterical, and hypochondriacal symptoms. *Arch. Gen. Psychiatry* 37: 51–59.

Sheehan, D. V., Raj, A. B., Harnett-Sheehan, K. et al. 1993. The relative efficacy of high-dose buspirone and alprazolam in the treatment of panic disorder: A double-blind placebo–controlled study. *Acta Psychiatr. Scand.* 88: 1–11.

Sholomskas, D. E., Wickamaratne, P. J., Dogolo, L. et al. 1993. Post-partum onset of panic disorder: A coincidental event? *J. Clin. Psychiatry* 54: 476–480.

Siegel, L., Jones, W. C. & Witson, J. O. 1990. Economic and life consequences experienced by a group of individuals with panic disorder. *J. Anx. Dis.* 4: 201–211.

Simon, G., Ormel, J., Von Korff, M. et al. 1995. Health care costs associated with depressive and anxiety disorders in primary care. *Am. J. Psychiatry* 152: 352–357.

Skodol, A. E., Oldham, J. M., Hyler, S. E. et al. 1995. Patterns of anxiety and personality disorder comorbidity. *J. Psychiatric Res.* 29: 361–374.

Skre, I., Onstad, S., Torgersen, S. et al. 1993. A twin study of DSM-III-R anxiety disorders. *Acta Psychiatr. Scand.* 88: 85–92.

Smail, P., Stockwell, T., Canter, S. et al. 1984. Alcohol dependence and phobic states. I: A prevalence study. *Br. J. Psychiatry* 144: 53–57.

Starcevic, J. 1991. Should postattack phenomena be included in the definition and description of a panic attack. *Am. J. Psychiatry* 148: 1752–1753.

Starcevic, J., Kellner, R. & Uhlenhuth, E. H. 1992. Panic disorder and hypochondriacal fears and beliefs. *J. Affect. Dis.* 24: 73–85.

Starkman, M. N., Zelnick, T. C., Nesse, R. M. et al. 1985. Anxiety in patients with pheochromocytomas. *Arch. Int. Med.* 145: 248–252.

Stein, M. B. & Asmundson, G. J. G. 1994. Autonomic function in panic disorder: Cardiorespiratory and plasma catecholamine responsivity to multiple challenges of the autonomic nervous system. *Biol. Psychiatry* 36: 548–558.

Stein, M. B., Chartier, M. & Walker, J. R. 1993a. Sleep in nondepressed patients with panic disorder: I. Systematic assessment of subjective sleep quality and sleep disturbance. *Sleep* 16: 724–726.

Stein, M. B., Enns, M. W. & Kryger, M. H. 1993b. Sleep in nondepressed patients with panic disorder: II. Polysomnographic assesment of sleep architecture and sleep continuity. *J. Affect. Dis.* 28: 1–6.

Stein, M. B., Millar, T. W., Larsen, D. K. et al. 1995a. Irregular breathing during sleep in patients with panic disorder. *Am. J. Psychiatry* 152: 1168–1173.

Stein, M. B., Shea, C. A. & Uhde, T. W. 1989. Social phobic symptoms in patients with panic disorder: Practical and theoretical implications. *Am. J. Psychiatry* 146: 235–238.

Stein, M. B. & Uhde, T. W. 1988. Thyroid indices in panic disorder. *Am. J. Psychiatry* 145: 745–747.

Stein, M. B., Walker, J. R., Anderson, G. et al. 1995b. Childhood physical and sexual abuse in patients with anxiety disorders and in a community sample. *Am. J. Psychiatry* 153: 275–277.

Stewart, R. S., Devous, M. D., Rush, A. J. et al. 1988. Cerebral blood flow changes during sodium-lactate-induced panic attacks. *Am. J. Psychiatry* 145: 442–449.

Swales, P. J. & Sheikh, J. I. 1992. Hysterectomy in patients with panic disorder. *Am. J. Psychiatry* 149: 846–847.

Targum, S. D. 1991. Panic attack frequency and vulnerability to anxiogenic challenge studies. *Psychiatry Res.* 36: 75–83.

Targum, S. D. & Marshall, L. E. 1989. Fenfluramine provocation of anxiety in patients with panic disorder. *Psychiatry Res.* 28: 295–309.

Taylor, C. B., Russiter, E. M. & Agras, W. S. In Press. Utilization of health care services by patients with anxiety and depression disorders.

Telch, M. J., Lucas, J. A. & Nelson, P. 1989. Non-clinical panic in college students: An investigation of prevalence and symptomatology. *J. Abn. Psychol.* 98: 300–306.

Telch, M. J., Lucas, J. A., Schmidt, N. B. et al. 1993. Group cognitive-behavioral treatment of panic disorder. *Behav. Res. Ther.* 31: 279–287.

Tesar, G. E. 1990. High-potency benzodiazepines for short-term management of panic disorder: The U.S. experience. *J. Clin. Psychiatry* 51 (Suppl. 4–10): Discussion 50–53.

Tesar, G. E., Rosenbaum, J. F., Pollack, M. H. et al. 1987. Clonazepam versus alprazolam in the treatment of panic disorder: Interim analysis of data from a prospective, double-blind, placebo-controlled trial. *J. Clin. Psychiatry* 48 (Suppl): 16–21.

Thyer, B. A., Parrish, R. T., Curtis, G. C. et al. 1985. Ages of onset of DSM-III anxiety disorders. *Compr. Psychiatry* 26: 113–122.

Tiffon, L., Coplan, J. D. & Papp, L. A. 1994. Augmentation strategies with tricyclic or fluoxetine treatment in seven partially responsive panic disorder patients. *J. Clin. Psychiatry* 5: 66–69.

Torgersen, S. 1983. Genetic factors in anxiety disorders. *Arch. Gen. Psychiatry* 40: 1085–1089.

Tweed, J. L., Schoenbach, V. J., George, L. K. et al. 1989. The effects of childhood parental death and divorce on the six-month history of anxiety disorders. *Br. J. Psychiatry* 154: 823–828.

Uhde, T. W., Boulenger, J., Roy-Byrne, P. P. et al. 1985. Longitudinal course of panic disorder: Clinical and biological considerations. *Prog. Neuro-Psychopharmacol. Biol. Psychiat.* 9: 39–51.

Uhde, T. W. & Kellner, C. W. 1987. Cerebral ventricular size in panic disorder. *J. Affect. Disorders* 12: 175–178.

van Den Hout, M. A., van der Molen, G. M., Griez, E. et al. 1987. Reduction of CO_2-induced anxiety in patients with panic attacks after repeated CO_2 exposure. *Am. J. Psychiatry* 144: 788–791.

van Vliet, I. M., Westenberg, H. G. M. & den Boer, J. A. 1993. MAO inhibitors in panic disorder: Clinical effects of treatment with biofaramine. *Psychopharmacology* 112: 483–489.

Vieland, V. J., Hodge, S. E., Lish, J. D. et al. 1993. Segregation analysis of panic disorder. *Psychiatr. Genetics* 3: 63–71.

Villeponteaux, V. A., Lydiard, R. B., Laraia, M. T. et al. 1992. The effects of pregnancy on preexisting panic disorder. *J. Clin. Psychiatry* 53: 201–203.

von Korff, M., Shapiro, S., Burke, J. D. et al. 1987. Anxiety and depression in a primary care clinic. *Arch. Gen. Psychiatry* 44: 152–156.

von Korff, M. R., Eaton, W. W. & Keyl, P. M. 1985. The epidemiology of panic attacks and panic disorder: Results of three community surveys. *Am. J. Epidemiol.* 122: 970–981.

Wang, Z. W., Crowe, R. R. & Noyes, R. 1992. Adrenergic receptor genes as candidate genes for panic disorder: A linkage study. *Am. J. Psychiatry* 149: 470–474.

Waziri, R. 1990. Psychosurgery for anxiety and obsessive-compulsive disorders. In *Handbook of Anxiety*, Vol. 4, eds. R. Noyes, M. Roth, G. D. Burrows, pp. 519–535, Elsevier, Amsterdam.

Weilburg, J. B., Schachter, S., Worth, J. et al. 1995. EEG abnormalities in patients with atypical panic attacks. *J. Clin. Psychiatry* 56: 358–362.

Weissman, M. M, Klerman, G. L., Markowitz, J. et al. 1989. Suicidal ideation and suicide attempts in panic disorder and attacks. *N. Engl. J. Med.* 321: 1209–1213.

Westling, B. E. & Öst, L-G. 1993. Relationshipo between panic attack symptoms and cognition in panic disorder patients. *J. Anx. Dis.* 7: 181–194.

Westphal, C. 1872. Die agoraphobie: eine neuropathische Erscheinung. *Arch. Psychiatr. Nervenkr.* 3: 138–161.

Wheeler, E. O., White, P. D., Reed, E. W. et al. 1950. Neurocirculatory asthenia (anxiety neurosis, effort syndrome, neurasthenia): A twenty-year follow-up study of one hundred and seventy-three patients. *JAMA* 142: 878–888.

Williams, J. B. W., Gibbon, M., First, M. B. et al. 1992b. The Structured Clinical Interview for DSM-III-R (SCID): II. Multisite test-retest reliability. *Arch. Gen. Psychiatry* 49: 630–636.

Williams, J. B. W., Spitzer, R. L. & Gibbon, M. 1992a. International reliability of a diagnostic intake procedure for panic disorder. *Am. J. Psychiatry* 149: 560–562.

Williams, S. L. & Zane, G. 1989. Guided mastery and stimulus exposure treatments for severe performance anxiety in agoraphobics. *Behav. Res. Ther.* 27: 237–245.

Winokur, G. 1990. The concept of secondary depression and its relationship to comorbidity. *Psychiatr. Clin. N. Am.* 13: 567–584.

Wittchen, H-U. & Essau, C. A. 1993. Epidemiology of panic disorder: Progress and unresolved issues. *J. Psychiatr. Res.* 27 (Suppl. 1): 47–68.

Wittchen, H-U. 1988. Natural course and spontaneous remissions of untreated anxiety disorders: Results of the Munich Follow-up Study. In *Panic and Phobias: Treatments and Variables Affecting Course and Outcome*, eds. I. Hand, H-U. Wittchen, pp. 3–17, Springer-Verlag, New York.

Wolfe, B. E. & Maser, J. D. 1994. *Treatment of Panic Disorder: A Consensus Development Conference.* American Psychiatric Press, Washington, DC.

Woodman, C. L. 1993. The genetics of panic disorder and generalized anxiety disorders. *Ann. Clin. Psychiatry* 5: 231–240.

Woodman, C. L., Noyes, R., Ballenger, J. C. et al. 1994. Predictors of response to alprazolam and placebo in patients with panic disorder. *J. Affect. Dis.* 30: 5–13.

Woodruff, R. A., Guze, S. B. & Clayton, P. J. 1972. Anxiety neurosis among psychiatric outpatients. *Compr. Psychiatry* 13: 165–170.

Woods, S. W., Charney, D. S., Goodman, W. K. et al. 1988a. Carbon dioxide-induced anxiety: Behavioral, physiologic, and biochemical effects of carbon dioxide in patients with panic disorders and healthy subjects. *Arch.. Gen. Psychiatry* 45: 43–52.

Woods, S. W., Charney, D. S., McPherson, C. A. et al. 1987. Situational panic attacks: Behavioral, physiologic, and biochemical characterization. *Arch. Gen. Psychiatry* 44: 365–375.

Woods, S. W., Koster, K., Krystal, J. K. et al. 1988b. Yohimbine alters regional cerebral blood flow in panic disorder. *Lancet* 2: 678.

World Health Organization (WHO). 1978. *Mental Disorders: Glossary and Guide to their Classification in Accordanced with the Ninth Revision of the International Classification of Diseases.* World Health Organization, Geneva.

World Health Organization (WHO). 1993. *The ICD-10 Classification of Mental and Behavioral Disorders: Diagnostic Criteria for Research.* World Health Organization, Geneva.

Yeragani, V. K., Balon, R., Pohl, R. et al. 1990. Decreased R-R variance in panic disorder patients. *Acta Psychiatr. Scand.* 81: 554–559.

Zandbergen, J. 1992. *Respiratory Regulation and Consequences of CO_2 Changes in Panic Disorder.* CIP-Data Koninklijke Bibliotheek, Den Haag.

Zitrin, C. M., Klein, D. F. & Woerner, M. G. 1983. Treatment of phobias. I: Imipramine and placebo. *Arch. Gen. Psychiatry* 40: 125–138.

Zung, W. W. K. 1971. A rating instrument for anxiety disorders. *Psychosomatics* 12: 371–379.

4

Social phobia

Definition

Social phobia is an unreasonable fear of embarrassing oneself in social or performance situations. In its milder or more circumscribed forms, it causes people to avoid activities such as speaking or eating in public that are an important part of social functioning. In its more severe and generalized forms, it imposes crippling restrictions that result in social isolation and loneliness. It is perhaps the most prevalent and disabling of the anxiety disorders yet is responsive to treatment. Still, few persons seek this treatment, viewing their problem as a form of shyness or inherent weakness to be endured. Added to this, mental health professionals have, until recently, been slow to diagnose and treat the condition.

Descriptions of social anxiety and phobias date from antiquity. Hippocrates had a patient, described by Burton (1621), who 'through bashfulness, suspicion, and timorousness, will not be seen abroad; . . . his hat still in his eyes, he will neither see, nor be seen by his good will. He dare not come in company, for fear he should be misused, disgraced, overshoot himself in gesture of speech, or be sick; he thinks every man observes him . . .'. Social phobia was first described in the USA by Beard (1879) and in France by Janet (1903). The disorder was later separated from other phobias by Marks & Gelder (1966) and Marks (1970). These authors included 'fears of eating, drinking, shaking, blushing, speaking, writing or vomiting in the presence of other people' as well as more general fears of initiating conversations or dating, and they identified the core feature as a fear of appearing ridiculous to others.

In certain situations social phobics fear embarrassment or humiliation and experience physiological symptoms, such as palpitations, blushing, sweating, and trembling. The activities they fear range from single performance situations, such as public speaking, to many or all social encounters.

Feared causes of embarrassment are varied but include awkward or inappropriate behavior (e.g., saying the wrong thing, stammering) and outward signs of anxiety (e.g., blushing, sweating, trembling). As a result, they avoid feared activities and restrict their lives.

Diagnostic criteria

Social phobia first appeared in the classification of mental disorders in 1980. According to DSM-III, it was 'a persistent, irrational fear of, and compelling desire to avoid, a situation in which the individual is exposed to possible scrutiny by others and fears that he or she may act in a way that will be humiliating or embarrassing' (American Psychiatric Association, 1980). Examples included fears of speaking or performing in public, using public bathrooms, eating in public, and writing in the presence of others. DSM-III specified that social phobics usually had only one fear but the DSM-III-R definition was expanded to include multiple fears, and a generalized subtype – persons who fear most social situations – was identified (American Psychiatric Association, 1987).

The DSM-IV criteria are shown in Table 4.1 (American Psychiatric Association, 1994). Consistent with the disorder's early onset, provision has been made in DSM-IV to diagnose social phobia in children, and avoidant disorder, an earlier childhood category, has been eliminated (Strauss & Last, 1993). When the diagnosis is made in children there must be evidence of age-appropriate social relationships. Also, in children, fear may be expressed behaviorally in the form of crying, tantrums, freezing, or shrinking in social situations. The ICD-10 criteria, shown in Table 4.2, are close to those found in DSM-IV; however, the former specify anxiety symptoms and the latter emphasize cognitive manifestations (World Health Organization, 1993).

Reliability and validity

Reliability

The interrater agreement for DSM-III-R social phobia has ranged from fair to excellent (kappa values 0.47 to 0.79) (DiNardo et al., 1983, 1993; Mannuzza et al., 1989; Onstad et al., 1991; Williams et al., 1992). The lowest kappas were found in a study of all psychiatric disorders in which base rates were low (Williams et al., 1992). Studies from anxiety clinics have yielded higher values. Mannuzza et al. (1989) found good agreement for

Table 4.1. *DSM criteria for social phobia*

A. A marked and persistent fear of one or more social or performance situations in which the person is exposed to unfamiliar people or to possible scrutiny by others. The individual fears that he or she will act in a way (or show anxiety symptoms) that will be humiliating or embarrassing
B. Exposure to the feared social situation almost invariably provokes anxiety, which may take the form of a situationally bound or situationally predisposed panic attack
C. The person recognizes that the fear is excessive or unreasonable
D. The feared social or performance situations are avoided or else are endured with intense anxiety or distress
E. The avoidance, anxious anticipation, or distress in the feared social or performance situation(s) interferes significantly with the persons normal routine, occupational (academic) functioning, or social activities or relationships, or there is marked distress about having the phobia
F. In individuals under age 18 years, the duration is at least 6 months
G. The fear or avoidance is not due to the direct physiological effects of a substance (e.g., a drug of abuse, a medication) or a general medical condition and is not better accounted for by another mental disorder (e.g., panic disorder with or without agoraphobia, separation anxiety disorder, body dysmorphic disorder, a pervasive developmental disorder, or schizoid personality disorder)
H. If a general medical condition or another mental disorder is present, the fear in criterion A is unrelated to it (e.g., the fear is not of stuttering, trembling in Parkinson's disease, or exhibiting abnormal eating behavior in anorexia nervosa or bulimia nervosa)
Specify: **Generalized** type (fears include most social situations)

Reprinted with permission from American Psychiatric Association (1994).

current (0.68) but poor agreement for past (0.33) social phobia. With respect to individual fears, Fyer et al. (1989) found good agreement for four but only fair to poor agreement for six others. In the study by Mannuzza et al. (1989), criterion ambiguity was a major source of disagreement and discrepancies occurred on ratings of impairment. Similarly, DiNardo et al. (1993) reported excellent agreement for social phobia as a principal diagnosis but only good agreement for an additional diagnosis. With additional diagnoses, interviewers sometimes differed about whether social phobia was independent or an associated feature of another disorder.

Validity

Social phobia is a valid clinical entity that differs from agoraphobia (Persson & Nordlund, 1985; Mannuzza et al., 1990). These two disorders are characterized by multiple phobias and, in many instances, panic attacks. Both have an early onset and follow a chronic course (Thyer et al., 1985; Öst, 1987). Beyond this there are differences, the most important

Table 4.2. *ICD-10 criteria for social phobia*

A. Either of the following must be present:
   1. marked fear of being the focus of attention, or fear of behaving in a way that will be embarrassing or humiliating
   2. marked avoidance of being the focus of attention, or of situations in which there is fear of behaving in an embarrassing or humiliating way
   These fears are manifested in social situations, such as eating or speaking in public, encountering known individuals in public, or entering or enduring small group situations (e.g., parties, meetings, classrooms).
B. At least two symptoms of anxiety in the feared situation, as defined under criterion B for agoraphobia,[a] must have been manifested at some time since the onset of the disorder, together with at least one of the following symptoms:
   1. blushing or shaking
   2. fear of vomiting
   3. urgency or fear of micturition or defecation
C. Significant emotional distress is caused by the symptoms or by the avoidance, and the individual recognizes that these are excessive or unreasonable
D. Symptoms are restricted to or predominate in the feared situations or contemplation of the feared situations
E. The symptoms listed in criteria A and B are not the result of delusions, hallucinations, or other disorders such as organic mental disorders, schizophrenia and related disorders, mood disorders, obsessive-compulsive disorder, and are not secondary to cultural beliefs

[a]See Chapter 3. Reprinted with permission from WHO (1993).

being the social phobic's fear of embarrassment or humiliation. Agoraphobics, by contrast, fear an inability to get to safety in case of incapacitation. In addition, social phobics more often have observable manifestations of anxiety with the potential for embarrassment, and they more often have avoidant personality traits than do agoraphobics (Amies et al., 1983; Jansen et al., 1994; Noyes et al., 1995).

Further validation comes from family studies showing that relatives of agoraphobics have an increased risk of agoraphobia but not social phobia, and that relatives of social phobics have an increased risk of social phobia but not agoraphobia (Noyes et al., 1986; Fyer et al., 1993). Also, biological challenge and treatment studies suggest differences (Papp et al., 1988). Patients with social phobia show a lower rate of panic in response to lactate challenge than those with panic or agoraphobia (Liebowitz et al., 1985a), and social phobic patients are less responsive to tricyclic antidepressants than patients with panic or agoraphobia (Liebowitz et al., 1985b).

Social phobics are also distinct from specific phobics. Specific phobics have an earlier onset in childhood (Marks & Gelder, 1966; Thyer et al.,

Table 4.3. *DSM-IV Criteria for Avoidant Personality Disorder*

A pervasive pattern of social inhibition, feelings of inadequacy, and
hypersensitivity to negative evaluation, beginning by early adulthood and present
in a variety of contexts, as indicated by four (or more) of the following:
(1) avoids occupational activities that involve significant interpersonal contact,
      because of fears of criticism, disapproval, or rejection
(2) is unwilling to get involved with people unless certain of being liked
(3) shows restraint within intimate relationships because of the fear of being
      shamed or ridiculed
(4) is preoccupied with being criticized or rejected in social situations
(5) is inhibited in new interpersonal situations because of feelings of inadequacy
(6) views self as socially inept, personally unappealing, or inferior to others
(7) is unusually reluctant to take personal risks or to engage in any new activities
      because they may prove embarrassing

Reprinted with permission from American Psychiatric Association (1994).

1985). These phobias often result from traumatic experiences and involve
fear of physical injury from exposure to a feared object (e.g., animals,
storms). Symptom profiles distinguish social and specific phobics as well
(Cameron et al., 1986).

As currently defined, social phobia is difficult to separate from avoidant
personality disorder, a pervasive pattern of social inhibition, feelings of
inadequacy, and hypersensitivity to criticism (American Psychiatric Association, 1987) (Table 4.3). This disorder was first described by Millon (1969)
and, subsequently, introduced into DSM-III. Millon described active
avoidance of relationships due to fear and hypersensitivity rather than to
disinterest that is characteristic of schizoid personality disorder. In DSM-
IV, the generalized subtype of social phobia and avoidant personality
disorder both include fear of embarrassment, avoidance of social situations, and impairment in social functioning. Studies have shown a high
degree of overlap, and comparisons of social phobics with and without
avoidant personality disorder have shown only differences in severity
(Herbert et al., 1992; Holt et al., 1992a; Turner et al., 1992). As a consequence, some authors have suggested combining the categories or redefin-
ing them to sharpen the distinction (Schneier et al., 1991).

Measurement

Structured interviews

A series of structured clinical interviews that include social phobia have
been revised for DSM-IV. The Anxiety Disorders Interview Schedule,

Revised Version (ADIS-IV) is a structured interview designed specifically for anxiety disorders (Brown et al., 1994a). The ADIS-IV calls for ratings of fear and avoidance in a number of social situations. It elicits information about important clinical features including the history of the disorder, extent of avoidance, situational and cognitive cues, etc. Global ratings of severity on 9-point linear scales are made, and these are used to determine the predominant disturbance when more than one disorder coexists. The ADIS-IV was developed for use in anxiety clinic populations but it includes screening for other major disorders. It takes two and a half hours and should be administered by experienced clinicians.

Another structured interview developed specifically for anxiety disorders is the Schedule for Affective Disorders and Schizophrenia-Lifetime Anxiety Version (SADS-LA) (Mannuzza et al., 1986). A DSM-IV revision of this instrument is in progress. The SADS-LA includes detailed assessment of many individual symptoms and yields diagnoses according to several classification systems. It elicits information about subthreshold symptoms and syndromes and about relationships between coexisting disorders. Ratings of fear in, and avoidance of, various social situations are included. The SADS-LA provides coverage of most psychiatric disorders but is lengthy and awkwardly worded. This instrument was designed for use in research involving anxiety disorders and the relationships between them.

Other structured interviews include the Structured Clinical Interview for DSM-IV (SCID), the Composite International Diagnostic Interview (CIDI) developed from the Diagnostic Interview Schedule, and the Schedule for Clinical Assessment in Neuropsychiatry (SCAN) developed from the Present State Examination (Robins et al., 1988; Page, 1991; Wing et al., 1991; First et al., 1995). These instruments have been revised in accordance with current DSM and ICD criteria and screen for all psychiatric disorders. The SCID is modeled after the typical clinical interview and employs open-ended questions, requiring professional interviewers. The CIDI, on the other hand, relies on closed-ended questions and may be administered by lay interviewers. Unlike other diagnostic instruments, the SCAN rates symptoms independent of classification. A computer system generates diagnoses so clinician judgment is applied to symptoms not disorders. These and other instruments are reviewed by Page (1991).

Symptom rating scales

Two observer-rated scales, the Brief Social Phobia Scale (BSPS) and the Liebowitz Social Anxiety Scale (LSAS), were designed to measure severity

Table 4.4. *The Brief Social Phobia Scale*

Instructions: It is recommended that the interviewer give a copy of this scale to
the client for the interview. The time period will cover the previous week, unless
otherwise specified (e.g., at the initial evaluation interview, when it could be the
previous month).

Part I. Fear/Avoidance
 How much do you fear and avoid the following situations? Please give separate
 ratings for fear and avoidance.

	Fear rating	*Avoidance rating*
	0 = None	0 = Never
	1 = Mild	1 = Rare
	2 = Moderate	2 = Sometimes
	3 = Severe	3 = Frequent
	4 = Extreme	4 = Always
	Fear (F)	Avoidance (A)
1. Speaking in public or in front of others	___	___
2. Talking to people in authority	___	___
3. Talking to strangers	___	___
4. Being embarrassed or humiliated	___	___
5. Being criticized	___	___
6. Social gatherings	___	___
7. Doing something while being watched (this does not include speaking)	___	___

Part II. Physiological (P)
 When you are in a situation that involves contact with other people, or when
 you are thinking about such a situation, do you experience the following
 symptoms?

	0 = None
	1 = Mild
	2 = Moderate
	3 = Severe
	4 = Extreme
8. Blushing	___
9. Palpitations	___
10. Trembling	___
11. Sweating	___

$F =$ $A =$ $P =$ Total $=$

Source: Davidson et al. (1991). © 1991 Physicians Postgraduate Press. Reprinted
with permission.

of symptoms in patients diagnosed with social phobia (Liebowitz, 1987; Davidson et al., 1991). The Brief Social Phobia Scale (Table 4.4) calls for ratings of fear (0 none to 4 extreme), avoidance (0 never to 4 always), and autonomic symptoms (0 none to 4 extreme) that occur in social situations. It yields scores for fear, avoidance, and physiological change as well as a total score. This brief 11-item measure has acceptable psychometric properties and appears sensitive to change with treatment (Davidson et al., 1991, 1993c).

The Liebowitz Social Anxiety Scale contains 24 items that are rated for fear (0 none to 3 severe) and avoidance (0 never to 3 usually). The item list is comprehensive and includes both performance and interactional situations. The scale has demonstrated good clinical utility and criterion validity (Holt et al., 1992a,b; Brown et al., 1995). It has been used in treatment trials to measure change (Greist et al., 1995). The items assess four dimensions: interaction with strangers, formal performance/center of attention, eating and drinking while being observed, and behavior at parties and other informal situations (Starkin et al., 1990).

The Fear Questionnaire (FQ) is a brief, self-rated measure that is frequently used for research and clinical purposes (Marks & Mathews, 1979). The scale contains 17 phobic items that are rated on 9-point, linear scales of avoidance (0 would not avoid it to 8 always avoid it). Three subscales have five items each: social phobia, agoraphobia, and blood/injury phobia. The scale has acceptable psychometric properties and is sensitive to change (Lelliott, 1988; Oei et al., 1991). Also, normative values for the general population are available (Mizes & Crawford, 1986). A recent study showed that the subscales correctly identified social and agoraphobic patients (Cox et al., 1991).

Several self-administered scales have been designed specifically for social phobia. One is the Social Phobia and Anxiety Inventory (SPAI). This is an empirically derived inventory that includes assessment of somatic symptoms and cognitions as well as avoidance and escape behaviors (Turner et al., 1989). It contains social phobic and agoraphobic subscales and includes ratings of response to strangers, authority figures, the opposite sex, and people in general (Turner and Beidel, in press). It is capable of distinguishing social phobics from normals and persons with other anxiety disorders and has proven sensitive to change with treatment (Beidel et al., 1993). A version of the scale has been developed for children (Beidel et al., 1995).

The Social Avoidance and Distress (SAD) and Fear of Negative Evaluation (FNE) scales have frequently been used in studies of social anxiety (Watson & Friend, 1969). The SAD contains statements about anxiety and avoidance in situations involving social interaction (e.g., I try to avoid situations which force me to be very sociable). The FNE includes items about expected negative evaluation by others (e.g., If someone is evaluating me I tend to expect the worse). An abbreviated version has been developed which uses 5-point Likert-type scales. These scales may not be suitable for subject selection and outcome assessment of social phobia (Turner et al., 1987).

The newest self-rated instruments are the Social Interaction Anxiety Scale (SIAS) and the Social Phobia Scale (SPS) (Heimberg et al., 1992). These are companion measures designed to assess separate domains of social anxiety. The SPS elicits information about situations involving scruitiny by others (e.g., speaking in front of a group) and the SIAS records responses during social interaction (e.g., speaking with someone in authority). Both scales are reliabable (Mattick & Clark, 1989) and correlate with other measures of social phobia. They have been used to distinguish patients with social phobia from those with other anxiety disorders and social phobia subtypes (Brown et al., 1994b). They are also sensitive to change with treatment.

Epidemiology

Prevalence

Social phobia is, perhaps, the most prevalent of the anxiety disorders (reviewed by Chapman et al., 1995; Walker & Stein, 1995); however, general population estimates have varied according to the criteria used. The National Comorbidity Survey (NCS) reported a lifetime prevalence of 13.3% and 12-month rate of 7.9% (Kessler et al., 1994). Lower estimates from the ECA study were based on narrow DSM-III criteria (Schneier et al., 1992; Davidson et al., 1993a). Persons in the ECA sample who claimed fears without impairment closely resembled those meeting full criteria, leading Davidson et al. (1994) to conclude that clinically significant social phobia affects over 10% of the population. The prevalence of social phobia in children averaged 1.4% in several studies (Anderson et al., 1987; Rey et al., 1992). Among the elderly, rates of social phobia are lower than for younger adults (Flint, 1994).

The most widely feared social situation is public speaking. In one community survey, nearly a third claimed much more nervousness about speaking in front of an audience than other people (Stein et al., 1994a). Table 4.5 shows frequency of fear in a variety of performance and interactive situations. The high rate of speaking fear suggests that it may differ

Table 4.5. *Nervousness in social situations as reported in the Winnipeg Area Study*

	Much more nervous than other people (%)	Somewhat more nervous than other people (%)
Public speaking (large audience)	31.0	24.0
Speaking in front of small group	6.9	18.0
Dealing with people in authority	3.6	19.7
Speaking to strangers or meeting new people	3.0	10.7
Attending social gatherings	1.3	13.2
Writing in front of other people	1.1	4.0
Eating in front of other people	0.8	6.3
At least one situation	33.3	27.6
At least one situation other than public speaking	12.7	32.5

Source: Modified from Stein et al. (1994a). © 1994, American Psychiatric Association. Reprinted with permission.

qualitatively from other social fears. Many persons experience anxiety in specialized performance situations. For example, 16.1% of music students and faculty reported that performance anxiety had interfered with their careers (Wesner et al., 1990). As social fears differ from phobias in degree, prevalence estimates are strongly influenced by the threshold used for diagnoses (Pollard & Henderson, 1988).

In clinical populations social phobia comprises 8–13% of the anxiety disorders seen and is less common than panic disorder or agoraphobia (Liebowitz et al., 1985b). Also, in clinical samples there is a slight preponderance of men (48–60%) (Schneier et al., 1992). The majority of social phobics who obtain treatment have been ill more than 10 years (Marks & Gelder, 1966; Schneier et al., 1991); however, most never seek treatment. In one epidemiological study, 19.6% sought treatment for emotional problems but only 5.4% consulted a mental health professional for social phobia (Davidson et al., 1993c). This low rate may reflect fear of treatment that involves social interaction.

Risk factors and comorbidity

Social phobia is more prevalent among women, the female to male ratio being about 3 to 2 (Bourdon et al., 1988; Chapman et al., 1995). Rates are

Table 4.6. *Lifetime rates of comorbid psychiatric disorders in social phobia*

	Social phobia N = 361 (%)	No social phobia N = 13 176 (%)	Adjusted odds ratio
Simple phobia	59.0	13.2	9.2
Agoraphobia	44.9	6.1	11.8
Alcohol abuse	18.8	12.2	2.2
Major depression	16.6	4.0	4.4
Drug abuse	13.0	5.0	2.9
Dysthymia	12.5	3.1	4.3
Obsessive-compulsive	11.1	2.5	4.4
Panic disorder	4.7	1.3	3.2

Source: Modified from Schneier et al. (1992). © 1992, American Medical Association. Reprinted with permission.

also higher among those who are younger, unmarried, less educated, have lower income, less stable employment, and lower socioeconomic status (Schneier et al., 1992; Davidson et al., 1993c). Comorbidity is high among social phobics and some of these demographic differences are related to coexisting disorders (Schneier et al., 1992). Social phobia is also associated with conduct disturbances, poor grades in school, poor work performance, reduced social interaction and support, impaired physical health, and increased health care utilization (Davidson et al., 1993c, 1994).

Lifetime comorbid disorders occurred in 69% of social phobics in the ECA study (Schneier et al., 1992). As is shown in Table 4.6, agoraphobia is the most frequent comorbid anxiety disorder of importance. Degonda & Angst (1993) found that 45% of social phobics in the community had coexisting agoraphobia. Rates for the most common disorders were 30–60% for agoraphobia, 20–35% for major depressive disorder, and 5–36% for alcohol use disorders (Schneier et al., 1992). Most comorbid disturbances have their onset after that of social phobia (mid-teens) which suggest that this disorder may be a risk factor for other disturbances.

Family and twin studies

Family studies indicate that social phobia is familial and that the disorder breeds true (Reich & Yates, 1988). In the only blind, direct-interview study, Fyer et al. (1993) found an increased prevalence of social phobia among the relatives of social phobic probands compared to relatives of never ill probands (16% vs. 5%). They did not find the prevalence of other anxiety disorders increased. In an extension of this study, Mannuzza et al. (1995) found social phobia more common among the relatives of probands with the generalized form than among relatives of probands with the non-generalized form of social phobia (16% versus 6%). These findings, together with family studies showing no increase in social phobia among relatives of simple phobics and agoraphobics, support the present classification (Noyes et al., 1986; Fyer et al., 1990); however, the familial risk is only modest, suggesting that non-familial factors are also important in the aetiology (Fyer et al., 1993).

Twin studies have consistently found greater concordance for shyness and social fears among monozygotic than dizygotic twins (Torgersen, 1979, 1983; Plomin & Daniels, 1986). These studies relied upon self-report data from non-patient subjects who may or may not have met DSM criteria. As an example, Torgersen (1979) found greater similarity with respect to fears of working, writing, trembling, or eating in front of others among monozygotic than among dizygotic twins. Similarly, Horn et al. (1976) reported greater correlations between monozygotic than dizygotic twins on ratings of sociability and social presence.

In a study of over 2000 personally interviewed female twins from a population-based registry, Kendler et al. (1992) examined the contribution of genetic and environmental factors to four types of phobias. For social phobics, the pairwise concordance was 24.4% for monozygotic and 15.3% for dizygotic twins. The best fitting etiologic model indicated that a third of the variance could be attributed to genetic factors and two-thirds to environmental influences. Kendler et al. (1992) concluded that genetic factors play a significant role in the etiology of social phobia but that, as with phobias in general, the individual-specific environment accounts for twice as much of the variance. Social phobia, according to these authors, falls midway between agoraphobia (most heritable) and simple phobias (least heritable).

Etiology and pathogenesis

Biologic factors

Neuroanatomical localization

No structural factors or regional blood flow abnormalities have been found in the brains of generalized social phobics by means of magnetic resonance imaging or spectroscopy (Potts et al., 1994; Stein et al., 1996). One study, using localized proton magnetic resonance spectroscopy, found significantly lower N-acetylaspartate ratios in cortical and subcortical regions (Davidson et al., 1993b). At present, these findings, even if replicated, are difficult to interpret.

Neuroendocrine systems

No differences in stress hormone levels have been found between social phobics and healthy controls. Urinary cortisol and post-dexamethasone blood cortisol, as well as levels of thyroid-stimulating hormone and thyroid hormones, have all been normal (Tancer et al., 1990; Potts et al., 1991; Uhde et al., 1994).

Public speaking increases plasma epinephrine levels transiently in normal persons (Dimsdale & Moss, 1980). Moreover, some social phobic symptoms are suggestive of the increased catecholamine output that often occurs in feared situations (Papp et al., 1988). As yet, few peripheral abnormalities have been found. A finding of blunted growth hormone response to clonidine challenge, which suggested a down regulation of post-synaptic alpha-2-noradrenergic receptors, could not be replicated (Tancer, 1993; Tancer et al., 1993). In social phobics, plasma norepinephrine and epinephrine levels have been in the normal range (Stein et al., 1994a), and lymphocyte beta-adrenergic receptors have not differed from normals in density or affinity (Stein et al., 1993a). Also, infusions of epinephrine have not elicited the symptoms of social phobia (Papp et al., 1988). A study that compared social phobics with normal subjects while giving a speech found no differences in heart rate, plasma epinephrine, norepinephrine, or cortisol (A. Levin, unpublished results, cited by Schneier & Liebowitz, 1990). Naftolowitz et al. (quoted by Tancer, 1993) reported similar findings. Thus, an elevation of peripheral epinephrine does not appear to account for phobic symptoms.

Neurotransmitter systems

The serotonergic system, challenged with fenfluramine, and the dopaminergic system, challenged with levodopa, have responded in social phobics as they have in normals (Tancer, 1993). There have also been no abnormalities in platelet serotonin transporter density or affinity (Stein et al., 1995).

Neuropeptide Y has anxiolytic effects when centrally administered to animals; however, plasma levels of neuropeptide Y have not been altered in generalized social phobics (Stein et al., 1996). Additionally, during caffeine challenge, three of 11 social phobics experienced panic attacks but their symptoms were unlike those that occurred naturally (Tancer, 1993). Thus, the adenosine system does not appear to play a major role in social phobia. Finally, sodium lactate, that induces attacks in a high proportion of panic disorder patients, caused a panic attack only in one of 15 patients (Liebowitz et al., 1985c).

Physiological reactivity

During mild challenges in the laboratory, such as listening to repetitive tones, patients with social phobia exhibit elevated electrodermal activity and delayed habituation compared to patients with simple phobia and normal subjects (Lader & Wing, 1964). These findings have not been replicated with patients diagnosed according to the more rigorous criteria of DSM-III or IV. Another study compared the response of volunteers who were shy and tense in social situations and control subjects to angry and happy faces. No differences between the groups were found in skin conductance or eye blink rate (Merckelbach et al., 1988). In generalized social phobics, Stein et al. (1984b) found increased blood pressure in response to the Valsalva maneuver and exaggerated vagal withdrawal in response to isometric exercise, but normal cardiovascular responses to other autonomic function tests.

During exposure to specific feared situations, social phobics showed increases in heart rate, respiration, and skin conductance (Johansson & Öst, 1982; Lande, 1982; Brady, 1984). Increased heart rate, followed by a slow return to baseline, has also been observed in social phobics during exposure and public speaking (Beidel et al., 1985; Turner et al., 1986; Heimberg & Barlow, 1988).

Social phobics rated themselves on the Pittsburgh Sleep Quality Index as having sleep disturbances. It took them longer to fall asleep and they experienced more nocturnal interruptions (Stein et al., 1993b); however, on polysomnograms no abnormalities in the sleep architecture were found (Brown et al., 1994c).

In summary, most studies indicate an absence of central or peripheral abnormalities in social phobics with the exception of an exaggerated autonomic response to feared social situations. Some of the discrepancies between studies may be explained on the basis of patient selection. Only more recent studies separated those with generalized social phobia from those with circumscribed phobias, such as fear of public speaking. The latter, when it occurs alone, is phenomenologically close to specific phobias and shows a unique pattern of heart rate acceleration during exposure to feared situations (Heimberg et al., 1990a). Thus, psychobiological differences that have not yet been explored may exist between subgroups of social phobics.

Psychological factors

Normal social anxiety and fears

As noted above, there is evidence for both genetic and environmental contributions to social phobia (reviewed by Rosenbaum et al., 1994). Shyness appears to be similar in this regard. The question is, then, what etiological factors are important and how do they interact? According to evolutionary theory, a predisposition to fears is inherited, and fears of biological value to early humans are, as a result of transmission, more readily acquired (Seligman, 1971). One such preparedness fear is that of angry or critical facial expressions (Ohman, 1986). This fear is invoked when a face is turned toward the subject and depends upon eye contact. It is a fear that contains elements of negative scrutiny and, like fears of its kind, is easily elicited but slowly extinguished.

Perhaps for evolutionary reasons we are sensitive to anger, criticism, and other forms of social disapproval. Social anxiety and fear are prevalent in the population and, at certain points in the life cycle, are especially prominent. For example, fear of strangers is an expected occurrence in infants, age 4–9 months, that gradually disappears near the end of the second year (Marks, 1987). This fear is stronger in girls than in boys, and identical twins resemble one another more than non-identical twins. Social phobia develops during another period of relatively intense social anxiety; it often begins in middle to late adolescence, a period when social embarrassment and lack of social confidence are common. Social phobia may evolve from normal anxiety that is intensified by the social expectations of that period (Amies et al., 1983).

Temperament

Recent work has focused on temperamental differences that might form the basis of vulnerability to social phobia and, perhaps, other anxiety disorders. Temperament refers to stable response dispositions that are evident early in life and that influence later personality development. One such temperamental category, known as behavioral inhibition, is characterized by a consistent tendency to display fear and to withdraw from novel or unfamiliar settings, people or objects. Kagan (1989) and colleagues have studied behavioral inhibition that occurs in about 15% of infants and children (Kagan et al., 1989). Characteristic behaviors that can be identified in the laboratory at an early age persist in school age children (Rosenbaum et al., 1994). The physiological correlates of behavioral inhibition, that reflect a low threshold for arousal and sympathetic activation, are consistent with hypothesized neurophysiological mechanisms.

A series of studies have linked this temperamental pattern to risk for anxiety disorders (Rosenbaum et al., 1991a). Rosenbaum et al. (1988) found behavioral inhibition in 70–85% of children whose parents had panic disorder but in only 15% of children whose parents had not had panic or agoraphobia (30% of these parents also had social phobia). Also, behaviorally inhibited children had increased rates of anxiety and phobic disorders compared to normal controls (Beiderman et al., 1990). When reassessed after 3 years, more anxiety disorders had emerged among the behaviorally inhibited children (Beiderman et al., 1993). Finally, when the parents of behaviorally inhibited children were examined, they were found to have higher rates of both child and adult anxiety disorders (Rosenbaum et al., 1991b). They had higher risks for social phobia and for avoidant and overanxious disorders of childhood. These results suggest that early behavioral inhibition may set the stage for the later development of social anxiety and fears. Research on the origins of shyness has reached similar conclusions concerning the role of temperament (reviewed by Bruch & Cheek, 1995).

Childhood environment

The role of early environmental factors in the development of social phobia has received little study; however, three investigations of perceived parental attitudes and rearing practices have reported consistent findings (Parker, 1979; Arrindell et al., 1983, 1989). Social phobics rated both parents as having been more rejecting and lacking in emotional warmth than did normal controls. Also, social phobics rated their parents as having been more rejecting and stricter than did agoraphobics. According to Arkin et al. (1986), such attitudes may contribute to social fear and avoidance. A child who is punished when his or her behavior does not live up to high parental standards, and who is not rewarded when it does, may acquire a fear of failure. Of course, behavioral inhibition in a child may influence early parent–child interaction; also, recall of parental behavior may be distorted by the current emotional state.

Bruch et al. (1989) reported similar findings but from a different perspective. They found social phobics more likely to recall avoidant and socially fearful behavior in their mothers. These mothers were seen as having been unsociable, socially isolated, and inclined to overvalue the opinions of others. The social phobics in this study appeared to have modeled the behavior of their parents and to have developed the disorder through vicarious learning. When Bruch et al. (1989) compared generalized and non-generalized social phobics to normal controls, they found that those with both subtypes reported greater parental concern with the opinions of others, but only those with the generalized subtype reported social isolation and a lack of family sociability (Bruch & Heimberg, 1994).

Personality

The generalized subtype of social phobia is intimately associated with avoidant personality disorder as previously described. A variety of factors may contribute to the development of avoidant traits and, in some instances, limited social skills or attractiveness may be important (Herbert et al., 1992); however, the socially inhibited behavior that is designed to protect the individual from embarrassment or disapproval, appears to defeat its purpose. Such persons appear aloof, socially awkward and uninteresting and, as a result, do not obtain the response from others that they seek. In order to avoid criticism, they may inhibit the expression of emotions, but this self-protective reticence isolates them further. In addition, avoidant persons describe a self-consciousness and preoccupation with their performance that, in social settings, diverts their attention and reduces their spontaneity.

Adverse events

The role of adverse events in the development of social phobia has scarcely been examined. Data from the ECA study show that such factors may be important. Davidson et al. (1993c) reported that maternal psychiatric disorder and separation or divorce of parents before age 10 years were more frequent in social phobics. No differences were observed between social phobics and normals with respect to paternal psychiatric illness, parental alcohol abuse, early parental death, parental poverty, or physical or sexual abuse. The finding of separation from a parent at an early age is not specific in that there are similar findings for persons with panic and agoraphobia. There is evidence that negative peer relations are associated with shyness (Bruch & Cheek, 1995). It is not clear whether the neglect, rejection and victimization contributes to or results from shyness.

Although the role of adverse events in social phobia has not received much attention, traumatic conditioning experiences appear important in the genesis of social anxiety (reviewed by Mineka & Zinbarg, 1995). Specific phobias often result from experiences involving perceived physical danger, and in similar fashion, social phobias may follow events involving perceived social danger (i.e., defeat, separation, alienation). In support of this, Öst & Hagdahl (1981) reported that 58.1% of social phobics had had traumatic experiences that contributed to the development of their disorder. Similarly, Townsley (1992) elicited traumatic conditioning experiences from 44% of social phobics compared to 20% of normal controls. This author found a higher rate of adverse experiences among discrete social phobics (56%) and a lower rate among generalized phobics (40%).

Cognitive pattern

Social phobia appears to develop in persons who respond to performance or social interactive situations with negative cognitions. These cognitions represent distortions or exaggerations of actual danger or the likelihood of negative evaluation (Beck & Emery, 1985; Stopa & Clark, 1993). Such persons have an expectation of embarrassment or humiliation, and this results in autonomic arousal. With arousal comes anxiety that may interfere with performance even to the point of completely interrupting it. The result is a vicious cycle that serves to maintain an abnormal response to social situations. Whether the cognitive pattern is a cause or a result of the pathological process has yet to be determined. This important aspect of the disorder is reviewed in detail by Stopa & Clark (1993).

Clinical picture

Clinical characteristics

Many social phobics experience difficulty in one or more circumscribed situations. Theirs is a discrete form of the disorder. They are not bothered by most social encounters, but their distress and impairment in specific situations may be great. The most common situations are speaking in public, eating in public, writing in public, and using public restrooms (Pollard & Henderson, 1988). In such settings, phobic persons fear that their behavior or some outward sign of anxiety will lead to embarrassment or humiliation. Consequently, they have a strong urge to avoid or escape from these feared situations. Some avoid getting up to speak for fear of saying something stupid or mispronouncing a word. Others are concerned that their voice might become unsteady, their hands might tremble, or their mind might go blank, causing them to forget what they had intended to say. Often, the larger the audience or the more formal the setting, the greater the fear. Many social phobics avoid public speaking; for some this is an inconvenience but for others it means failure to advance, even job loss, when this activity is an important part of employment.

Some social phobics are afraid of eating or drinking in front of others. They fear that their hands will shake as they hold their fork or cup, causing food to spill (Marks, 1987). Others feel a lump in their throat and fear choking on food thereby making a spectacle of themselves. Still others are afraid they may vomit or lose control of their bowels in response to eating. This fear tends to increase in crowded restaurants, but some are bothered by eating at home if friends are invited in, and a few are even uncomfortable eating in front of their family. As eating serves an important social function, avoidance of eating in public may restrict social life and interfere with a career, where business is transacted over meals, for example.

Persons who are afraid of writing in front of others often fear poor penmanship, misspelled words, or trembling that may cause embarrassment. According to Marks (1987), fear of trembling or shaking may cause persons to avoid handling money in front of others, avoid writing on the blackboard in front of the class, or putting together packages on an assembly line. Those who fear using public restrooms are afraid they will be unable to urinate, leading not only to physical distress but to embarrassment. Their difficulty, which is greatest in crowded restrooms, may extend to private ones as well. Such fears may lead to travel restrictions and medical complications (Brandt et al., 1994).

Persons with generalized social phobia are bothered by many or most social situations, especially those involving social interaction (Amies et al., 1983). In conversation with others, these persons may fear saying something embarrassing or not knowing what to say. Some are comfortable with persons they know well but are distressed by, and avoid, small and large social gatherings. Others are bothered by interaction with persons in authority, persons of the opposite sex, or persons who are assertive or opinionated (Liebowitz et al., 1985b). Still others are bothered by situations in which they might be an object of scrutiny, such as walking in front of others, dancing, or entering a room in which others are already seated. In such settings social phobics often fear awkward or uncontrolled movements.

In phobic situations, or in anticipation of them, social phobics experience anxiety together with autonomic symptoms (Rapee, 1995). This

anxiety is often marked and, in some individuals, reaches panic proportions. Often it interferes with or even disrupts their behavior. In feared
situations patients, often find that their concentration is impaired and that
they are unable to think. Their movements may become awkward or jerky,
or they may temporarily find themselves frozen or unable to move. Typical
somatic symptoms include palpitations, sweating, trembling and blushing
(Amies et al., 1983; Solyom et al., 1986). Commonly one or more of these
symptoms becomes the focus of fearful preoccupation. For many social
phobics, they are the dreaded outward signs of anxiety (e.g., blushing) that
others might see. Consequently, in phobic situations, the patient's attention becomes narrowly focused upon physiological activation; symptoms
then become warning signals of impending danger, thus generating more
anxiety. Patients describe a vicious cycle in which perceived threat leads to
anxiety, and anxiety increases the perception of threat.

Cognitively, generalized social phobics are fearful of criticism or disapproval, have low self-esteem, and evaluate themselves negatively (Nichols,
1974). They are often preoccupied with potential criticism or feelings of
inadequacy, and view themselves as socially inept or inferior to others, all
avoidant personality characteristics (Table 4.2). False beliefs, according to
Beck & Emery (1985), lead socially phobic individuals to respond to social
stimuli in a maladaptive fashion. These include the idea that others hold a
low opinion of them, that approval is essential to their well-being, that
appearing anxious is shameful, and that performance is the basis of self-
esteem. Phobic persons become preoccupied with misperceived threats and
this draws attention away from persons with whom they are interacting.
Some show a more damaging pattern of social inhibition and unwillingness
to become involved in relationships based on such beliefs.

The behavior of social phobics is characterized by poor performance and
avoidance of phobic situations. Their performance in social settings is
impaired, although usually not to the degree that they think. Some appear
to lack social skills, and this lack may contribute to their anxiety. Others
have anxiety that interferes with otherwise adequate skills. These patients,
once treated, interact normally in the absence of interfering anxiety. Regardless of its source, phobic avoidance may be limited or extensive,
leading to restrictions in dating, educational attainment, marriage, and
career achievement (Schneier et al., 1994). Some social phobics avoid social
situations while others are inhibited within them; they enter social situations but leave quickly, avoid eye contact, limit interaction, or otherwise
disengage themselves from their social surroundings.

Subtypes

A generalized subtype was introduced in DSM-III-R for individuals with fears of all or most social situations. This is distinguished from more discrete or circumscribed phobias of public speaking, eating in public, etc. (Mannuzza et al., 1995). Studies have shown that persons with both sub-types experience social anxiety and fear negative evaluation, but that generalized social phobics have a more severe disorder (Heimberg et al., 1990a; Gelernter et al., 1992; Levin et al., 1993;). Also, their phobias are more severe and they perform less well in social situations. They tend to be younger, to have less education, and are less likely to be employed. In contrast, discrete social phobics are distinguished by marked autonomic reactivity in phobic situations. Speaking phobics, for example, may experience a 20 beat-per-minute increase in heart rate in response to behavioral challenge (Heimberg et al., 1990a).

Paruresis is a disturbance characterized by an inability to urinate in public places (Williams & Degenhardt, 1952). This difficulty is increased by lack of privacy, presence of strangers, and close proximity of others which evokes self-consciousness and anxiety along with autonomic arousal. Sympathetic activation increases contraction of the internal and external urethral sphincters that must be relaxed for urination. The disorder is associated with a low pressure/low flow voiding pattern (Barnes et al., 1985). Estimates of prevalence among college students range from 7% to 32% in men and from 14% to 20% in women. Behavior therapy techniques have shown promise but pharmacotherapy has been discouraging (Zgourides, 1987; Hatterer et al., 1990).

Pattern of morbidity

As social phobia typically begins in the teen years, it may adversely influence psychological development, including the formation of intimate relationships and the attainment of educational and career goals. Its impact is evident from epidemiological studies (Schneier et al., 1992; Davidson et al., 1993c, 1994). Compared to persons without the disorder, social phobics in the community have worse school performance and complete fewer years of education (Last & Strauss, 1990). Also, they more often have poor grades, have to repeat years, and are expelled from school. Fewer than half completed high school (Davidson et al., 1994). Social phobics more often see themselves as lacking social support and as having few close friends. Also, fewer than half marry (Davidson et al., 1994).

Impairment also extends to employment and economic status (Schneier et al., 1994). Social phobics are more often absent from work, had more often been terminated, and are less often employed. They are also more often financially dependent; 22% were receiving welfare assistance or disability compensation (Schneier et al., 1992). In addition, these persons have more chronic medical problems, more sick days, more medical and mental health visits, and more use of psychotropic drugs (Davidson et al., 1994). Comorbid disorders contributed to this morbidity, but the impairment seen in subthreshold cases is comparable to that for social phobics meeting criteria.

Secondary social phobia

Social phobia may develop in association with other mental and physical disorders. In such instances, symptoms begin after the onset of the primary disorder and fear of embarrassment is focused upon one or more manifestations of that disorder. An example is social phobia secondary to panic disorder with or without agoraphobia (Liebowitz et al., 1985c). Although many patients with panic disorder are embarrassed by their disorder, a few fear embarrassment related to having panic attacks in public. Fear and avoidance of situations where panic attacks might be witnessed – secondary social phobia – may contribute to the disability.

Secondary social phobia may occur with almost any mental disorder, especially those with visible manifestations that might lead to embarrassment, such as obsessive-compulsive disorder or anorexia nervosa. In these instances, fear of embarrassment might be related to rituals or eating behaviors. Also, depression may be a cause of secondary social phobia. In one study, a substantial minority of patients with major depression had social phobic symptoms (Dilsaver et al., 1992). These symptoms coincided with or began after the onset of depressive symptoms and resolved with successful treatment. Fear of embarrassment was related to the manifestations (e.g., social withdrawal, impaired concentration) of depression and contributed to impairment caused by the mood disorder.

Social phobia may develop in response to physical illness as well. Data from the ECA study showed a relationship between neurological disorders (e.g., Parkinson's disease, epilepsy) and social phobia (Davidson et al., 1993c). This is consistent with an association between social phobia and Parkinson's disease in clinical samples (Stein et al., 1990a). In this instance, Stein et al. (1990a) found social phobia in 17% of patients with Parkinson's disease and social phobic symptoms in an additional 13%. Social phobia

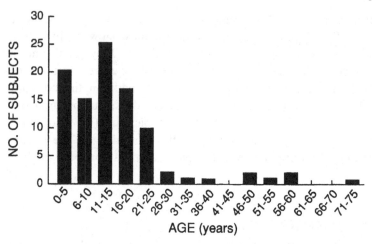

Figure 4.1 Age at onset of social phobia in subjects without agoraphobia or simple phobia (*n* = 106). From Schneier et al. (1992). © 1992, American Medical Association. Reprinted with permission.

arising from disfiguring or disabling physical conditions, such as stuttering, spasmodic torticollis, etc. was described in a series of cases by Oberlander et al. (1994). These patients had typical social phobic symptoms except that the focus of their attention was an aspect of their condition and the onset followed that of the disability.

Natural history

Onset

Social phobia typically has its onset in the mid to late teens (Marks & Gelder, 1966; Thyer et al., 1985; Mannuzza et al., 1990; Schneier et al., 1992). Figure 4.1 shows an age of onset distribution from the ECA study in which the mean was 15.5 years. Social phobia occurs in children and, in this age group, increases in frequency with age (Francis et al., 1992; Rey et al., 1992). The onset tends to be gradual, occurring over months or years (Marks, 1987). Usually there is no precipitant, although on occasion an embarrassing incident will serve as a trigger (e.g., vomiting in front of others). In some cases, social sensitivity that existed from early childhood increases to a point of full-blown disorder after puberty. Social phobics who seek treatment often delay the initial contact for many years (Marks & Gelder, 1966; Amies et al., 1983). Some seek help when personal aspirations are challenged, while others obtain treatment for comorbid conditions, such as major depression or alcohol dependence (Degonda & Angst, 1993).

Course and outcome

Social phobia appears to follow a chronic, unremitting course; however, the data with respect to natural history are quite limited (Liebowitz et al., 1985b; Solyom et al., 1986). Studies of social phobics in the community have found considerable chronicity. For example, Degonda & Angst (1993) observed that, after 10 years, 41% still reported significant fear and avoidance and, for the group as a whole, interpersonal sensitivity had even increased. Social phobics in the ECA study had a mean 19.4 years of illness (Davidson et al., 1993a). Of these, only 27% had recovered, meaning that their symptoms had remitted for at least 6 months and that, at the time of interview, they fell below the diagnostic threshold.

Data from a 5-year follow-up of social phobics who had been treated in anxiety clinics showed that the great majority remained significantly impaired despite treatment (Reich et al., 1994). Only 11% had achieved complete, and 25% partial, remissions over that interval. Follow-ups of pharmacologically and behaviorally treated social phobics have indicated that, despite improvement, symptoms tend to persist and, in some instances, require additional treatment (Tyrer & Steinberg, 1975; Versiani et al., 1988; Wlazlo et al., 1990; Mersch et al., 1991; Sutherland et al., 1994; Noyes & Holt, 1996). Heimberg et al. (1993) found that, with newer psychological techniques, the outcome of treated patients may be better. They found that after 5 years social phobics who had received cognitive-behavioral group therapy were doing better than those who had received educational-supportive group therapy. The average cognitive-behavioral patient was barely symptomatic, while the average educational-supportive patient showed a need for further treatment.

Predictors of outcome

Davidson et al. (1993a) subjected likely variables to a logistic regression analysis and identified three predictors of recovery in a community sample, these being later age of onset, higher level of education, and absence of psychiatric comorbidity. Similarly, Van Ameringen et al. (1991) found that onset before age 15 years and duration of more than 15 years defined a more severe disorder. In a clinical population, Reich et al. (1994) were unable to find any demographic or illness variables that predicted outcome after 5 years; however, their patients were a heterogeneous group and included those who met criteria for social phobia regardless of the primary diagnosis. In a treatment study, favorable outcome was predicted by a lower initial Liebowitz Social Anxiety Scale score (Sutherland et al., 1994).

Complications

Alcohol and drug dependence

Alcohol dependence may develop as a complication of social phobia (Kushner et al., 1990; Heckelman & Schneier, 1995). Early observations of an association between this disorder and alcoholism have been confirmed in subsequent clinical and community studies (Mullaney & Trippett, 1979; Smail et al., 1984). In the ECA study, 18% of social phobics had abused alcohol, their risk being roughly double that of persons without social phobia (Schneier et al., 1992). Treated populations have yielded similar findings. Schneier et al. (1989), for example, found that 16% of social phobics had a history of alcoholism. In addition, drug abuse has been found in 13% of social phobics from the community but has not been common in clinical populations (Amies et al., 1983; Schneier et al., 1992).

Among social phobics, alcohol dependence often occurs as a direct complication of the disorder (Kushner et al., 1990). This conclusion is supported by studies reporting high rates of self-medication with alcohol and an onset of alcoholism after that of social phobia (Stravynski et al., 1986; Turner et al., 1986; Chambless et al., 1987; Schneier et al., 1989). Many authors, beginning with Quitkin et al. (1972), have emphasized the importance of treating anxiety disorders in order to prevent relapse of alcohol or drug dependence. In this instance, social phobia may interfere with alcohol rehabilitation, an intervention that relies upon group participation and public speaking. On the other hand, social phobic symptoms may develop as a consequence of alcoholism and disappear with cessation of drinking (Heckelman & Schneier, 1995). In either case, social phobia tends to be more severe in patients with coexisting alcoholism, and alcoholism is more severe with comorbid anxiety disorders (Ross et al., 1988; Schneier et al., 1989).

Major depressive disorder

Several studies have indicated that major depressive disorder is an important complication of social phobia. Rates of depression have ranged from

35% to 50%, somewhat lower than those reported for panic disorder and agoraphobia (Sanderson et al., 1990; Stein et al., 1990b; Van Ameringen et al., 1991). The observation that social phobia begins before major depressive disorder in most cases suggests that it is the cause of subsequent depression, but a common predisposing factor remains a possibility (Schneier et al., 1992). Several studies have shown that, when social phobia and panic disorder or agoraphobia coexist, the likelihood of major depressive disorder becomes especially high (Stein et al., 1990b; Reiter et al., 1991; Noyes et al., 1992). Patients with this combination of disorders may have a constellation of features (e.g., dysfunctional attitudes, lack of assertiveness) that makes them especially susceptible to depression.

Suicide

Clinical and epidemiological studies have found increases in suicide attempts among social phobics ranging from 12% to 20% lifetime (Amies et al., 1983; Schneier et al., 1992; Cox et al., 1994). Comorbidity accounts for most, but not all, of the increase compared to persons without social phobia (Schneier et al., 1992). Specifically, social phobics who had attempted suicide reported more past treatment for depression than those who had not (Cox et al., 1994). Suicidal ideation is also frequent in association with comorbid depression. Thiry-four per cent of a treated sample reported suicidal ideation in the past year and, in a community sample, those with depression more frequently thought about death or wanted to die. Thus, social phobia is associated with suicidal ideation and attempts, often in association with depression.

Differential diagnosis

Agoraphobia

Agoraphobia is a syndrome of multiple fears, some of which involve social situations such as crowded stores, restaurants, etc. Other agoraphobic fears such as travel, bridges, tunnels, etc. may or may not involve public scrutiny (American Psychiatric Association, 1994). Social phobics more often have fears of interacting with persons in authority or those of the opposite sex. They more often report fears of being watched, criticized or teased, or of speaking, eating, writing, etc. in front of other people (Amies et al., 1983). Also, agoraphobics are bothered by confinement and fear of being unable to get to safety in case of a panic attack, whereas social phobics are bothered by the scrutiny of others and embarrassment resulting therefrom. Agoraphobics are often comforted by the presence of a safe person and, in their company, can enter phobic situations. Social phobics are more comfortable when alone.

Patients with panic disorder experience panic attacks as do some patients with social phobia; however, panic patients often have spontaneous or unprovoked attacks while social phobics do not. Also, the occurrence of panic is unpredictable even among agoraphobics. The situation that provokes an attack one time may not do so the next. Social phobics have a more predictable phobic response, which may include panic in comparable situations. Social phobics more often focus upon symptoms that they feel invite the scrutiny of others (e.g., blushing, sweating, trembling); panic and agoraphobic patients more often report cardiovascular symptoms (i.e., shortness of breath, chest pain, dizziness) (Amies et al., 1983).

Of course, social phobia and agoraphobia often coexist and, when a patient qualifies, both diagnoses should be made. In a few instances, social phobia develops in response to panic disorder. It is common for panic patients to be concerned about embarrassment should their panic attacks be witnessed. When fear of embarrassment leads to avoidance of social situations and impairment beyond that expected of panic disorder alone, then a secondary diagnosis of social phobia should be considered. In such instances, the onset of social phobia follows the development of spontaneous panic attacks; otherwise, social phobia usually has an earlier onset (Mannuzza et al., 1990).

Avoidant and schizoid personality disorder

The distinction between social phobia and avoidant personality disorder is difficult, because as presently defined, there is extensive overlap of characteristic features. Personality disorders are recognized as long-standing, pervasive patterns of maladaptive behavior; the behavior in this case is social avoidance. Most patients with the generalized subtype of social phobia also qualify for avoidant personality disorder and should receive both diagnoses (American Psychiatric Association, 1994). Persons with avoidant personality disorder may have less interest in social interaction, but when social isolation is accompanied by anhedonia, then schizoid personality disorder may be present. Some have suggested that persons with avoidant personality have fewer social skills and less anxiety in social situations than typical social phobics.

Individuals with personality disorders belonging to the schizoid cluster (i.e., schizoid, paranoid, schizotypal) and persons with pervasive developmental disorder avoid social situations but do so because of a lack of interest in them. In the case of persons with paranoid personality disorder, this avoidance is prompted by a belief that the motives of others are not well intentioned. Social phobics have a capacity for and interest in social contact and suffer loneliness related to its avoidance; schizoid individuals, by contrast, prefer to be alone. DSM-IV, in fact, specifies that children who qualify for the diagnosis of social phobia must have at least one age-appropriate, social relationship outside the immediate family (American Psychiatric Association, 1994).

Performance anxiety

Fear of social situations, especially public speaking, is extremely prevalent in the general population. Persons with performance anxiety or stage fright should not be given a diagnosis of social phobia unless their anxiety leads to significant distress or causes definite impairment (American Psychiatric Association, 1994). This determination is difficult in cases where avoidance, of for example public speaking, does not interfere because a person's job does not require it. Just the same, one should probably be considered phobic if he or she is unable to engage in activities that are important and expected of most people, such as public speaking, eating in public, etc.

Secondary social phobia

Social anxiety and avoidance are associated features of many mental disorders, for example schizophrenia and major depressive disorder. According to DSM-IV, if these symptoms occur only during the course of another mental disorder and are better explained by that disorder, then an additional diagnosis of social phobia should not be made (American Psychiatric Association, 1994). If, on the other hand, social anxiety and avoidance are not explained by the underlying disorder and make a significant contribution to impairment, then a secondary diagnosis may be warranted. This is a departure from DSM-IV which, in these instances, calls for a diagnosis of social phobia, not otherwise specified. Similarly, physical conditions may be associated with increased social anxiety and avoidant behavior (e.g., essential tremor, stuttering, Parkinson's disease). Here again, if the social anxiety is excessive and represents a major source of impairment, a secondary diagnosis (i.e., social phobia) may be warranted.

Body dysmorphic disorder

Body dysmorphic disorder, or dysmorphophobia, is a disturbance characterized by preoccupation with a defect in appearance that is imagined or exaggerated. Persons with this disorder often avoid social situations fearing that others will react negatively to their appearance. Unlike social phobics, who recognize that their fear is excessive, persons with body dysmorphic disorder are convinced about what distresses them and are little comforted by being alone. In contrast, the social phobic is embarrassed by outward manifestations of anxiety that they believe others may see.

Treatment

Management

Effective pharmacological and psychological treatments of social phobia are available. At present, phenelzine is the pharmacological treatment of choice, and cognitive-behavioral group treatment is the psychological treatment of choice for the generalized subtype (Juster et al., 1994; Heimberg & Juster, 1995; Potts & Davidson, 1995). These treatments appear to be about equally effective and, when combined, may work better than either treatment alone. Evidence favoring such combined treatment is presently lacking so that clinical judgment, treatment availability, and patient preference must be considered. Medication may, by reducing anxiety, improve patient adherence to psychological treatment; psychological treatment may, on the other hand, improve the stability of treatment gains over the long run.

Treatment must take the individual characteristics of the social phobic and available treatment resources into account. Discrete phobics (e.g., public speaking, musical performing) who encounter phobic situations only occasionally may benefit from single doses of a beta-blocking drug (e.g., propranolol 40 mg) or a benzodiazepine (e.g., alprazolam 0.5 mg) taken an hour or more before their performance. They should then be encouraged to expose themselves to public speaking (e.g., toastmasters club) or performance situations and, as their comfort increases, to phase out medication (Agras, 1990). Discrete social phobics also respond to exposure-based therapy.

Generalized social phobics or those with avoidant personality traits are more apt to benefit from medication taken on a regular basis. While phenelzine has established efficacy, the dietary restrictions (i.e., tyramine-free diet) and the risk of hypertensive crises are difficult for some patients to tolerate. Tricyclic antidepressants appear to lack efficacy and benzodiazepines have dependence potential (Liebowitz et al., 1985b). Patients who take benzodiazepines before social encounters to increase their comfort may develop psychological dependence. The daily dose of phenelzine is similar to that used for depression but the dose of serotonin reuptake inhibitors may be higher than that for depression (e.g., fluoxetine 40–80 mg). The latter are well tolerated but often associated with sexual dysfunction.

Cognitive-behavioral therapy should be started at the same time medication is begun. Conducting this treatment in groups appears to be ideal because the group provides controlled exposure to a social situation in which feared activities can be rehearsed (e.g., conversation with someone of the opposite sex) and negative cognitions examined. This therapy combines exposure and cognitive restructuring, techniques that interact to give a superior result. Because of the unpredictable nature of social interactions, graded exposure (i.e., gradually increasing intensity) may be difficult to arrange, and patients may avoid cues in social situations. Consequently, patient effort and therapist guidance are especially important in this treatment endeavor.

Pharmacological treatment

Beta-blocking drugs

The sympathetic activation that occurs in performance and competitive situations is mediated by beta-adrenergic receptors, and their peripheral manifestations (e.g., dry mouth, palpitations, sweating, blushing, tremor) may be reversed by beta-blocking drugs. For example, the cardiovascular reaction to public speaking, including tachycardia and increased systolic blood pressure, may be blocked by these agents (Taggart et al., 1973). On account of this, beta-adrenergic antagonists have been tried in situations where excessive physiological arousal might have a detrimental effect on performance (Liebowitz et al., 1985b). Most studies compared the effect of single doses of drug or placebo on ratings of subjective distress and objective performance. Some found drug superior to placebo but others did not. In several studies, musicians reported feeling less anxious while performing on a beta-blocking drug (Noyes, 1988). Performance on stringed instruments, as assessed by blind raters, was superior on drug in some studies but this advantage tended to disappear after the first session.

The widespread use of beta-blocking drugs among professional musicians suggests efficacy. In one survey 27% of musicians reported occasional use (Fishbein et al., 1988).

Trials of beta-blocking drugs in social phobics have been disappointing. Falloon et al. (1981) found propranolol no better than placebo in a small number of social phobics who were also receiving social skills training. Although an open trial with atenolol was promising, the drug failed to show superiority in a placebo-controlled trial (Liebowitz et al., 1992). Nevertheless, social phobics of the discrete subtype (e.g., speaking or performing in public) may benefit from 20–80 mg propranolol taken an hour before speaking or performing. A fall in resting heart rate is an indicator of peripheral beta-blockade that correlates with relief of anxiety.

Benzodiazepines and azapirones

Open trials with high-potency benzodiazepines – alprazolam and clona-zepam – in social phobic patients were promising and led to controlled trials. The first of these, by Gelernter et al. (1991), showed alprazolam (mean 4.2 mg daily) to be more effective than placebo. Alprazolam was as beneficial as cognitive-behavioral therapy but less effective than phenelzine; however, when the drugs were discontinued, most patients on alprazolam relapsed whereas those on phenelzine maintained their improvement.

Convincing evidence for the efficacy of clonazepam came from a pla-cebo-controlled trial by Davidson et al. (1993c). In this study, 75 social phobics received clonazepam (mean 2.4 mg daily) or placebo. Response rates were 78% for clonazepam and 20% for placebo. Statistically signifi-cant effects were found as early as the first week on a global improvement measure and the second week using the Brief Social Phobia Scale (Figures 4.2 and 4.3). As a group, patients on clonazepam were improved to the point that their mean social phobia score was close to that for the normal population. Clonazepam was said to be well tolerated, the most frequent side-effects being unsteadiness 30%, dizziness 29%, lack of orgasm 23%, bad taste 14%, and blurred vision 12%. When clonazepam was rapidly tapered (over 2 weeks) and discontinued, 74% of subjects relapsed.

Open trials of buspirone, an azapirone, show that this drug has modest efficacy in social phobia (Munjack et al., 1991; Schneier et al., 1993). Munjack et al. (1991) reported that nine of 17 patients experienced at least moderate improvement after 8 weeks, and Schneier et al. (1993) found eight of 17 patients much improved after 12 weeks on a mean of 46 mg daily. A higher proportion of patients able to tolerate 45 mg or more daily (67%) were much improved.

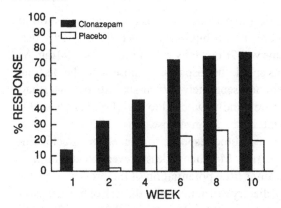

Figure 4.2 Response rates in patients with social phobia: Clonazepam versus placebo. From Davidson et al. (1994).* © 1994, Physicians Postgraduate Press. Reprinted with permission.
*Last observations were carried forward. All comparisons were statistically significant at $p < 0.02$.

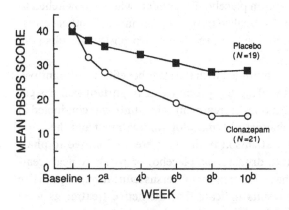

Figure 4.3 Efficacy of clonazepam: Davidson Brief Social Phobia Scale (DBSPS). [a]$p < 0.02$; [b]$p < 0.01$. (From Davidson et al. (1994). © 1994, Physicians Postgraduate Press. Reprinted with permission.

Monoamine oxidase inhibitors

Studies in which phenelzine, a monoamine oxidase inhibitor, proved beneficial for mixed phobic and atypical depressives led to its trial in social phobia (Liebowitz et al., 1988). Three controlled studies have shown phenelzine to be superior to placebo (Gelernter et al., 1991; Liebowitz et al., 1992; Versiani et al., 1992). In one of these, the overall response rate (among those who completed the trial) was 64% for patients receiving phenelzine compared to 23% for those on placebo. As a group, patients showed substantial reductions not only in fear but in avoidance of social activities. The mean dose of phenelzine was 76 mg daily with a range of 45–90 mg. As the number of subjects was small, the response of those with the discrete subtype could not be examined separately. When six patients, who had responded to phenelzine, were blindly switched to placebo after 16 weeks, two relapsed but four maintained their response.

Versiani et al. (1992) compared the response to phenelzine, moclobemide, and placebo in a 16 week trial. Moclobemide is a reversible inhibitor of monoamine oxidase that causes little potentiation of the presser response to tyramine. Consequently, dietary restrictions and the risk of hypertensive crises are less than with phenelzine or tranylcypromine. After 8 weeks, both active drugs were more effective than placebo, and patients on phenelzine were somewhat better than those receiving moclobemide. By 16 weeks further improvement had occurred in the moclobemide group, and by that time, 73% of subjects on phenelzine and 54% on moclobemide were much improved compared to 12% on placebo. Responders who were switched to placebo tended to relapse. Controlled trials of brofaromine, another reversible monoamine oxidase inhibitor, have also shown positive results (van Vliet et al., 1992).

These favorable results, combined with the clear benefits from cognitive-behavioral treatment of social phobia, prompted an important well-designed study comparing these modes of treatment. This study was conducted in two sites, one which emphasizes pharmacological treatment and the other psychological treatment. Patients at both sites were randomized to pharmacological treatment (i.e., drug versus placebo) or psychological treatment (i.e., cognitive behavioral treatment versus education, supportive treatment). Preliminary results indicate that the active treatments were about equally effective with a slight edge going to phenelzine on some measures (M. R. Liebowitz, personal communication).

Serotonin reuptake inhibitors

Open trials indicate that the serotonin reuptake inhibitors, fluoxetine and sertraline, may be useful for social phobia (Van Ameringen et al., 1993, 1994). Ten of 16 patients treated with fluoxetine (mean 54 mg daily) responded to the drug (Van Ameringen et al., 1993). Similarly, 16 of 22 social phobics given sertraline (mean 148 mg daily) responded. The most common adverse effects were gastrointestinal distress followed by increased nervousness and insomnia. In a controlled trial, van Vliet et al. (1994) found fluvoxamine, in a daily dose of 150 mg, superior to placebo. Given the opportunity to continue medication after the trial, 14 of 16 elected to do so.

Psychological treatment

A number of psychological treatments have been employed for social phobia, and some have proven more effective than others. The literature is growing rapidly in this area, and a number of reviews are available (Heimberg, 1993; Donohue et al., 1994; Heimberg & Juster, 1995; Juster et al. in press). Although many important questions remain and more research needs to be done, cognitive-behavioral group treatment has emerged as the treatment of choice (Heimberg & Juster, 1994); however, other approaches have application and should be considered in overall treatment planning.

Social skills training

Some social phobics have adequate skills for interacting but anxiety interferes. Others lack skills and become anxious in situations where their awkwardness is exposed (Stravynski et al., 1982). To correct such deficits, social skills training was developed. Such training takes an educational approach. Targeted behaviors (e.g., conversing with others) are introduced, modeled by the therapist, then rehearsed by the patient. The therapist provides feedback and reinforcement, and the patient practices until he or she becomes skillful. Although a number of studies suggest benefit, they have mostly lacked controlled comparisons (Wlazlo et al., 1990; Donohue et al., 1994). Also, attempts to show that skills training preferentially helped those with skills deficits have only been partly successful (Trower et al., 1978; Öst et al., 1981).

Exposure in vivo

Freud observed that therapy for phobias makes little progress until the patient exposes him or herself to phobic situations. Exposure is now a well-established treatment for phobic disorders. It involves making a list of feared situations and establishing a hierarchy of the most feared to the least. Then, under the support and guidance of the therapist, a patient exposes himself to the least feared situation until he becomes comfortable before moving to the next. The patient is encouraged to remain in each situation until his or her anxiety declines, and in so doing, he or she learns to confront the situation without discomfort. In this way, negative reinforcement that maintains the disorder (i.e., relief of anxiety on leaving situations) is removed and anxiety extinguished. Application of this technique to social phobia has been recent, but a series of studies have shown exposure to be superior to relaxation training or information plus self-exposure instructions (Heimberg & Barlow, 1991; Hope et al., 1993).

Butler et al. (1984) compared exposure alone, exposure plus anxiety management (i.e., relaxation training, distraction techniques, rational self-talk), and wait-list condition in social phobics. Patients met with a therapist weekly for 7 weeks after which both exposure groups were significantly improved. After 6 months, the exposure plus anxiety management patients were doing better than those who had received exposure alone, which suggests that exposure by itself might not be the most effective approach. In doing this research, Butler (1985) observed several difficulties in carrying out exposure in social phobics. She noted that, because social situations are variable and unpredictable, it may be hard to arrange repetition of situations that have gradually increasing difficulty. In addition, she observed that many social encounters are brief and do not allow the required length of exposure. Finally, socially phobic individuals are preoccupied with the presumed negative evaluation of others but receive little feedback with which to correct misperceptions (Hope et al., 1990).

Exposure plus cognitive restructuring

Treatments designed to modify maladaptive cognitions were shown to have a beneficial effect in social phobics, and this led to trials in which exposure and cognitive restructuring were combined (Emmelkamp et al., 1985; Mattick et al., 1989). Mattick & Peters (1988) compared exposure to exposure plus cognitive restructuring which they integrated with exposure procedures. Although patients who received exposure improved, those receiving the combined treatment did better. At follow-up, only 14% of patients who received the combined treatment reported avoidance of the target phobia, compared to 48% of the exposure only patients. In a second study, Mattick et al. (1989) again showed the advantage of combining exposure and cognitive restructuring over either treatment alone. Patients who received the combination showed significant reductions not only in phobic avoidance but also in negative self-evaluation and maladaptive beliefs.

Heimberg et al. (1985, 1990b) developed a cognitive-behavioral group treatment. In groups, patients receive exposure to social situations in a controlled manner. Their cognitive-behavioral group treatment is administered in 12 weekly, two-and-a-half hour sessions in groups of six (Heimberg & Juster, 1994; Heimberg et al., 1995). In the course of the treatment patients are taught the cognitive-behavioral model and shown how cognitive restructuring is achieved. They learn how to identify negative cognitions, how to challenge the logic behind these cognitions, and how to replace them with rational alternatives. Patients then confront feared situations, first as they are simulated in the group and then as homework assignments. While completing behavioral tasks (e.g., conversing with someone, giving a talk), patients are asked to monitor their anxiety and cognitions. At the same time they are encouraged to practice remaining in feared situations and using newly-formulated positive cognitions. Detailed descriptions of this technique are available (Bulter & Wells, 1995).

The results of cognitive-behavioral group treatment have been quite favorable (Heimberg & Juster, 1994). For example, in a study comparing this treatment with group therapy that provided only education and support, 75% of the cognitive-behaviorally treated patients were clinically improved compared to 40% of patients receiving the control treatment. At 5 year follow-up, similar proportions of patients continued to show improvement and, on average, the cognitive-behaviorally treated patients showed few remaining symptoms while the control group treated patients were rated as requiring further treatment. Thus, exposure appears to be most effective when combined with cognitive restructuring, as in this group treatment (Donohue et al., 1994; Heimberg & Juster, 1994).

Pharmacological versus psychological and combined treatments

Several studies have compared the efficacy of pharmacological and cognitive-behavioral interventions or a combination of the two (Falloon et al., 1981; Clark & Agras, 1991; Gelernter et al., 1991; Turner et al., 1994; M. R. Liebowitz et al., personal communication). In reviewing four of these, Heimberg (1993) noted that little could be concluded except that cognitive-behavioral treatment appears to be as effective as pharmacological therapy. With two exceptions, these studies used drugs (i.e., propranolol, atenolol and buspirone) that were less effective than phenelzine. The two studies that examined combined psychological and pharmacological interventions did not show added effectiveness (Falloon et al., 1981; Clark & Agras, 1991). Here too, both employed relatively ineffective drugs and treated small samples.

The most recent study comparing phenelzine, placebo, cognitive-behavioral treatment, and psychological placebo therapy (i.e., education and group support) is nearing completion. As previously described this large study was conducted in two sites known for their expertise and research in pharmacological and psychological therapies. Over 130 patients were enrolled in this study which lasted 12 weeks. Patients who responded to acute treatment were followed for 6 months on maintenance treatment, then for 6 months maintenance free (i.e., no treatment). Preliminary results indicate that the active treatments were about equally effective at the end of the acute phase.

Enormous progress has been made in the diagnosis and treatment of social phobia since its first appearance in the official classification less than two decades ago. The development of effective treatment for such a widespread and disabling condition is a great triumph.

References

Agras, W. S. 1990. Treatment of social phobias. *J. Clin. Psychiatry* 51 (Suppl. 10): 52–55.

American Psychiatric Association. 1980. *Diagnostic and Statistical Manual of Mental Disorders*, Third Edition, American Psychiatric Association, Washington, DC.

American Psychiatric Association. 1987. *Diagnostic and Statistical Manual of Mental Disorders*, Third Edition, Revised, American Psychiatric Association, Washington, DC.

American Psychiatric Association. 1994. *Diagnostic and Statistical Manual of Mental Disorders*, Fourth Edition, American Psychiatric Association, Washington, DC.

Amies, P. L., Gelder, M. G. & Shaw, P. M. 1983. Social phobia: A comparative clinical study. *Br. J. Psychiatry* 142: 174–179.

Anderson, J. C., Williams, S., McGee, R. et al. 1987. DSM–III disorders in preadolescent children. *Arch. Gen. Psychiatry* 44: 69–76.

Arkin, R. M., Lake, E. A. & Baumgardner, A. H. 1986. Shyness and self-presentation. In *Shyness: Perspectives on Research and Treatment*, eds. W. H. Jones, J. M. Cheek, S. R. Briggs, Plenum Press, New York.

Arrindell, W. A., Emmelkamp, P. M. G., Monsma, A. et al. 1983. The role of perceived parental rearing practices in the aetiology of phobic disorders: A controlled study. *Br. J. Psychiatry* 143: 183–187.

Arrindell, W. A., Kwee, M. G. T., Methorst, G. J. et al. 1989. Perceived parental rearing styles of agoraphobic and socially phobic inpatients. *Br. J. Psychiatry* 155: 526–535.

Barnes, J. C., Harrison, G. & Murray, K. 1985. Low pressure/low flow voiding in younger men: Psychological aspects. *Br. J. Urology* 57: 414–417.

Beard, G. M. 1879. Morbid fear as a symptom of nervous disease. *Hos. Gaz.* 6: 305–308.

Beck, A. T. & Emery, G. 1985. *Anxiety Disorders and Phobias: A Cognitive Perspective*. Basic Books, New York.

Beidel, D. C., Turner, S. M. & Cooley, M. R. 1993. Assessing reliable and clinically significant change in social phobia: Validity of the Social Phobia and Anxiety Inventory. *Behav. Assess.* 8: 331–337.

Beidel, D. C., Turner, S. M. & Dancu, C. V. 1985. Physiological, cognitive, and behavioral aspects of social anxiety. *Behav. Res. Ther.* 23: 109–117.

Beidel, D. C., Turner, S. M. & Morris, T. L. 1995. A new inventory to assess childhood social anxiety and phobia: The Social Phobia and Anxiety Inventory for Children. *Psychol. Assess.* 7: 73–79.

Biederman, J., Rosenbaum, J. F., Bolduc-Murphy, E. A. et al. 1993. A 3-year follow-up of children with and without behavioral inhibition. *J. Am. Acad. Child Adolesc. Psychiatry* 32: 814–821.

Biederman, J., Rosenbaum, J. F., Hirshfeld, D. R. et al. 1990. Psychiatric correlates of behavioral inhibition in young children of parents with and without psychiatric disorders. *Arch. Gen. Psychiatry* 47: 21–26.

Bourdon, K. H., Boyd, J. H., Rae, D. S. et al. 1988. Gender differences in phobias: Results of the ECA community survey. *J. Anx. Disorders* 2: 227–241.

Brady, J. P. 1984. Social skill training for psychiatric patients. I. Concepts, methods and clinical results. *Am. J. Psychiatry* 141: 333–340.

Brandt, G. T., Norwood, A. E. & Ursano, R. J. 1994. Urosepsis: An unusual presentation of social phobia. *Am. J. Psychiatry* 151: 1520.

Brown, E. J., Heimberg, R. G. & Juster, H. R. 1995. Social phobia subtype and avoidant personality disorder: Effect on severity of social phobia, impairment, and outcome of cognitive-behavioral treatment. *Behav. Ther.* 26: 467–486.

Brown, E. J., Turovsky, J., Heimberg, R. G. et al. 1994b. Validation of the Social Interaction Anxiety Scale and the Social Phobia Scale across the anxiety disorders. (submitted)

Brown, T. A., DiNardo, P. A. & Barlow, D. H. 1994a. Anxiety Disorders Interview Schedule for DSM-IV (ADIS-IV). Graywinds, Albany, New York.

Brown, T. M., Black, B. & Uhde T. W. 1994c. The sleep architecture of social phobia. *Biol. Psychiatry* 35: 420–421.

Bruch, M. A., Heimberg, R. G., Berger, P. et al. 1989. Social phobia and perceptions of early parental and personal characteristics. *Anx. Res.* 2: 57–65.

Bruch, M. A. & Cheek, J. M. 1995. Developmental factors in childhood and adolescent shyness. In *Social Phobia: Diagnosis, Assessment, and Treatment*, eds. R. G. Heimberg, M. R. Liebowitz, D. A. Hope, F. R. Schneier, pp. 163–182, Guilford Press, New York.

Bruch, M. A. & Heimberg, R. G. 1994. Differences in perception of parental and personal characteristics between generalized and nongeneralized social phobics. *J. Anx. Dis.* 8: 155–168.

Burton, R. 1621. *The Anatomy of Melancholy.* Eleventh Edition (1813), p. 272, Volume 1, London.

Butler, G. 1985. Exposure as a treatment for social phobia: Some instructive difficulties. *Behav. Res. Ther.* 23: 651–657.

Butler, G., Cullington, A., Munby, M. et al. 1984. Exposure and anxiety management in the treatment of social phobia. *J. Consult. Clin. Psychol.* 52: 642–650.

Butler, G. & Wells, A. 1995. Cognitive-behavioral treatments: Clinical applications. In *Social Phobia: Diagnosis, Assessment, and Treatment*, eds. R. G. Heimberg, M. R. Liebowitz, D. A. Hope, F. R. Schneier, pp. 310–333, Guilford Press, New York.

Cameron, O. B., Thyer, B. A. & Nesse, R. M. 1986. Symptom profiles of patients with DSM-III anxiety disorders. *Am. J. Psychiatry* 143: 1132–1137.

Chambless, D. L., Cherney, J., Caputo, G. C. et al. 1987. Anxiety disorders and alcoholism: A study with inpatient alcoholics. *J. Anx. Dis.* 1: 9–40.

Chapman, T. F., Mannuzza, S. & Fyer, A. J. 1995. Epidemiology and family studies of social phobia. In *Social Phobia: Diagnosis, Assessment, and Treatment*, eds. R. G. Heimberg, M. R. Liebowitz, D. A. Hope, F. R. Schneier, pp. 21–40, Guilford Press, New York.

Clark, D. B. & Agras, W. S. 1991. The assessment and treatment of performance anxiety in musicians. *Am. J. Psychiatry* 148: 598–605.

Cox, B. J., Direnfeld, D. M. & Swinson, R. P. 1994. Suicidal ideation and suicide attempts in panic disorder and social phobia. *Am J. Psychiatry* 151: 882–886.

Cox, B. J., Swinson, R. P. & Shaw, B. F. 1991. Value of the Fear Questionnaire in differentiating agoraphobia and social phobia. *Br. J. Psychiatry* 159: 842–845.

Davidson, J. R. T., Hughes, D. C., George, L. K. et al. 1993a. The epidemiology of social phobia: Findings from the Duke Epidemiological Catchment Area Study. *Psychol. Med.* 23: 709–718.

Davidson, J. R. T., Hughes, D. C., George, L. K. et al. 1994. The boundary of social phobia: Exploring the threshold. *Arch. Gen. Psychiatry* 51: 975–983.

Davidson, J. R. T., Krishnan, K. R. R., Charles, H. C. et al. 1993b. Magnetic resonance spectroscopy in social phobia: Preliminary findings. *J. Clin. Psychiatry* 54: 19–25.

Davidson, J. R. T., Potts, N. L. S., Richichi, E A.. et al. 1993c. Treatment of social phobia with clonazepam and placebo. *J. Clin. Psychopharmacol.* 13: 423–428.

Davidson, J. R. T., Potts, N. L. S., Richichi, E. A. et al. 1991. The Brief Social Phobia Scale. *J. Clin. Psychiatry* 52 (Suppl. 11): 48–51.

Davidson, J. R. T., Tupler, L. A., & Potts, N. L. S. 1994. Treatment of social phobia with benzodiazepines. *J. Clin. Psychiatry*, 56: 28–32.

Degonda, M. & Angst, J. 1993. The Zurich study XX. Social phobia and agoraphobia. *Eur. Arch. Psychiatry Clin. Neurosci.* 243: 95–102.

Dilsaver, S. C., Oamar, A. B. & Del Medico, J. J. 1992. Secondary social phobia in patients with major depression. *Psychiatr. Res.* 44: 33–40.

Dimsdale, J. E. & Moss, J. 1980. Short-term catecholamine response to psychological stress. *Psychosom. Med.* 42: 493–497.

DiNardo, P. A., Moras, K., Barlow, D. H. et al. 1993. Reliability of DSM-III-R anxiety disorder categories using the Anxiety Disorders Interview Schedule-Revised (ADIS-R). *Arch. Gen. Psychiatry* 50: 241–256.

DiNardo, P. A., O'Brien, G. T. & Barlow, D. H. 1983. Reliability of DSM-III-R anxiety disorder categories using a new structured interview. *Arch. Gen. Psychiatry* 40: 1070–1074.

Donohue, B. C., Van Hasselt, V. B. & Hersen, M. 1994. Behavioral assessment and treatment of social phobia. *Behav. Modification* 18: 262–288.

Emmelkamp, P. M. G., Mersch, P. P., Vissia, E. et al. 1985. Social phobia: A comparative evaluation of cognitive and behavioral interventions. *Behav. Res. Ther.* 23: 365–369.

Falloon, I. R. H., Lloyd, G. G. & Harpin, R. E. 1981. The treatment of social phobia: Real life rehearsal with nonprofessional therapist. *J. Nerv. Ment. Dis.* 169: 180–184.

First, M. B., Spitzer, R. L., Gibbon, M. et al. 1995. *Structured Clinical Interview for DSM-IV – Patient Edition (SCID)*, Biometrics Research Department, New York State Psychiatric Institute, New York.

Fishbein, M., Middlestadt, S. E., Oltati, J. et al. 1988. Medical problems among ICSOM musicians: Overview of a national survey. *Med. Problems Performing Artists* 3: 1–8.

Flint, A. J. 1994. Epidemiology and comorbidity of anxiety disorders in the elderly. *Am. J. Psychiatry* 151: 640–649.

Francis, G., Last, C. G. & Strauss, C. C. 1992. Avoidant disorder and social phobia in children and adolescents. *J. Am. Acad. Child Adolescent Psychiatry* 31: 1086–1089.

Fyer, A. J., Mannuzza, S., Chapman, T. F. et al. 1993. A direct interview family study of social phobia. *Arch. Gen. Psychiatry* 50: 286–293.

Fyer, A. J., Mannuzza, S., Gallops, M. S. et al. 1990. Familial transmission of simple phobias and fears. *Arch. Gen. Psychiatry* 47: 252–256.

Fyer, A. J., Mannuzza, S., Martin, L. Y. et al. 1989. Reliability of anxiety assessment. II. Symptom agreement. *Arch. Gen. Psychiatry* 46: 1102–1110.

Gelernter, C. S., Stein, M. B., Tancer, M. E. et al. 1992. An examination of syndromal validity and diagnostic subtypes in social phobia and panic disorder. *J. Clin. Psychiatry* 53: 23–27.

Gelernter, C. S., Uhde, T. W., Cimbolic, P. et al. 1991. Cognitive-behavioral and pharmacological treatments of social phobia: A controlled study. *Arch. Gen. Psychiatry* 48: 938–945.

Greist, J. H., Kobak, K. A., Jefferson, J. W. et al. 1995. Epidemiology and family studies of social phobia. In *Social Phobia: Diagnosis, Assessment, and Treatment*, eds. R. G. Heimberg, M. R. Liebowitz, D. A. Hope, F. R. Schneier, pp. 185–201, Guilford Press, New York.

Hatterer, J. A., Gorman, J. M., Fyer, A. J. et al. 1990. Pharmacotherapy of four men with paruresis. *Am. J. Psychiatry* 147: 109–111.

Heckelman, L. R. & Schneier, F. R. 1995. Diagnostic issues. In *Social Phobia: Diagnosis, Assessment, and Treatment*, eds. R. G. Heimberg, M. R. Liebowitz, D. A. Hope, F. R. Schneier, pp. 3–20, Guilford Press, New York.

Heimberg, R. G. 1993. Specific issues in the cognitive-behavioral treatment of social phobia. *J. Clin. Psychiatry* 54: 36–45.

Heimberg, R. G. & Barlow, D. H. 1991. New developments in cognitive-behavioral therapy for social phobia. *J. Clin. Psychiatry* 52: 21–30.

Heimberg, R. G. & Barlow, D. H. 1988. Psychosocial treatments for social phobia. *Psychosomatics* 29: 27–37.

Heimberg, R. G., Becker, R. E, Goldfinger, K. et al. 1985. Treatment of social phobia by exposure, cognitive restructuring, and homework assignments. *J. Nerv. Ment. Dis.* 173: 236–245.

Heimberg, R. G., Dodge, C. S., Hope, D. A. et al. 1990b. Cognitive behavioral treatment of social phobia: Comparison to a credible placebo control. *Cognitive. Ther. Res.* 14: 1–23.

Heimberg, R. G., Hope, D., Dodge, C. et al. 1990a. DSM-III-R subtypes of social phobia: Comparison of generalized social phobics and public speaking phobics. *J. Nerv. Ment. Dis.* 173: 172–179.

Heimberg, R. G. & Juster, H. R. 1994. Treatment of social phobia in cognitive-behavioral groups. *J. Clin. Psychiatry* 55 (Suppl. 6): 38–46.

Heimberg, R. G. & Juster, H. R. 1995. Cognitive-behavioral treatments: Literature review. In *Social Phobia: Diagnosis, Assessment, and Treatment*, eds. R. G. Heimberg, M. R. Liebowitz, D. A. Hope, F. R. Schneier, pp. 261–309, Guildford Press, New York.

Heimberg, R. G., Juster, H. R., Hope, D. A. et al. 1995. Cognitive behavioral group treatment for social phobia: Description, case presentation, and empirical support. In *Social Phobia: Clinical and Research Persepctives*, ed. M. B. Stein, pp. 293–321, American Psychiatric Press.

Heimberg, R. G., Mueller, G. P., Holt, C. S. et al. 1992. Assessment of anxiety in social interaction and being observed by others: The Social Interaction Anxiety Scale and the Social Phobia Scale. *Behav. Ther.* 23: 53–73.

Heimberg, R. G., Salzman, D. G., Holt, C. S. et al. 1993. Cognitive behavioral group treatment for social phobia: Effectiveness at five-year follow-up. *Cognitive Ther. Res.* 17: 325–339.

Herbert, J. D., Hope, D. A. & Bellock, A. S. 1992. Validity of the distinction between generalized social phobia and avoidant personality disorder. *J. Abn. Psychol.* 101: 332–339.

Holt, C. S., Heimberg, R. G. & Hope, D. A. 1992a. Avoidant personality disorder and the generalized subtype of social phobia. *J. Abn. Psychol.* 101: 318–325.

Holt, C. S., Heimberg, R. G., Hope, D. A. & Liebowitz, M.R. 1992b. Situational domains of social phobia. *J. Anx. Dis.* 6: 63–77.

Hope, D. A., Holt, C. S. & Heimberg R. G. 1993. Social phobia. In *Handbook of Effective Psychotherapy*, ed. T. R. Giles, pp. 227–251. Plenum Press, New York.

Hope, D. A., Rapee, R. M., Heimberg, R. G. et al. 1990. Representations of the self in social phobia: Vulnerability to social threat. *Cognitive Ther. Res.* 14: 177–189.

Horn, K. M., Plomin, R. & Rosenman, R. 1976. Heritability of personality traits in adult male twins. *Behav. Genet.* 6: 17–30.

Janet, P. 1903. *Les Obsessions et la Psychasthenie*. Alcan, Paris.

Jansen, M. A., Arntz, A., Merckelbach, H. et al. 1994. Personality disorders and features in social phobia and panic disorder. *J. Abn. Psychology* 103: 391–395.

Johansson, J. & Öst, L. G. 1982. Perception of autonomic reactions and actual heart rate in phobic patients. *J. Behav. Assess.* 4: 133–143.

Juster, H. R., Heimberg, R. G. & Holt, C. S. In Press. Social phobia: Diagnostic issues and review of cognitive-behavioral treatment strategies. In *Progress in Behavioral Modification*, eds. M. Hersen, R. Eisler, and P. Miller. Cole Publishing, Pacific Grove, CA.

Juster, H. R., Heimberg, R. G. & Holt, C. S. 1994. Social phobia: Diagnostic issues and review of cognitive-behavioral treatment strategies. In *Progress in Behavior Modification*, eds. M. Hersen, R. Eisler, P. Miller, Sycamore Publishing Company, Sycamore, IL.

Kagan, J. 1989. Temperamental contributions to social behavior. *Am. Psychol.* 44: 668–674.

Kagan, J., Reznick, J. S. & Gibbons, J. 1989. Inhibited and uninhibited types of children. *Child Dev.* 60: 838–845.

Kendler, K., Neale, M., Kessler, R. et al. 1992. The genetic epidemiology of phobias in women: The interrelationship of agoraphobia, social phobia, situational phobia and simple phobia. *Arch. Gen. Psychiatry* 49: 273–281.

Kessler, R. C., McGonagle, D. K., Zhao, S. et al. 1994. Lifetime and 12-month prevalence of DSM-III-R psychiatric disorders in the United States: Results from the National Comorbidity Survey. *Arch. Gen. Psychiatry* 51: 8–19.

Kushner, M. G., Shear, K. J. & Beitman, B. D. 1990. The relation between alcohol problems and the anxiety disorders. *Am. J. Psychiatry* 147: 685–695.

Lader, M. H. & Wing, L. 1964. Habituation and psycho-galvanic reflex in patients with anxiety states and in normal subjects. *J. Neurol. Neurosurg. Psychiatr.* 27: 210–218.

Lande, S. D. 1982. Physiological and subjective measures of anxiety during flooding. *Behav. Res. Ther.* 20:472–490.

Last, C. G. 1993. Social and simple phobias in children. *J. Anx Disorders* 7: 141–152.

Last, C. G. & Strauss, C. C. 1990. School refusal in anxiety–disordered children and adolescents. *J. Am. Acad. Child Adol. Psychiatry* 29: 31–35.

Lelliott, P. 1988. Marks and Mathews Fear Questionnaire. In *Dictionary of Behavioral Assessment Techniques*, eds. M. Hersen, A. S. Bellack, pp. 293–304, Pergamon Press, New York.

Levin, A. P., Saoud, J. B., Strauman, T. et al. 1993. Responses of 'generalized' and 'discrete' social phobics during public speaking. *J. Anxiety Disord.* 7: 207–222.

Liebowitz, M. R. 1987. Social phobia. In *Modern Problems of Pharmacopsychiatry: Anxiety*, eds. D. F. Klein, J. M. Gorman, A. F. Fyer et al., pp. 141–173, Karger, Basel, Switzerland.

Liebowitz, M. R., Gorman, J. M., Fyer, A. J. et al. 1985b. Social phobia: Review of a neglected anxiety disorder. *Arch. Gen. Psychiatry* 42: 729–736.

Liebowitz, M. R., Quitkin, F. M., Stewart, J. W. et al. 1988. Antidepressant specificity in atypical depression. *Arch Gen Psychiatry* 45: 129–137.

Liebowitz, M. R., Schneier, F. R., Campeas, R. et al. 1992. Phenelzine vs. atenolol in social phobia: A placebo-controlled comparison. *Arch. Gen. Psychiatry* 49: 290–300.

Liebowtiz, M. R., Fyer, A. J. Gorman, J. M. et al. 1985a. Specificity of lactate infusions in social phobia versus panic disorders. *Am. J. Psychiatry* 142: 947–950.

Mannuzza, S., Fyer, A. J., Martin, M. S. et al. 1989. Reliability of anxiety assessment. I. Diagnostic agreement. *Arch. Gen. Psychiatry* 46: 1093–1101.

Mannuzza, S., Schneier, F. R., Chapman, T. F. et al. 1995. Generalized social phobia: Reliability and validity. *Arch. Gen. Psychiatry* 52: 230–237.

Mannuzza, S., Fyer, A. J., Liebowitz, M. R. et al. 1990. Delineating the boundaries of social phobia: Its relationship to panic disorder and agoraphobia. *J. Anxiety Disord.* 4: 41–59.

Manuzza, S., Fyer, A. J., Klein, D. F. et al. 1986. Schedule for Affective Disorders and Schizophrenia – Lifetime, Anxiety (SADS-LA): Rational and conceptual development. *J. Psychiatr. Res.* 20: 317–325.

Marks, I. M. 1970. The classification of phobic disorders. *Br. J. Psychiatry* 116: 377–386.

Marks, I. M. 1987. *Fears, Phobias, and Rituals: Panic, Anxiety, and Their Disorders*, pp. 362–371, Oxford University Press, London.

Marks, I. M. & Mathews, A. M. 1979. Brief standard self–rating for phobic patients. *Behav. Res. Ther.* 17: 263–267.

Marks, I. M. & Gelder, M. G. 1966. Different ages of onset in varieties of phobia. *Am. J. Psychiatry* 123: 218–221.

Mattick, R. P. & Clark, J. C. 1989. Development and validation of measures of social phobia, scrutiny fear, and social interaction anxiety.

Mattick, R. P. & Peters, L. 1988. Treatment of severe social phobia: Effects of guided exposure with and without cognitive restructuring. *J. Consult. Clin. Psychol.* 56: 251–260.

Mattick, R. P., Peters, L. & Clark, J. C. 1989. Exposure and cognitive restructuring for social phobia: A controlled study. *Behav. Ther.* 20: 3–23.

Merckelbach, H., Van Hout, W., Van Den Hout, M. A. et al. 1988. Psychophysiological and subjective reactions of social phobias and normals to facial stimuli. *Behav. Res. Ther.* 3: 289–294.

Mersch, P. P. A., Emmelkamp, P. M. G. & Lips, C. 1991. Social phobia: Individual response patterns and the long-term effects of behavioral and cognitive interventions: A follow-up study. *Behav. Res. Ther.* 29: 357–362.

Millon, T. 1969. *Modern Psychopathology: A Biosocial Approach to Maladaptive Learning and Functioning*, pp. 231–233, Saunders, Philadelphia, PA.

Mineka, S. & Zinbarg, R. 1995. Conditioning and ethological models of social phobia. In *Social Phobia: Diagnosis, Assessment, and Treatment*, eds. R. G. Heimberg, M. R. Liebowitz, D. A. Hope, pp. 134–162, Guilford Press, New York.

Mizes, J. S. & Crawford, J. 1986. Normative values on the Marks and Mathews' Fear Questionnaire: A comparison as a function of age and sex. *J. Psychopathol. Behav. Assess.* 8: 253–262.

Mullaney, J. A. & Trippett, C. J.. 1979. Alcohol dependence and phobias: Clinical description and relevance. *Br. J. Psychiatry* 135: 563–573.

Munjack, D. J., Bruns, J., Baltazar, P. L. et al. 1991. A pilot study of buspirone in the treatment of social phobia. *J. Anxiety Disord.* 5: 87–98.

Nichols, K. A. 1974. Severe social anxiety. *Br. J. Med. Psychol.* 47: 301–306.

Noyes, R. 1988. Beta-blocking drugs in anxiety disorders. In *Handbook of Anxiety Disorders*, eds. C. G. Last, M. Hersen, pp. 219–234, Pergamon Press, New York.

Noyes, R., Crowe, R. R., Harris, E. L. et al. 1986. Relationship between panic disorder and agoraphobia: A family study. *Arch. Gen. Psychiatry* 43: 227–232.

Noyes, R. & Holt, C. S. 1996. Natural course of anxiety disorders. In *Long-Term Treatments of Anxiety Disorders: Psychological and Pharmacological Approaches*, eds. M. Mavissakalian, R. F. Prien, American Psychiatric Press, Washington, DC.

Noyes, R., Woodman, C. L., Garvey, M. J. et al. 1992. Generalized anxiety disorder versus panic disorder: Distinguishing characteristics and patterns of comorbidity. *J. Nerv. Ment. Dis.* 180: 369–379.

Noyes, R., Woodman, C. L., Holt, C. S., et al. 1995. Avoidant personality traits distinguish social phobia from panic disorder. *J. Nerv. Ment. Dis.* 183: 145–153.

Oberlander, E. L., Schneier, F. R. & Liebowitz, M. R. 1994. Physical disability and social phobia. *J. Clin. Psychopharmacol.* 14: 136–143.

Oei, T. P. S., Moylan, A. & Evans, L. 1991. Validity and clinical utility of the Fear Questionnaire for anxiety disorder patients. *Psychological Assess.* 3: 391–397.

Öhman, A. 1986. Face the beast and fear the face: Animal and social fears as prototypes for evolutionary analyses of emotion. *Psychophysiology* 23: 123–145.

Onstad, S. I., Torgersen, S. & Kringlen, E. 1991. High interrater reliability for the Structured Clinical Interview for DSM-III-R, Axis I (SCID-I). *Acta Psychiatr. Scand.* 84: 167–173.

Öst, L-G. 1987. Age of onset in different phobias. *J. Abnorm. Psychol.* 96: 223–229.

Öst, L-G. & Hagdahl, K. 1981. Acquisition of phobias and anxiety response patterns in clinical patients. *Behav. Res. Ther.* 16: 439–447.

Öst, L-G., Jerremalm, A. & Johansson, J. 1981. Individual response patterns and effects of different behavioral methods in the treatment of social phobia. *Behav. Res. Ther.* 19: 1–16.

Page, A. C. 1991. An assessment of structured diagnostic interviews for adult anxiety disorders. *Int. Rev. Psychiatry* 3: 265–278.

Papp, L. A., Gorman, J. M. & Liebowitz, M. R. 1988. Epinephrine infusions in patients with social phobia. *Am. J. Psychiatry* 145: 733–736.

Parker, G. 1979. Reported parental characteristics of agoraphobics and social phobics. *Br. J. Psychiatry* 135: 555–560.

Persson, G. & Nordlund, C. L. 1985. Agoraphobics and social phobics: Differences in background factors, syndrome profiles and therapeutic response. *Acta Psychiat. Scand.* 71: 148–159.

Pittman, R. N., Rabin R. A. & Molinoff, P. B. 1984. Desensitization of beta-adrenergic receptor-coupled cyclase activity. *Behav. Pharmacol.* 22: 3579–3584.

Plomin, R. & Daniels, D. 1986. *Shyness: Perspectives on Research and Treatment*, eds. W. H. Jones, J. M. Cheek, S. R. Briggs, pp. 63–90, Plenum Press, New York.

Pollard, C. M. & Henderson, J. G. 1988. Four types of social phobia in a community sample. *J. Nerv. Ment. Dis.* 176: 440–449.

Potts, N. L. S. & Davidson, J. R. T. 1995. Pharmacological treatments: Literature review. In *Social Phobia: Diagnosis, Assessment, and Treatment*, eds. R. G. Heimberg, M. R. Liebowitz, D. A. Hope, F. R. Schneier, pp. 334–365, Guilford Press, New York.

Potts, N. L. S., Davidson, J. R. T. & Krishnan, R. R. 1990. Levels of urinary free cortisol in social phobia. *J. Clin. Psychiatry* 52 (Suppl. 11): 41–42.

Potts, N. L. S., Davidson, J. R. T., Krishnan, R. R. et al. 1994. Magnetic resonance imaging in social phobia. *Psychiatry Res.* 52: 35–42.

Quitkin, F. M., Rifkin, A., Kaplan, J. et al. 1972. Phobic anxiety syndrome complicated by drug dependence and addiction: A treatable form of drug abuse. *Arch. Gen. Psychiatry* 27: 159–162.

Rapee, R. M. 1995. Descriptive psychopathology of social phobia. In *Social Phobia: Diagnosis, Assessment, and Treatment*, eds. R. G. Heimberg, M. R. Liebowitz, D. A. Hope, F. R. Schneier, pp. 41–66, Guilford Press, New York.

Reich, J. H., Goldenberg, L., Vasile, R. et al. 1994. A prospective follow-along study of the course of social phobia. *Psychiatry Res.* 54: 249–258.

Reich, J. H. & Yates, W. R.1988. Family history of psychiatric disorders in social phobia. *Compr. Psychiatry* 29: 72–75.

Reiter, S. R., Otto, M. W., Pollack, M. H. et al. 1991. Major depression in panic disorder patients with comorbid social phobia. *J. Affect. Dis.* 22: 171–177.

Rey, J. M., Plapp, J. M. & Wever, C. 1992. Epidemiology of anxiety disorders of childhood and adolescence. *Handbook of Anxiety*, Vol. 5, eds. G. D. Burrows, M. Roth, R. Noyes, pp. 309–328, Elsevier, Amsterdam.

Robins, L. N., Wing, J., Whittchen, H-U. et al. 1988. The Composite International Diagnostic Interview. *Arch. Gen. Psychiatry* 45: 1069–1077.

Rosenbaum, J. F., Biederman, J., Gersten, M. et al. 1988. Behavioral inhibition in children of parents with panic disorder and agoraphobia: A controlled study. *Arch. Gen. Psychiatry* 45: 463–470.

Rosenbaum, J. F., Biederman, J., Hirshfeld, D. R. et al. 1991a. Behavioral inhibition in children: A possible precursor to panic disorder or social phobia. *J. Clin. Psychiatry* 52 (Suppl. 11): 5–9.

Rosenbaum, J. F., Biederman, J., Hirshfeld, D. R. et al. 1991b. Further evidence of an association between behavioral inhibition and anxiety disorders: Results from a family study of children from a non-clinical sample. *J. Psychiatr. Res.* 25: 49–65.

Rosenbaum, J. F., Biederman, J., Pollock, R. A. et al. 1994. The etiology of social phobia. *J. Clin. Psychiatry* 55 (Suppl. 6): 10–16.

Ross, H. E., Glaser, F. B. & Germanson, T. 1988. The prevalence of psychiatric disorders in patients with alcohol and other drug problems. *Arch. Gen. Psychiatry* 45: 1023–1031.

Sanderson, W. C., DiNardo, P. A., Rapee, R. M. et al. 1990. Syndrome comorbidity in patients diagnosed with DSM-III-R anxiety disorder. *J. Abnorm. Psychol.* 99: 308–312.

Schneier, F. R., Heckelman, L. R., Garfinkel, R. et al. 1994. Functional impairment in social phobia. *J. Clin. Psychiatry.* 55: 322–331.

Schneier, F. R., Jihad, B. S., Campeas, R. et al. 1993. Buspirone in social phobia. *J. Clin. Psychopharmacol.* 13: 251–256.

Schneier, F. R., Johnson, J., Hornig, C. D. et al. 1992. Social phobia: Comorbidity and morbidity in an epidemiologic sample. *Arch. Gen. Psychiatry* 49: 282–288.

Schneier, F. R. & Liebowitz, M. R. 1990. Social phobia in adulthood. In *Handbook of Child and Adult Psychopathology*, eds. M. Hersen, C. G. Last, pp. 169–180, Pergamon Press, New York.

Schneier, F. R., Martin, L. Y., Liebowtiz, M. R. et al. 1989. Alcohol abuse and social phobia. *J. Anxiety Disord.* 3: 15–23.

Schneier, F. R., Spitzer, R. L., Gibbon, M. et al. 1991. The relationship of social phobia subtypes and avoidant personality disorder. *Compr Psychiatry* 32: 496–502.

Seligman, M. E. P. 1971. Phobias and preparedness. *Behav. Ther.* 2: 307–320.

Smail, P., Stockwell, T., Canter, S. et al. 1984. Alcohol dependence and phobic anxiety states, I. A prevalence study. *Br. J. Psychiatry* 144: 53–57.

Solyom, L., Ledwidge, B. & Solyom, C. 1986. Delineating social phobia. *Br. J. Psychiatry* 149: 464–470.

Spitzer, R. L., Williams, J. B., Gibbon, M. et al. 1992. Structured Clinical Interview for DSM-III-R (SCID): History, rationale, and description. *Arch. Gen. Psychiatry* 49: 624–629.

Starkin, S. L., Holt, C. S., Heimberg, R. G. et al. 1990. The Liebowitz Social Phobia Scale: An exploratory analysis of construct validity. *Presented at the Annual Meeting of the Association for the Advancement of Behavior Therapy*, Washington, DC.

Stein, M. B., Asmundson, G. J. G. & Chartier, M. 1994b. Autonomic responsivity in generalized social phobia. *J. Affect. Dis.* 31: 211–221.

Stein, M. B., Delaney, S. M., Chartier, M. J. et al. 1995. [3H] Paroxetine binding to platelets of patients with social phobia: Comparison to patients with panic disorder and healthy volunteers. *Biol. Psychiatry* 37: 224–228.

Stein, M. B., Hauger, R. L., Dhalla, K. S. et al. 1996. Plasma neuropeptide Y in anxiety disorders: Findings in panic disorder and social phobia. *Psychiatry Res.* 59: 183–188.

Stein, M. B., Heuser, I. J., Juncos, J. L. et al. 1990a. Anxiety disorders in patients with Parkinson's disease. *Am. J. Psychiatry* 147: 217–220.

Stein, M. B., Huzel, L. L. & Delaney, S. M. 1993a. Lymphocyte beta-adrenoreceptors in social phobia. *Biol. Psychiatry* 34: 45–50.

Stein, M. B., Kroft, C. D. L. & Walker, J. R. 1993b. Sleep impairment in patients with social phobia. *Psychiatry Res.* 49: 251–256.

Stein, M. B. & Leslie, W. D. 1996. A brain single photon-emission computer tomography (SPECT) study of generalized social phobia. *Biol. Psychiatry* 39: 825–828.

Stein, M. B., Tancer, M. E. & Gelernter, C. S. 1990b. Major depression in patients with social phobia. *Am. J. Psychiatry* 147: 637–639.

Stein, M. B., Walker, J. R. & Forde, D. R. 1994a. Setting diagnostic thresholds for social phobia: Considerations from a community survey of social anxiety. *Am. J. Psychiatry* 151: 408–412.

Stopa, L. & Clark, D. M. 1993. Cognitive process in social phobia. *Behav. Res. Ther.* 31: 255–267.

Strauss, C. C. & Last, C. G. 1993. Social and simple phobias in children. *J. Anxiety Disord.* 7: 141–152.

Stravynski, A., Lamontagne, Y. & Lavallee, Y. J. 1986. Clinical phobias and avoidant personality disorder among alcoholics admitted to an alcoholism rehabilitation setting. *Can. J. Psychiatry* 31: 714–719.

Stravynski, A., Marks, I. M. & Yale, W. 1982. Social skills problems in neurotic outpatients. *Arch. Gen. Psychiatry* 39: 1378–1385.

Sutherland, S. M., Davidson, J. R. T., Tupler, L. et al. 1994. Two year post-treatment follow-up of social phobia. *Presented at the Annual Meeting of the Anxiety Disorders Association of America*, Santa Monica, CA.

Taggart, P., Carruther, M. & Somerville, W. 1973. Electrocardiogram, plasma catacholamines and lipids, and their modification by oxprenolol when speaking before an audience. *Lancet* 2: 341–346.

Tancer, M.E. 1993. Neurobiology of social phobia. *J. Clin. Psychiatry* 54: 26–30.

Tancer, M. E., Stein, M. B., Gelernter, C. S. et al. 1990. The hypothalamic-pituitary-thyroid axis in social phobia. *Am. J. Psychiatry* 147: 929–933.

Tancer, M. E., Stein, M. B. & Uhde, T. W. 1993. Growth hormone response to intravenous clonidine in social phobia: Comparison to patients with panic disorder and health volunteers. *Biol. Psychiatry* 34: 591–595.

Thyer, B. A., Parrish, R. T., Curtis, G. C. et al., 1985. Ages of onset of DSM-III anxiety disorders. *Compr. Psychiatry* 26: 113–121.

Torgersen, S. 1979. The nature and origin of common phobic fears. *Br. J. Psychiatry* 134: 343–351.

Torgersen, S. 1983. Genetic factors in anxiety disorders. *Arch. Gen. Psychiatry* 40: 1085–1089.

Townsley, R. 1992. *Social Phobia: Identification of Possible Etiological Factors.* Doctoral dissertation, University of Georgia, Athens.

Trower, P., Yardley, K., Bryant, B. M. et al. 1978. The treatment of social failure. A comparison of anxiety reduction and skills-acquisition procedures on two social problems. *Behav. Modification* 2: 41–60.

Turner, S. M. & Beidel, D. C. In Press. *Social Phobia and Anxiety Inventory Manual.* Multi-Health Systems, Toronto.

Turner, S. M., Beidel, D. C., Dancu, C. V. et al. 1986. Psychopathology of social phobia and comparison to avoidant personality disorder. *J. Abn. Psychology* 4: 389–394.

Turner, S. M., Beidel, D. C. & Jacob, R. G. 1994. Social phobia: A comparison of behavior therapy and atenolol. *J. Consul. Clin. Psychol.* 62: 350–358.

Turner, S. M., Beidel, D. C. & Townsley, R. M. 1992. Social phobia: A comparison of specific and generalized subtypes and avoidant personality disorder. *J. Abnorm. Psychol.* 101: 326–331.

Turner, S. M., Biedel, D. C., Dancu, C. V. et al. 1989. An empirically derived inventory to measure social fears and anxiety: The Social Phobia and Anxiety Inventory. *Psychol. Assess.* 1: 35–40.

Turner, S. M., McCanna, M. & Biedel, D. C. 1987. Validity of the Social

Avoidance and Distress and Fear of Negative Evaluation Scales. *Behav. Res. Ther.* 25: 113–115.

Tyrer, P. & Steinberg, D. 1975. Symptomatic treatment of agoraphobia and social phobias: A follow-up study. *Br. J. Psychiatry* 127: 163–168.

Uhde, T. W., Tancer, M. E., Gelernter, C. S. et al. 1994. Normal urinary free cortisol and post-dexamethasone cortisol in social phobia: Comparison to normal volunteers. *J. Affect. Dis.* 30: 155–161.

Van Ameringen, M., Mancini, C., Styan, G. et al. 1991. Relationship of social phobia with other psychiatric illness. *J. Affect. Dis.* 21: 93–99.

Van Ameringen, M., Mancini, C. & Streiner, D. L. 1993. Fluoxetine efficacy in social phobia. *J. Clin. Psychiatry* 54: 27–32.

Van Ameringen, M., Mancini, C. & Streiner, D. L. 1994. Sertraline in social phobia. *J. Affect. Dis.* 31: 141–145.

van Vliet, I. M., den Boer, J. A. & Westernberg, H. G. M. 1994. Psychopharmacological treatment of social phobia: a double-clind, placebo controlled study with fluvoxamine. *Psychopharmacology* 115: 128–134.

Versiani, M., Mundim, F. D., Nardi, A. E. et al. 1988. Tranylcypromine in social phobia. *J. Clin. Psychopharmacol.* 8: 183–279.

Versiani, M., Nardi, A. E., Mundim, F. D. et al. 1992. Pharmacotherapy of social phobia: A controlled study with moclobemide and phenelzine. *Br. J. Psychiatry* 161: 353–360.

Walker, J. R. & Stein, M. B. 1995. Epidemiology of social phobia. In *Social Phobia: Clinical and Research Persepctives*, ed. M. B. Stein, American Psychiatric Press, Washington, DC.

Watson, P. & Friend, R. 1969. Measurement of social-evaluative anxiety. *J. Consult. Clin. Psychol.* 33: 448–457.

Wesner, R. B., Noyes, R. & Davis, T. L. 1990. The occurrence of performance anxiety among musicians. *J. Affect. Disord.* 18: 177–185.

Williams, G. W. & Degenhardt, B. T. 1952. Paruresis: A survey of a disorder of micturition. *J. Gen. Psychology* 51: 19–29.

Williams, J. B. W., Gibbon, M., First, M. B. et al. 1992. The Structured Clinical Interview for DSM-III-R (SCID). II. Multisite test-retest reliability. *Arch. Gen. Psychiatry* 49: 630–636.

Wing, J. K., Babor, T., Brugha, T. et al. 1990. SCAN: Schedule for Clinical Assessment in Neuropsychiatry. *Arch. Gen. Psychiatry* 47: 589–593.

Wlazlo, Z., Schroeder-Hartwig, K., Hand, I. et al. 1990. Exposure in vivo vs. social skills training for social phobia: Long-term outcome and differential effects. *Behav. Res. Ther.* 28: 181–193.

World Health Organization 1993. *The ICD-10 Classification of Mental and Behavioral Disorders: Diagnostic Criteria for Research*, World Health Organization, Geneva.

Zgourides, G. D. 1987. Paruresis: Overview and implications for treatment. *Psychol. Rep.* 60: 1171–1176.

5
Specific phobia

Definition

Specific phobias, formerly called simple phobias, are characterized by fears of objects or situations known by affected persons to be harmless. Despite this knowledge, phobic individuals regularly react with intense fear when confronted with a phobic stimulus. According to Miller et al. (1974), fears become a phobias when they exceed the demands of the situation, cannot be explained or reasoned away, are beyond voluntary control, lead to avoidance of feared situations, persist over an extended period, are maladaptive, and are not age- or stage-specific.

The term phobia is derived from the Greek word 'phobos', meaning fear. Since Hippocrates, abnormal fears have been described but the term phobia was not introduced until the nineteenth century. Freud separated common phobias from realistic fears, while Kraepelin combined phobic and obsessive fears in his textbook in 1913. Phobias did not achieve a separate diagnostic category in ICD until 1947 or in DSM until 1952. In the 1960s, Marks (1987) subdivided phobic disorders; and DSM-III extended the division, while ICD maintained fewer distinctions (American Psychiatric Association, 1980). As Marks (1987) pointed out, phobias can develop in response to almost any object or situation. Indeed, some psychiatric textbooks from the turn of the century list more than a hundred Greek-named phobias. For taxonomic reasons, phobias were grouped in clusters. Decisions had to be made, when fears were common (e.g., of darkness, animals), about which ones were to be included in the classification. Similarly, phobias that occur as part of other psychiatric disorders were excluded.

Specific phobias are focused upon, and restricted to, specific situations such as animals, heights, storms, darkness, closed places, airplanes, dentists or the sight of blood. In a person with an uncomplicated specific phobia,

Table 5.1. *DSM-IV criteria for specific phobia*

A. Marked and persistent fear that is excessive or unreasonable, cued by the presence or anticipation of a specific object or situation (e.g., flying, heights, animals, receiving an injection, seeing blood)
B. Exposure to the phobic stimulus almost invariably provokes an immediate anxiety response, which may take the form of a situationally bound or situationally predisposed panic attack. Note: In children, the anxiety may be expressed by crying, tantrums, freezing, or clinging
C. The person recognizes that the fear is excessive or unreasonable. Note: In children, this feature may be absent
D. The phobic situation(s) is avoided or else is endured with intense anxiety or distress
E. The avoidance, anxious anticipation, or distress in the feared situation(s) interferes significantly with the person's normal routine, occupational (or academic) functioning, or social activities or relationships, or there is marked distress about having the phobia
F. In individuals under age 18 years, the duration is at least 6 months
G. The anxiety, panic attacks, or phobic avoidance associated with the specific object or situation are not better accounted for by another mental disorder, such as obsessive compulsive disorder (e.g., fear of dirt in someone with an obsession about contamination), posttraumatic stress disorder (e.g., avoidance of stimuli associated with a severe stressor), separation anxiety disorder (e.g., avoidance of school), social phobia (e.g., avoidance of social situations because of fear of embarrassment), panic disorder with agoraphobia, or agoraphobia without history of panic disorder

Specify:
   Animal type
   Natural environment type (e.g., heights, storms, water)
   Blood–injection–injury type
   Situational type (e.g., airplanes, elevators, enclosed places)
   Other type (e.g., phobic avoidance of situations that may lead to choking, vomiting, or contracting an illness; in children, avoidance of loud sounds or costumed characters)

From the American Psychiatric Association (1994). Reprinted with permission.

other psychiatric problems are uncommon, and in absence of the phobic stimulus, there is usually no fear, anxiety or other problem (Marks, 1987).

Diagnostic criteria

DSM-IV lists seven criteria necessary to diagnose a specific phobia as outlined in Table 5.1 (American Psychiatric Association, 1994). A phobia is characterized by marked and persistent fear of clearly discernible, circumscribed objects or situations. Exposure to the phobic stimulus almost invariably provokes an immediate anxiety response. This response can take the form of a situationally bound or situationally predisposed panic attack. Adolescents or adults, but not necessarily children, need to recognize that their fear is excessive or unreasonable. Most often the phobic stimulus is avoided, although it is sometimes endured with dread. Fearful avoidance or anxious anticipation of encountering the phobic stimulus has to interfere significantly with the person's daily routine, occupational functioning, or social life, or the person has to be markedly distressed about having the phobia. Finally, the symptoms cannot be accounted for by another disorder.

Furthermore, DSM-IV lists five subtypes of phobias: (1) an animal type, (2) a natural environment type, e.g., fears of storms, water or heights, (3) a blood-injection-injury type, (4) a situational type, e.g., fears of tunnels, bridges, trains or elevators, and (5) an other type, e.g., fear and avoidance of stimuli that may lead to choking. DSM-IV differs from DSM-III-R mainly by requiring an individual below the age of 18 years to have had the fear at least 6 months (American Psychiatric Association, 1987). In addition, children are not required to see the fear as unreasonable.

The ICD-10 criteria, shown in Table 5.2, are similar, although less elaborate, than those of DSM-IV (World Health Organization, 1992). The main difference is that DSM-IV, but not ICD-10, requires recognition that the fear is unreasonable. In defending this exclusion from ICD-10, Tyrer (1989) argued that patients with specific phobias only present for treatment if they regard them as unreasonable. He also makes the point that some fears, while exaggerated, may be reasonable; for instance, a person who has been assaulted may be afraid to leave his or her house at night.

Reliability and validity

While 'pure' specific phobias are easily identified, studies differ in the assessment of reliability, even when the same instruments are used. Early assessments, using the Anxiety Disorder Interview Schedule (ADIS), showed very low reliability; however, the number of subjects was small (Barlow, 1985). With the revised ADIS and a larger number of patients, the reliability became very high (Di Nardo et al., 1993). Low reliability was found using the SADS-LA (Mannuzza et al., 1989), but high reliability was reported using the Munich Diagnostic Checklist (Hiller et al., 1990) and the Longitudinal Interval Follow-up Evaluation – Upjohn Version (LIFE-UP), an instrument for prospectively following the course of psychiatric disorders (Warshaw et al., 1994). Wide discrepancies in the prevalence of specific phobias at three sites in the Epidemiologic Catchment Area (ECA)

Table 5.2. *ICD-10 Criteria for Specific (isolated) Phobias*

A. Either of the following must be present:
  (1) marked fear of a specific object or situation not included in agoraphobia or social phobia
  (2) marked avoidance of a specific object or situation not included in agoraphobia or social phobia
  Among the most common objects and situations are animals, birds, insects, heights, thunder, flying, small enclosed spaces, the sight of blood or injury, injections, dentists, and hospitals
B. Symptoms of anxiety in the feared situation as defined in agoraphobia criterion B,* must have been manifest at some time since the onset of the disorder
C. Significant emotional distress is caused by the symptoms or by the avoidance, and the individual recognizes that these are excessive or unreasonable
D. Symptoms are restricted to the feared situation or contemplation of the feared situation. If desired, the specific phobias may be subdivided as follows:
  ___ animal type (e.g., insects, dogs)
  ___ nature-forces type (e.g., storms, water)
  ___ blood, injection, and injury type
  ___ situational type (e.g., elevators, tunnels)
  ___ other type

*Agoraphobia, Criterion B

At least two symptoms of anxiety in the feared situation must have been present together, on at least one occasion since the onset of the disorder, and one of the symptoms must have been from item (1) to (4) listed below:
Autonomic arousal symptoms
  (1) palpitations or pounding heart, or accelerated heart rate
  (2) sweating
  (3) trembling or shaking
  (4) dry mouth (not due to medication or dehydration)

Symptoms involving chest and abdomen
  (5) difficulty in breathing
  (6) feeling of choking
  (7) chest pain or discomfort
  (8) nausea or abdominal distress (e.g., churning in stomach)

Symptoms involving mental state
  (9) feeling dizzy, unsteady, faint or light-headed
  (10) feelings that objects are unreal (derealization), or that the self is distant or 'not really here' (depersonalization)
  (11) fear of losing control, 'going crazy', or passing out
  (12) fear of dying

General symptoms
  (13) hot flushes or cold chills
  (14) numbness or tingling sensations

From WHO (1993). Reprinted with permission.

study indicate that judgment about what constitutes a phobia may differ, even when raters are trained in using the same instrument – in this case the Diagnostic Interview Schedule (DIS) (Robins et al., 1984). Particularly striking were the discrepancies observed when diagnoses made by lay interviewers using the DIS were compared with those made by psychiatrists (Anthony et al., 1985). Aspects of the validity of specific phobia are discussed under Differential diagnosis.

Measurement

Questions relevant to diagnostic assessment are contained in the Schedule of Affective Disorders and Schizophrenia, Lifetime Anxiety Version (Mannuzza et al., 1986) and the Structured Clinical Interview for DSM-IV (Spitzer et al., 1992), but they are not detailed enough to permit quantitative assessments or measurement of change. The Fear Survey Schedule (FSS-III, Wolpe & Lang, 1964) lists 76 fears that are common in phobic patients. It contains five factors: social fears; fears of public places; fears of bodily injury, death, and illness; fears of sexual and aggressive acts; and fear of harmless animals. Test-retest reliability for the subscales is very high. The disadvantage of the scale is its length, which makes it less suitable for regular assessment of phobias. The Fear Questionnaire (FQ, Marks & Mathews, 1979), shown in Table 5.3, lists the main fear of a patient, in addition to 15 of the most common phobias. Further, it lists associated anxiety-depressive symptoms and provides a global rating of phobic symptoms. All items are rated for severity, ranging from zero to eight. The scale contains three factors: agoraphobia, social phobia and blood-injury phobia. Ratings on this scale were found to be reasonably stable over a 1-year period. Both the FSS and FQ can be used for assessing the type and severity of individual phobias as well as phobic disorders. A number of scales for rating specific fears – for instance, fear of spiders (Szymanski & O'Donahue, 1995) – have been developed for special patient populations but are too restricted for general clinical use.

Progress in treatment also has been assessed by means of psychophysiological and behavioral measures; however, good psychophysiological measures are difficult to identify, show great inter-individual variability and correlate poorly with subjective anxiety and behavioral change. They are, consequently, more useful in research than in clinical practice (Marks et al., 1971; Hoehn-Saric & McLeod, 1993). Behavioral tests that identify feared activities and rank them according to a hierarchy of severity have been used to test therapeutic progress, particularly in the treatment of

Table 5.3. *Fear questionnaire*

Choose a number from the scale below to show how much you would avoid each of the situations listed below because of fear or other unpleasant feelings. Then write the number you chose in the box opposite each situation.

0	1	2	3	4	5	6	7	8
Would not avoid it		Slightly avoid it		Definitely avoid it		Markedly avoid it		Always avoid it

1. Main phobia you want treated (describe in your own words) ____

2. Injections or minor surgery ____
3. Eating or drinking with other people ____
4. Hospitals ____
5. Traveling alone in busy streets ____
6. Walking alone in busy streets ____
7. Being watched or stared at ____
8. Going into crowded shops ____
9. Talking to people in authority ____
10. Sight of blood ____
11. Being criticized ____
12. Going alone far from home ____
13. Thought of injury or illness ____
14. Speaking or acting to an audience ____
15. Large open spaces ____
16. Going to the dentist ____
17. Other situations (describe) ____

Ag + BI + Soc = Total
2–16

Now choose a number from the scale below to show how much you are troubled by each problem listed, and write the number in the box opposite.

0	1	2	3	4	5	6	7	8
Would not avoid it		Slightly avoid it		Definitely avoid it		Markedly avoid it		Always avoid it

18. Feeling miserable or depressed ____
19. Feeling irritable or angry ____
20. Feeling tense or panicky ____
21. Upsetting thoughts coming into your mind ____
22. Feeling you or your surroundings are strange or unreal ____
23. Other feelings (describe) ____

Total ____

Table 5.3. *(cont.)*

How would you rate the present state of your phobic symptoms on the scale below?

0	1	2	3	4	5	6	7	8

No phobias present	Slightly disturbing/ not really disabling	Definitely disturbing/ disabling	Markedly disturbing/ disabling	Very disturbing/ disabling

Please circle one number between 0 and 8.

Source: Marks & Matthews (1979). © 1979, Elsevier Science Ltd. Reprinted with permission.

agoraphobia (Mathews et al., 1981). While they are useful in the assessment of a particular patient, they cannot, because of their individual construction, be used to compare patients.

Epidemiology

Prevalence

The prevalence of phobias can only be estimated approximately. There are several reasons for this. Older studies did not distinguish between different types of phobias. Clinical estimates are biased because few phobics seek help. Moreover, it is often difficult to draw the line between a fear that is an appropriate response to a frightening stimulus and a response pattern that is out of proportion, persistent and maladaptive. Also, it is difficult at times, to distinguish true phobias from phobia-like symptoms that belong to other disorders.

In children of all ages fears are common. In studies, reviewed by Silverman & Nelles (1990), the prevalence in children ranged from 8% to 43%, with girls exhibiting fears more frequently than boys. Prevalence of phobias was lower and ranged from 3% to 7%. A study using DSM-III criterion for phobias revealed a prevalence of 2.4% (Anderson et al., 1987).

In adults the estimated 6-month prevalence of simple phobias ranged between 4% and 7% (Marks, 1987). The National Comorbidity Survey established the lifetime prevalence at 11.3% and the 30-day prevalence at 5.5%. Lower prevalence rates were found in Florence, Italy (a lifetime prevalence of 0.63%), possibly because of hierarchical diagnostic rules, and

Table 5.4. *Specific unreasonable fears assessed in the interview with twins*

	% of sample endorsing this fear accompanied by interference	% with subtype of phobia endorsing this fear
Animal phobia		
Insects	1.0	9.4
Spiders	3.3	30.2
Mice	2.3	21.3
Snakes	5.5	50.6
Bats	1.6	14.8
Situational phobia		
Tunnels	2.9	23.8
Other closed places	3.7	30.6
Bridges	3.1	25.3
Airplanes	4.7	38.1
Other high places	7.4	60.0

Source: Modified from Kendler et al. (1992). © 1992, American Medical Association. Reprinted with Permission.

the fact that the diagnosticians were psychiatrists instead of lay interviewers (Faravelli et al., 1989). Table 5.4 shows the percentage of female twins who, when personally interviewed by clinicians, acknowledged the presence of specific phobias and claimed that these phobias caused interference with their lives (Kendler et al., 1992). While phobias – especially those for heights and snakes – were common, only about 10% felt they interfered with their lives.

Risk factors

Women have higher rates of phobias then men. In the ECA study, reviewed by McGlynn & McNeil (1990), the 6-month prevalence ranged from 2.3% to 7.3% in men and 6.6% to 15.7% in women. The prevalence also is higher in blacks than non-blacks and lower in college graduates (Brown et al., 1990).

Comorbidity

Comorbidity with other psychiatric disorders is not infrequent. In one survey, 40.2% of specific phobias started before other comorbid disorders. Among specific phobics, lifetime comorbidity included other anxiety disorders in 68.7% (44.5% social phobia, 27% agoraphobia, and 27% panic disorder), affective disorders in 46.8% (major depression 42.3% and dysthymia 15.8%), and substance use disorders in 39.4% (Magee et al., 1996). It appears that persons who develop other disorders are more likely to develop phobias as well. On the other hand, a considerable number of individuals with specific phobias remain free of other psychiatric disorders (Fyer et al., 1990). A large study of female twins showed comorbidity to be lower for animal and situational phobias than for other phobias (Kendler et al., 1992).

Family and twin studies

Based on the results of a family study, Fyer et al. (1990) concluded that specific phobia is a highly familial disorder that does not transmit risk for other phobic or anxiety disorders. An extended study by the same authors revealed further support for a specific familial contribution to simple or specific phobias (Fyer et al., 1995).

In a twin study, Torgersen (1979) found monozygotic twins more often concordant than dizygotic twins with respect to phobic fears, with the exception of separation fear. He concluded that genetic factors play a part in the development of phobic fears. Developmental factors further contributed to the vulnerability. Among monozygotic pairs, the second born (and shorter at birth) twin was also the more fearful, dependent, reserved and less self-confident in childhood. A large study in female twins indicated that genetic factors play a significant but by no means overwhelming role in the aetiology of phobias (Kendler et al., 1992). Among animal phobics, higher heritability and lower familial and environmental influences were aetiologically important. The opposite was true for situational phobias; moreover, environmental factors that specifically predisposed individuals to situational phobias were three times as important as environmental experiences that predisposed persons to all phobias (Kendler et al., 1992).

Etiology and pathogenesis

Biological factors

Certain childhood fears are part of normal development. As cognitive development advances, children first become anxious when separated from their mothers or when facing strangers; later, they become fearful of animals and, finally, of social situations. In general, these fears are transitory and can be regarded as adaptive and protective responses of the developing organism (Marks, 1987).

Even among adults, certain stimuli are more likely to trigger phobias. Darwin (1877) suggested that some childhood fears are innate and reflect past evolutionary dangers. Seligman (1971) hypothesized that humans, like animals, are 'prepared' to develop certain fears. Such genetic predispositions are well known in animals. For instance, monkeys fear snakes even if they have never been exposed to them. Behaviorists originally believed that the mind is a tabula rasa and that, with appropriate intervention, any stimulus might become a trigger for anxiety (Watson & Morgan, 1917). Several studies, however, strongly suggest that persons condition more easily to certain stimuli, for instance snakes and spiders, than to other more traumatic experiences, such as air raids (Rachman, 1977). The fact that humans are 'hardwired' to respond to certain situations with fear may explain the prominence of certain phobias. One also has to consider that persons may become sensitized to certain stimuli by frequent environmental exposure making them look 'prepared' (Marks, 1987; Davey, 1995).

Neuroanatomical localization

Recent imaging studies give some understanding of the brain areas involved when a person experiences phobic fears. Rauch et al. (1995) conducted the most sophisticated study to date of the neuroanatomy of simple phobias. Using positron emission tomography (PET) with $150\text{-}CO_2$, the investigators scanned patients with small animal phobias during exposure to a feared object and a control stimulus. Exposure to the feared object led to significant blood flow increases in the anterior cingulate cortices, insular cortex, anterior temporal cortex, posterior medial orbitofrontal cortex and thalamus, which suggest that the simple phobic state is mediated by paralimbic structures. A second study measured cerebral blood flow changes with PET in snake phobics after exposure to the phobic stimuli (Fredrikson et al., 1993). Patients exhibited blood flow increases in the visual association cortex and thalamus but not the prefrontal cortex. Mountz et al. (1989) also measured cerebral blood flow using PET in patients with simple animal phobias. Scans were taken during rest and immediately after exposure to the feared object. Cerebral blood flow decreased during confrontation, but this was attributed to hyperventilation. Similarly, another study that measured changes in blood flow while patients listened to a taped description of exposure to the phobic stimulus found only reduced flow (O'Carroll et al., 1993). Obviously, results of imaging studies are affected by scanning procedures, presentation of stimuli, and other concomitant conditions such as fatigue; however, two studies reported activation of the thalamus and one activation of the paralimbic structures during the challenge. Only one study reported activation of prefrontal regions, perhaps reflecting differences in cognitive processing of stimuli that in one case involved acute exposure (Fredrikson et al., 1993) and in another case prolonged exposure to a feared object (Rauch et al., 1995).

Learning and memory

Recent studies of learning and memory – described in greater detail in Chapter 1 – may explain the formation of bonds between certain stimuli and affective responses. Declarative memories that are descriptive of the stimulus are probably formed in the hippocampus, while affective memories are formed in the amygdala. Other areas of the brain, especially the prefrontal cortices, are also intimately involved in the generation and fixation of memories. The formation of memories is accomplished through neuronal change called long-term potentiation (LTP). LTP initiates a cascade of change that leads to synaptic alternation in the brain and to fixation of newly acquired memories. Norepinephrine as well as corticotropin-releasing hormone that are elevated during arousal, further potentiate the formation of LTP, thereby strengthening a memory and its affective response. Interestingly, habituation to a previously, but no longer, noxious stimuli does not occur passively. Habituation requires active change in systems that are involved in learning of the memory, in this case a phobic memory (Davis, 1992). This may explain why phobias do not weaken in the absence of exposure to the stimulus but remain unchanged until contact with the stimulus occurs. Only active learning through exposure, which convinces a person of the harmlessness of the stimulus, leads to a reduction of the fear response. Our present knowledge of acquisition of affective memories, however, fails to explain why a phobic person develops such excessive and persistent reactions, and why they develop only to some, but not other, fear-inducing situations.

Physiologic reactivity

Persons with uncomplicated specific phobias are generally anxious only when facing the feared stimulus. In contrast to other anxiety disorders, skin conductance shows few spontaneous fluctuations, and forearm blood flow is not elevated in phobic patients at rest. Their autonomic response resembles that of non-anxious controls as long as they are outside of the phobic situation (Hoehn-Saric et al., 1993). They habituate more rapidly than agoraphobics or social phobics (Lader et al., 1967), especially those with low anxiety levels and little social impairment (Lader et al., 1967). Some phobics exhibit a stronger startle response to loud noises, a response that diminishes with successful treatment (de Jong et al., 1993).

Specific phobias are not homogeneous (Himle et al., 1989) and subgroups may differ in their response to anxiety-provoking stimulations. Verburg et al. (1994) reported that animal phobics were not more vulnerable to CO_2 inhalation than controls, but that persons phobic of situations and natural phenomena, such as heights, thunderstorms or wind, reacted more strongly. The increase in subjective anxiety in the latter groups was comparable to that observed in panic disorder. Thus, some types of phobics have higher trait anxiety than normals or animal phobics.

When facing or imagining phobic stimuli, patients react physiologically with greater elevations in heart rate, blood pressure, forearm blood flow, skin conductance and respiration than they do to other frightening images (Geer, 1966; Hoehn-Saric et al., 1993; McNeil et al., 1993). The phobics' response also differs quantitatively from that of normals. When spider phobics were presented with slides of spiders, they showed a defensive response with acceleration of heart rate, cephalic vasoconstriction and increased palmar skin conductance. Controls showed an orienting response with heart rate deceleration, cephalic vasodilatation and an increase in skin conductance. Neutral slides elicited an orienting response from phobics but no response from controls (Hare & Blevings, 1975).

Patients with multiple phobias are generally more anxious than those with single phobias and have stronger heart rate responses to phobic stimuli (McNeil et al., 1993). Highly aroused subjects tend to show diffuse autonomic responding during acquisition conditioning and do not differentiate between reinforced and unreinforced cues. These subjects also fail to extinguish after multiple trials, which suggests that highly anxious individuals not only acquire fears easily but generalize those fears to irrelevant stimuli. Furthermore, they continue to react fearfully even in the absence of adverse consequences (Hugdahl et al., 1977).

Physiological and behavioral responses generally are poorly correlated. Subtypes that are fearful and socially anxious have more uniform expression of physiological responses, phobic imagery, and phobic behavior. Non-anxious individuals with single phobias tended to show weaker correlations between physiological and behavioral responses (McNeil et al., 1993). During treatment further dissociation often occurs. Although physiological, subjective and behavioral responses tend to change in the same direction, there may be little correspondence between the amount of change in each system. For instance, skin conductance may decrease while subjective fear and behavioral responses show little change (Mathews, 1971).

Neuroendocrine systems

Extensive neuroendocrine studies have been conducted by Curtis and associates. In one study (Curtis et al., 1976), patients with circumscribed phobias were treated with in vivo flooding and blood samples were drawn every 20 minutes during five sessions. The first, second and fifth sessions were control sessions, while flooding was carried out during the third and fourth sessions. Plasma cortisol secretion followed a general downward curve at each session. Cortisol levels were higher during the first and second sessions, which suggests a novelty effect. The authors concluded that adrenal activity is not ordinarily a part of the phobic reaction or that chronicity caused extinction of an earlier response. In another study (Curtis et al., 1978) involving flooding, the plasma cortisol response of phobic patients was inconsistent and showed marked individual variation. Only half of the patients responded with increased cortisol secretion in spite of high anxiety. Moreover, when a cortisol increase was associated with flooding, it usually occurred before, during and after the confrontation. During procedures, dental phobics were found to have increased salivary cortisol levels (Benjamin et al., 1992). Flooding led to elevations in growth hormone in some but not all phobic patients (Curtis et al., 1979). Thus, endocrine responses to phobic stimuli are more complex than peripheral physiological responses; they are highly variable and are not clearly related to the intensity of fear during exposure.

Neurotransmitter systems

Two studies (Arntz et al., 1993; Merckelbach et al., 1993) examined the relationship between phobias and the brain opiod system. The acquisition of an aversive response was not altered by the blockade of this system by naltrexone. Naltrexone brought out greater avoidance but did not affect emotional, cognitive and physiological responses. Thus, the opiod system may be involved in the expression of some specific phobias, but it is certainly not of major importance in its psychobiology.

Physiological response of blood-injury phobics

The physiological response of blood-injury phobics differs from that of other specific phobics. In contrast to the predominantly sympathetic response of other phobics, blood-injury phobics exhibit a biphasic physiological response. At first, they experience an increase in heart rate and in blood pressure followed by a sharp drop (Thyer et al., 1985; Marks, 1988). Some patients also hyperventilate before procedures, such as phlebotomy, thereby inducing hypocapnia and reduced cerebral blood flow (Foulds, 1993). Patients who faint or are on the edge of doing so develop massive bradycardia and a drop in blood pressure or both. Bradycardia may result in asystole accompanied by apnea that can last up to 25 seconds (Graham, 1961). Interestingly, patients with blood-injury phobia do not differ from normal subjects on cardiovascular or respiratory parameters during rest or physical challenges, such as the cold pressure test, Master's two-step test, or postural changes (Ruetz et al., 1967; Steptoe & Wardle, 1988). They respond as normal persons do, with increased heart rate to mental stressors, such as arithmetic or the Stroop color-card test (L-G. Öst, unpublished study, cited by Marks, 1988).

The biphasic response of patients with blood-injury phobia represents an initial sympathetic activation, followed by a sudden cessation of sympathetic activity accompanied by parasympathetic activation. The initial sympathetic activation manifests itself in increased heart rate and blood pressure, increased vasoconstriction and, possibly, epinephrine and norepinephrine excretion. The subsequent drop in heart rate probably results from a sudden increase in the cardiac vagal tone; the drop in blood pressure is associated with a sudden cessation in sympathetic impulses causing vasoconstriction (Wallin & Sundlof, 1982). Therefore, the bradycardia may be altered by atropine but not the hypotension. Marks (1988), pointing to the high familial incidence of blood-injury phobia, believes that it represents an inherited exaggeration of the autonomic response to injury.

Psychological factors

Several psychological theories have been used to explain the aetiology of phobias, and based on these theories, methods of treatment have been developed. Freud believed that phobias were not related to obvious stimuli but to hidden and unacceptable sources of anxiety, for instance, hatred toward a loved one. In the process of symptom formation, these sources were excluded from consciousness by repression and attached to the manifest phobic objects by displacement. Freud recognized that phobias do not yield to psychological exploration alone, but that treatment necessitates direct confrontation with the feared object (Hollander et al., 1988).

Aversive conditioning

Behaviorists regard phobias as the product of aversive conditioning. Based on such theory, Wolpe (1958) developed a treatment method using 'reciprocal inhibition'. He hypothesized that relaxation during mental visualization of phobic stimuli would reduce sympathetic and increase parasympathetic tone. As fear and relaxation are not compatible, a step-wise induction of feared stimuli should gradually lead to desensitization. However, phobias in children rarely follow traumatic events, although some early traumas may have been forgotten; traumatic events more frequently cause phobias in adults (Marks, 1987). Mowrer's two-factor theory states that phobias develop in two steps (Mowrer, 1960). First, fear is a classical conditioned response to a phobic stimulus. Subsequent avoidance behavior is anxiety-reducing and serves to prevent extinction from occurring. According to this theory, contact with the stimulus, as occurs in exposure therapy, is necessary for fear reduction and unlearning of the phobia.

Vicarious learning

More frequently phobias seem to be acquired through vicarious learning, particularly when children observe fears in adults. Modeling, which is based on social learning theory (Bandura, 1977), tries to undue such learned responses through examples (Bandura et al., 1977). Also, some phobias may be induced by information and instruction, although high authority of the inductor and anxious predisposition of the inductee appear to be prerequisites. For a more detailed discussion see Schneier et al. (1995).

Once a phobia is established, cognitive response patterns change. For example, a dichotic listening task requires that a person attend to one message to the exclusion of another and recognize the occurrence of target words appearing in both messages. A clinical phobic group recognized more phobia-relevant target words than a control group due to superior recognition of words that were anxiety generating (Burgess et al., 1981). Similar results were obtained in a study using masked and unmasked phobic stimuli. Recognition of a stimulus is made difficult when it is immediately followed by a masking stimulus. Animal phobics responded with greater skin conductance elevation to unmasked as well as masked phobic stimuli which suggests that phobic patients are sensitized to such a degree that they anticipate potentially threatening stimuli (Öhman et al., 1994).

Clinical picture

Persons with specific phobias react with fear to situations that they recognize as harmless. The intensity of their reaction varies from controllable discomfort to full panic with palpitations, shortness of breath, sweating, trembling and shaking and, in severe phobias, even incontinence or fainting. They may freeze or their behavior may become erratic. For instance, attempts to avoid feared animals while driving may lead to accidents. The fear generally subsides when the stimulus is removed. Uncomplicated specific phobics do not display other psychopathology and are not particularly anxious. Severe phobics, however, may develop anticipatory anxiety or anxiety in anticipation of encounters with the feared stimuli. If such stimuli are frequently present – for instance, birds or dogs on the street or thunderstorms during the warm season – the anticipatory anxiety may become confining. In one survey 25.5% of individuals with 'pure' phobias viewed themselves impaired, 30.3% sought help and 6.3% took medication (Magee et al., 1996). Thus, relatively few phobics seek treatment; instead the majority rearrange their lifestyle to accommodate their fears.

Individuals seeking treatment frequently have phobias involving dogs and cats, elevators, or transportation. They generally have multiple phobias and experience panic attacks in the presence of the feared objects or situations. Untreated individuals typically report only one phobia that is seldom complicated by panic attacks (Chapman et al., 1993). Phobics often seek treatment because changing circumstances force confrontations with a dreaded cue, because their lifestyle has become too restricted, or because they have learned about available treatment (McGlynn & McNeil, 1990). Persons with multiple phobias sometimes request help for phobias that cause problems but not for phobias they can avoid. For example, a priest, who fainted during mass and developed a fear of this religious observance, wanted to overcome this professionally incapacitating fear, but as he traveled rarely was not interested in the treatment of his fear of flying.

Subtypes

Animal phobias

Animal fears develop normally in children between the ages of 2 and 4 years then subside. Mild fears of animals are extremely common in adults but are rarely strong enough to be called phobias (Silverman & Nelles, 1990). Animal phobias generally begin in early childhood usually before ages 8–10 years. They occur predominantly in women and, untreated, remain stable or worsen with age. Patients generally come from stable families, but often they were fearful and shy as children. The mode of onset is usually unknown. In one study almost 70% of patients could not identify a cause for their fear, while the remainder recalled frightening encounters with animals or vicarious experiences (McNally & Steketee, 1985). Other surveys report larger proportions of cases that appear to result from conditioning (Öst et al., 1981). Animal phobias that have their onset in adulthood generally start with a traumatic experience such as a dog bite (Marks, 1987).

Animal phobias manifest themselves as isolated fears of animals, such as birds, cats, dogs, spiders, moths or bees. The sight of such animals evokes fear and leads to their avoidance. Contact with the animal evokes intense fear, distress, panic, sweating, and trembling. Sudden movements of the species are particularly frightening, and defensive or erratic movements by the phobic person may worsen the situation. A bee phobic, instead of being quiet, may wave his hands when he sees a bee, and this may result in his being stung. A driver, noticing a spider, may make defensive movements and loose control of his vehicle. Panic subsides when the stimulus is removed.

The degree of disability varies with the intensity of fear and how common is the species. Anticipatory anxiety may lead to avoidance that can approach the severity seen in agoraphobia. Marks (1987) described a woman who was so afraid of birds that she was unable to go out of her house. It can also, as mentioned, lead to uncontrolled responses. For instance, a woman who could not swim jumped from a boat into the water to avoid a spider (Marks, 1987). Often phobics fear the animal less than their reaction of panic with potential catastrophic consequence (e.g., causing an accident). Some patients are plagued by fear-related nightmares.

Other frequent phobias

Thunderstorm phobics anticipate bad weather and listen with fear to weather reports. They feel worse during seasons in which storms are frequent and long for the safer winter. During a thunderstorm, they may cover themselves with a blanket, hide in the cellar, turn off the electricity and use candles. They may even become incontinent as a result of the fear (Marks, 1987).

Claustrophobics fear closed places, such as tunnels and elevators. They avoid such places, and may, in a building, walk up and down ten floors rather than take an elevator. A medically important claustrophobia is the fear of being enclosed during medical procedures, particularly during magnetic resonance imaging (MRI) scans. Some patients refuse and others need heavy sedation to tolerate scanning procedures (Melendez & McCrank, 1993).

Fear of heights is common but is rarely incapacitating. Some fear traveling in buses, trains, boats or cars. After assaults exaggerated fears of going out, without other symptoms of posttraumatic stress disorder (PTSD), are common. This is discussed in greater detail in Chapter 6 on posttraumatic stress disorder. Fears of losing sphincter control may border on social phobia and obsessional preoccupation. Sexual anxiety or fear can lead to poor performance, failure of erection, premature ejaculation, anorgasmia, and vaginism. Fear of hospitals and of sick and dead persons may lead to embarrassing neglect of ill friends and relatives.

Blood-injury phobia

Blood injury phobia is probably a genetically determined autonomic response. This phobia has been reviewed by Marks (1987, 1988) and by Thyer et al. (1985). It has a high familial prevalence, with up to 68% of biological relatives affected. It is more frequently observed in monozygotic than dizygotic twins (Torgersen, 1979). Some patients, however, attribute the onset of their phobia to some traumatic event (Thyer et al., 1985). As normals also show mild vagal stimulation when seeing blood, the response of these phobics is not qualitatively different but is exaggerated. Blood-injury phobia has its onset in childhood. Mild fear of blood is common in children; 44% of 6 to 8-year-olds and 27% of 9 to 12-year-olds were found to be fearful of the sight of blood. Intense fear occurs only in 2–3% of children and adults, and is more frequent in women. Coexisting generalized anxiety is infrequent. The sight of blood or injury first leads to an increase in heart rate, followed by bradycardia, nausea, pallor, dizziness and, in more severe cases, fainting. For blood-injury phobics this can have serious consequences including avoidance of medical procedures, of pregnancy, or of entering a medical career. When such subjects must have blood taken, they should lie down to prevent fainting. In our experience, the blood pressure may drop precipitously even in the supine position. In contrast to other phobias, treatment using relaxation techniques may contribute to the drop of blood pressure. More effective are maneuvers involving heightening arousal by such means as tensing muscles and the stimulation of anger (Cohn et al., 1976; Öst & Sterner, 1987).

Phobia of dentistry

Fear of dentistry is common (Lindsay, 1983). A survey estimated that up to 40% of the population has some fears of dental interventions and sometimes avoid dentists but that only 5% have dental phobia (Kleinknecht et al., 1973). It usually starts in childhood or adolescence and may lead to disruptive behavior in children. In adults it leads to avoidance. Fear during dental procedures may be so intense that fainting occurs. Dental fears are more common in women and in persons who are introverted and neurotic, have less education and have made poorer progress in school. In addition, comorbidity with other anxiety disorders, depression, personality disorders, high levels of somatization and generalized phobic avoidance are frequent (Roy-Byrne et al., 1994). In treatment, educational pre-exposure, a gradual approach using reassurance, and peer modeling by video tape have been found useful (Marks, 1987).

Choking phobia

Some persons have an exaggeration of the normal protective gag reflex such that they are unable to brush their teeth or button their collars without gagging. At times smells and sights that are vaguely associated with unpleasant oral experiences may become triggers. Many patients are men who had a childhood onset. They are also prone to fears of dental procedures and social fears, being afraid of eating in the company of people not acquainted with their condition. This can lead to serious restrictions in social intercourse. Choking phobias can also be acquired suddenly after choking on food, and this is more often seen in women than men (McNally, 1994). A hypersensitive gag reflex has to be distinguished from dysphagia, a medical condition, and from globus hystericus. Treatment with exposure and learning to tolerate foreign objects in the mouth, while relaxing the jaws and tongue, is recommended (Marks, 1987).

Eating phobia

Eating phobias can overlap with hypersensitivity of the gag reflex, leading to a fear of choking. Solid food is more feared than soft food. This condition may lead to weight loss. Treatment includes training to tolerate solid food by gradually increasing it during meals. Another type of eating phobia is food aversion, which entails repugnance toward certain types of food, usually meat and greasy foods. Such foods cause nausea, retching, and, perhaps, vomiting. It usually starts in childhood or adolescence but also can be a conditioned response to chemotherapy. The reduction of food odors in cancer wards can diminish such food aversion. Some concentration camp survivors are unable to eat meat because the smell of it reminds them of the crematoria. Another type of food phobia is caused by severe allergic reactions to food that causes angioedema in the throat. The swelling of mucous membranes in the throat causes difficulties breathing, and if untreated, can lead to death. While such patients have reason to fear their condition, they may become unreasonably fearful and avoid safe food to the point of serious weight loss. Reeducation and gradual retraining can lead to the removal of this condition (Marks, 1987).

Flying phobia

Ten per cent of the general population avoids flying, and 20% of those who fly have substantial anxiety during the flight. Some fear that they might crash and die, others fear heights, confinement or instability of the aircraft (Greist & Greist, 1981). Treatment consists of graded exposure or desensitization in phantasy. Some airlines have programmes that combine teaching, relaxation and gradual exposure to the aircraft. They finish the course with a celebration or 'champagne' flight.

Space phobia

Space phobia is fear of falling in the absence of visuospatial support (Marks & Bebbington 1976; Marks, 1981). It usually occurs in patients with diverse neurological or cardiovascular disorders and mostly in elderly women. While space phobia is initiated by some unsteadiness, the fear related to it is greatly exaggerated. Sufferers, for instance, may be unable to cross a room except on their hands and knees or close to the wall. Marks (1987) described a patient who could hardly walk but could ride a bicycle. Space phobia starts late in life and is resistant to treatment. Sometimes mechanical devices, for example, a banister in a strategic place, may reduce the fear.

Phobias in childhood

Fears and phobias in children have a symptomatology similar to that of adults except that children often do not regard their fears as unreasonable (Silverman & Nelles, 1990). Fears in children are often transitory, lasting from one to several weeks. In some children, however, fears persist or change with age and cognitive sophistication into more realistic fears. Lasting fears may reflect higher trait anxiety. Children with phobias are more likely to improve than adults with phobias; however, in more than half of the children, the phobias, while improved, persist. When treated, phobias improve faster in younger than in older children, but even with treatment, 7% of children retain severe phobias. Phobias of animals, thunder and injections tend to persist into adulthood. The effect of phobias on the child depends on their severity. A child with a severe dog phobia may become practically housebound and neglect social activities and school. Severe phobias, even when they last a short time, may have a negative effect on the child's development.

Treatment of children with phobias requires the participation of parents. Often children reflect the fears of a parent, and improvement in the parent leads to improvement in the child (Windheuser, 1977). Important also is the assessment of secondary gain. Relaxation, cognitive coping, exposure, modeling and the treatment of coexisting fears in parents have been found to be effective (Silverman et al., 1990).

Natural history

Onset

The onset of phobias varies greatly and can be observed from childhood to old age. Animal and blood-injury phobias, and fears of thunderstorms generally start in childhood (Marks, 1987). In a large survey, Magee et al. (1996) placed the average onset of phobia at age 15 years.

Course and outcome

Some childhood fears, such as fears of animals, persist into adulthood; however, most phobic children develop into normal adults (Marks, 1987). Untreated, phobias generally remain unchanged or worsen with time. Motivated individuals may treat their phobias by themselves. Marks (1987) quotes the German poet, Goethe, who conquered his fear of heights by climbing the steeples of churches. Such determination, however, is uncommon. While childhood fears tend to fade with age, fears that persist, or are acquired in adulthood remain chronic. Particularly resistant to change are phobias that start in old age. Under severe stress, such as imprisonment, neurotic symptoms, including phobias, tend to disappear but reemerge after life has returned to normal (Kral, 1951).

Predictors of outcome

Good outcomes of treated phobic disorders have been associated with shorter duration, inner conflict as a cause of fear, being stressed at the onset, lower levels of free anxiety, greater need for success and less avoidance, better relationship between parents during childhood, higher social class, need for order, and greater satisfaction at work (Persson et al., 1984). Poor outcomes of exposure treatment were found in older patients and in patients who had a greater number of phobics in their family (Cameron et al., 1986). Patients with immature defense styles, particularly those using projection, had less favorable outcomes (Muris & Herckelbach, 1996). Thus, healthier personality, lower levels of anxiety, higher motivation, development of the phobia during a period of stress and younger age are all favorable predictors.

Complications

Phobias may be a minor nuisance or may severely restrict a person's life. Fear of medical procedures may delay necessary treatment of illnesses; fear of traveling may adversely affect a person's professional development; fears of gagging may restrict social life. Phobias that place limitations on social life may also affect other family members and cause conflict. In children, severe phobias may retard psychosocial development.

Differential diagnosis

There are rarely difficulties in diagnosing a 'pure' specific fear. Specific phobias need to be distinguished from realistic fears, such as the fear of going into an unsafe neighborhood at night or the fear of driving after one has had several accidents. Specific fears differ from agoraphobia by being circumscribed, while agoraphobia tends to generalize to all situations in which panic attacks have occurred. Moreover, phobic stimuli almost invariably elicit fear reactions in specific phobics, while they often, but not invariably, cause panic attacks in agoraphobics. The specific phobic fears facing a phobic object or situation; the agoraphobic fears having a panic attack in certain situations.

Social phobia is characterized by fear of situations in which a person feels scrutinized, irrespective of the importance of the situation. Obsessional fears generally focus on violence, dirt, contamination or neglect and often involve ritualistic undoing. PTSD is characterized by intrusive memories of a traumatic experience which cause fear. While triggers that cause fear in PTSD patients can generalize, they remain conceptually linked to the original trauma. For example, a soldier traumatized in battle may react with panic to the sound of a backfiring car. School phobia, a childhood disturbance, may have diverse causes, ranging from a true phobia – such as fear of ringing the school bell – to fear of failure, fear of a particular teacher or of schoolmates, or to an excuse to avoid the boredom of school.

At times, temporal lobe epilepsy causes ictal fear that is characterized by sudden onset and a repetitious clinical picture. One patient hallucinated snakes and felt terrified by them each time she had a seizure; however, this disorder is rarely stimulus specific and causes clouding or loss of consciousness. Rarely, temporal lobe seizures can be followed by days of fear during which the person is in a postictal state (Marks, 1987).

Treatment

Management

The most important ingredient in the treatment of phobias is motivation. Highly motivated individuals quickly overcome even severe phobias, whereas unmotivated persons rarely loose them. For instance, a well-known scientist overcame his fear of flying because he wanted to attend international meetings. He also overcame his fear of tunnels because the drive from home to his work place went through a tunnel. On the other hand, he never overcame his fear of driving because he was always chauffeured. In a motivated person, it suffices to encourage a programme of gradual exposure to the feared object or situation within a safe environment. Obviously, if a dog phobic encounters a vicious dog, it will only deepen his fear, whereas playing with a mild-mannered small dog may decrease it. Very early Kraepelin (1915) observed that once phobics realize that they can overcome their fear, they actively approach the feared situation and undo the phobia with little help.

Reasons for seeking professional help vary. Patients may seek treatment when they move to an environment where feared animals are frequent, for instance, from the city to the country. Others may come on the insistence of family members who have been affected by the patient's fear. Some seek help with a phobia after other problems, such as depression, had brought them to the psychiatrist. A number of techniques have been developed that help patients expose themselves systematically to feared situations. Medications are of minor value in the treatment of specific phobias but they can be useful in initiating the desensitization process in very anxious individuals.

Pharmacotherapy

Benzodiazepines have been found useful in patients who fear the initial exposures. Marks et al. (1972) found that diazepam was more effective than placebo when given 4 but not 1 hour before exposure. In another study animal phobics were exposed to the feared stimuli for 10 minutes after single doses of a beta-blocker, tolamolol, a benzodiazepine, diazepam, or placebo. Tolamolol abolished tachycardia but not avoidance or anxiety, whereas diazepam reduced avoidance but not tachycardia (Bernadt et al., 1980). The medications had little effect on subjective fear. Thus, beta-blockers have not been found very useful (Fagerstrom et al., 1985). Alcohol may reduce anxiety but was not found effective in a study of animal phobics (Thyer & Curtis, 1984). Imipramine, effective in the treatment of panic attacks, was not superior to placebo in specific phobics (Zitrin et al., 1983). Thus, with the exception of benzodiazepines, medications have little use in the treatment of specific phobias. The disadvantage of benzodiazepines is that some patients, while gaining situational relief, lose motivation for overcoming their phobias. Some flight phobics regularly use benzodiazepines before flights and are unwilling to fly without them.

Psychotherapy

Exposure in vivo

The preferred treatment of simple phobias is direct or, when this is not possible, imaginary exposure through behavior therapy (Marks, 1987). Behavioral techniques help the patient expose himself or herself to feared situations thereby learning that these situations need not be feared. Before exposure, a detailed description of the circumstances that trigger fear is obtained. Then, a fear and avoidance hierarchy or individualized list of increasingly distressing phobic situations is developed in collaboration with the patient. In the process, patients may rate fear and avoidance on 100 point scales. Important also is a functional analysis that identifies potential antecedents and consequences that may serve to maintain phobic behavior, such as secondary gain. Designing successful exposure-based treatment often requires much creativity. Hierarchies need to be individually tailored, and different approaches may be used for patients who react more behaviorally as opposed to those who react more physiologically. Cognitive aspects also need to be assessed. One has to elicit the nature of patients' worries. For instance, does a flight phobic worry about a possible crash, about his or her body's reactions or about an embarrassing loss of control (Schneier et al., 1995)?

Exposure is usually conducted gradually, step-by-step from the least distressing to the most feared confrontation. The oldest method, systematic desensitization by reciprocal inhibition, starts with relaxation (Wolpe, 1958). Then, the therapist induces vivid imaginations of feared situations, starting with the least distressing item in the hierarchy, until anxiety occurs. The patient signals such anxiety by raising a finger. When this occurs, imaging is replaced by relaxation. The image is then reintroduced until no anxiety is experienced. At this point the patient is instructed to move to the next item in the hierarchy. Treatment is based on the assumption that a gradual approach permits anxiety reduction at each step, and therefore, encourages facing greater challenges with subsequent exposures. The disadvantage of systematic desensitization is that not all patients learn to relax sufficiently and some are unable to visualize feared situations. Moreover, live exposure has been found to be more effective than imaginary exposure (Crowe et al., 1972). A snake phobic, for instance, may be exposed to a black and white photograph of a snake, then to a colored photograph, a stuffed snake, a live snake in a cage and finally encouraged to hold a harmless snake. Anxiety may be reduced faster when the patient has some control of the degree of exposure (McGlynn et al., 1995).

Modifications of exposure

Exposure therapy may be gradual or intensive. The most intensive approach is flooding, which involves exposing the patient all at once to his or her greatest fear in the expectation that prolonged exposure will lead to anxiety reduction. Flooding is very anxiety provoking and does not necessarily yield better results than a more gradual approach.

Participant modeling is also useful. The therapist first models the desired behavior by making contact with the feared stimulus and then asks the patient to do the same (Bandura et al., 1977). Marks (1987) quotes a successful application of modeling. When Queen Elizabeth feared the extraction of a painful tooth, the Bishop of London called a surgeon and had one of his teeth extracted in the presence of Her Majesty. His example encouraged the Queen to submit to the operation.

While in vivo or real life exposure is the preferable approach, it is not always possible. In this case, imaginary techniques may be used. For example, a person afraid of lightening may practice anxiety reduction in phantasy by imagining increasingly fearful situations. The hierarchy may start with therapist-assisted imagination of a weather report announcing a thunderstorm and end with the imagination of lightening striking a lightening rod loudly, but harmlessly. The use of computer-generated virtual reality for phobic conditions that do not permit direct exposure is promising. Virtual reality integrates real-time computer graphics, body tracking devices, visual display, and other sensory input devices that immerse a subject in a computer-generated environment. While the method is technically complex and needs further perfection, it has been successfully used for fears of heights, elevators and flying (Rothbaum et al., 1996).

In addition, self-exposure techniques in which persons learn to practice exposure by themselves should be taught and monitored (Ghosh et al., 1988). Here, as with therapist-assisted techniques, the exposure needs to be long enough for anxiety reduction to occur during the session.

Treatment outcome

Clinical observation indicates that patients who, after exposure feel no relief and remain convinced that the next exposure will be equally horrible, do not improve with treatment. Improvement occurs only when sessions end with anxiety reduction and a feeling of accomplishment and mastery (Bandura et al., 1977). A good therapist–patient relationship contributes to the outcome, particularly of exposure in vivo. The relationship alone does not extinguish the phobia, exposure does (Watson, 1973).

While specific phobias respond well to behavioral interventions, treatment is not always effective. A significant proportion of patients experience only moderate improvement and another 25–50% of patients drop out of therapy (Schneier et al., 1995). Poor results are obtained when secondary gain outweighs the benefits of treatment, when the potential gain of therapy is low, when avoidance is high, and when elderly persons who have acquired fears are treated. Poor outcomes are also seen when phobias are part of more complex psychiatric illnesses (Kraepelin, 1915).

Other psychotherapies also have been found effective as long as they lead patients to expose themselves to the feared situation. Schneier and colleagues (1995) concluded that 'the patient will benefit from any form of support and persuasion enabling him or her to tolerate sustained exposure'.

References

American Psychiatric Association. 1980. *Diagnostic and Statistical Manual of Mental Disorders*, Third Edition. American Psychiatric Association,

Washington, DC.

American Psychiatric Association. 1987. *Diagnostic and Statistical Manual of Mental Disorders*, Third Edition, Revised. American Psychiatric Association, Washington, DC.

American Psychiatric Association. 1994. *Diagnostic and Statistical Manual of Mental Disorders*, Fourth Edition, American Psychiatric Association, Washington, DC.

Anderson, J. C., Williams, D., McGee, R. et al. 1987. DSM-III disorders in pre-adolescent children: Prevalence in a large sample from the general population. *Arch. Gen. Psychiatry*. 44: 69–76.

Anthony, J. C., Folstein, M., Romanoski, A. J. et al. 1985. Comparison of the lay Diagnostic Interview Schedule and a standardized psychiatric diagnosis. *Arch. Gen. Psychiatry* 42: 667–675.

Arntz, A., Merckelbach, H. & de Jong, P. J. 1993. Opioid antagonist affects behavioral effects of exposure in vivo. *J. Consult. Clin. Psychol.* 61: 865–870.

Bandura, A. 1977. *Social Learning Theory*. Prentice-Hall, Englewood Cliff, NJ.

Bandura, A., Adams, N. E. & Beyer, J. 1977. Cognitive processes mediating behavioral change. *J. Pers. Soc. Psychol.* 35: 125–139.

Barlow, D. H. 1985. The dimensions of anxiety disorders. In *Anxiety and the Anxiety Disorders*, eds. A. H. Tuma, and J. Maser, pp. 479–500, Lawrence Erlbaum, Hillsdale, NJ.

Benjamins, C., Asscheman, H. & Schuurs, A. H. B. 1992. Increased salivary cortisol in severe dental anxiety. *Psychophysiology* 29: 302–305.

Bernadt, M. W., Silverstone, T. & Singleton, W. 1980. Beta-adrenergic blockade in phobic subjects. *Br. J. Psychiatry* 137: 452–457.

Brown, D. R., Eaton, W. W. & Sussman, L. 1990. Racial differences in prevalence of phobic disorders. *J. Nerv. Ment. Dis.* 178: 434–441.

Burgess, I. S., Jones, L. M., Robertson, S. A. et al. 1981. The degree of control exerted by phobic and non-phobic verbal stimuli over the recognition behaviour of phobic and non-phobic subjects. *Behav. Res. Ther.* 19: 233–243.

Cameron, O. G., Thyer, B. A., Feckner, S. et al. 1986. Behavior therapy of phobias: Predictors of outcome. *Psychiat. Res.* 19: 245–246.

Chapman, T. F., Fyer, A. J., Mannuzza, S. et al. 1993. A comparison of treated and untreated simple phobia. *Am. J. Psychiatry* 150: 816–818.

Cohn, C. K., Kron, R. E. & Brady, J. P. 1976. A case of blood-illness phobia treated behaviorally. *J. Nerv. Ment. Dis.* 162: 65–68.

Crowe, M. J., Marks, I. M., Agras, W. S. et al. 1972. Time-limited desensitization, implosion and shaping for phobic patients. *Behav. Res. Ther.* 10: 319.

Curtis, G. C., Buxton, M., Nesse, R. M. et al. 1976. 'Flooding in vivo' during the circadian phase of minimal cortisol secretion: Anxiety and therapeutic success without adrenal cortical activation. *Biol. Psychiatry* 11: 101–107.

Curtis, G. C., Nesse, R. M., Buxton, M. et al. 1978. Anxiety and plasma cortisol at the crest of the circadian cycle: Reappraisal of a classical hypothesis. *Psychosom. Med.* 40: 368–378.

Curtis, G. C., Nesse, R. M., Buxton, M. et al. 1979. Plasma growth hormone: Effect of anxiety during flooding in vivo. *Am. J. Psychiatry* 136: 410–413.

Darwin, C. 1877. A biographical sketch of an infant. *Mind* 2: 285–294.

Davey, G. C. L. 1995. Preparedness and phobia: Specific evolved associations or a generalized expectancy bias? *Behav. Brain Sci.* 18: 289–325.

Davis, M. 1992. The role of the amygdala in fear-potentiated startle: Implications for animal models of anxiety. *TIPS* 13: 35–41.

de Jong, P. J., Arntz, A. & Merckelbach, H. 1993. The startle probe response as an instrument for evaluating exposure effects in spider phobia. *Adv. Behav. Res. Ther.* 15: 301–316.

Di Nardo, P. A., Moras, K., Barlow, D. H. et al. 1993. Reliability of DSM-III-R anxiety disorder categories: Using the Anxiety Disorders Interview Schedule-Revised (ADIS-R). *Arch. Gen. Psychiatry* 50: 251–256.

Fagerstrom, K. O., Hugdahl, K. & Lundstrom, N. 1985. Effect of beta-receptor blockade on anxiety with reference to the three-systems model of phobic behavior. *Neuropsychobiology* 13: 187–193.

Faravelli, C., Guerrini Degl'Innocenti, B. & Giardinelli, L. 1989. Epidemiology of anxiety disorders in Florence. *Acta Psychiatr. Scand.* 79: 308–312.

Foulds, J. 1993. Cerebral circulation during treatment of blood-injury phobia: A case study. *Behav. Psychother.* 21: 137–146.

Fredrikson, M., Wik, G., Greitz, T. et al. 1993. Regional cerebral blood flow during experimental phobic fear. *Psychophysiology* 30: 126–130.

Fyer, A. J., Mannuzza, S., Gallops, M. S. et al. 1990. Familial transmission of simple phobias and fears: A preliminary report. *Arch. Gen. Psychiatry* 47: 252–256.

Fyer, A. J., Mannuzza, S., Chapman, T. F. et al. 1995. Specificity in familial aggregation of phobic disorders. *Arch. Gen. Psychiatry* 52: 564–573.

Geer, H. 1966. Fear and autonomic arousal. *J. Abnorm. Psychol.* 4: 253–255.

Ghosh, A., Marks, I.M. & Carr, A. C. 1988. Therapist contact and outcome of self-exposure treatment for phobias: Controlled study. *Br. J. Psychiatry* 152: 234–238.

Graham, D. T. 1961. Prediction of fainting in blood donors. *Circulation* 3: 901–906.

Greist, J. H. & Greist, G. L. 1981. *Fearless Flying: A Passenger Guide to Modern Airline Travel.* Nelson Hall, Chicago.

Hare, R. D. & Blevings, G. 1975. Defensive responses to phobic stimuli. *Biol. Psychol.* 3: 1–13.

Hiller, W., von Bose, M., Dichtl, G. et al. 1990. Reliability of checklist-guided diagnoses for DSM-IIIR affective and anxiety disorders. *J. Affect. Disord.* 20: 235–247.

Himle, J. A., McPhee, K., Cameron, O. G. et al. 1989. Simple phobia: Evidence for heterogeneity. *Psychiatry Res.* 28: 25–30.

Hoehn-Saric, R. & McLeod, D. R. 1993. Somatic manifestations of normal and pathological anxiety. In *Biology of Anxiety Disorders*, eds., R. Hoehn-Saric, D. R. McLeod, pp. 177–222, American Psychiatric Press, Washington DC.

Hollander, E., Liebowitz, M. R. & Gorman, J. M. 1988. Anxiety disorders. In *Textbook of Psychiatry*, eds. J. A. Talbott, R. E. Hales, S. C. Yudofsky, American Psychiatric Press, Washington, DC.

Hugdahl, K., Fredrikson, M. & Ohman, A. 1977. 'Preparedness' and 'arousability' as determinants of electrodermal conditioning. *Behav. Res. Ther.* 15: 345–353.

Kendler, K. S., Neale, M. C., Kessler, R. C. et al. 1992. The genetic epidemiology of phobias in women: The interrelationship of agoraphobia, social phobia, situational phobia, and simple phobia. *Arch. Gen. Psychiatry* 49: 273–281.

Kleinknecht, R. A., Klepac, R. K. & Alexander, L. D. 1973. Origin and characteristics of fear of dentistry. *J. Am. Dent. Assoc.* 86: 824–847.

Kraepelin, E. 1915. *Psychiatrie.* Johann A. Barth, Leipzig.

Kral, V. A. 1951. Psychiatric observations under severe chronic stress. *Am. J. Psychiatry* 108: 185–192.

Lader, M. H., Gelder, M. G. & Marks, I. M. 1967. Palmar skin conductance measures as predictors of response to desensitization. *J. Psychosom. Res.* 11: 283–290.

Lindsay, S. J. E. 1983. Fear of dental treatment. In *Contributions to Medical Psychology III*, ed. S. Rachman, Pergamon, Oxford.

Magee, W. J., Eaton, W. W., Wittchen, H. U. et al. 1996. Agoraphobia, simple phobia, and social phobia in the National Comorbidity Survey. *Arch. Gen. Psychiatry* 53: 159–168.

Mannuzza, S., Fyer, A. J., Klein, .F. et al. 1986. Schedule for affective disorders and schizophrenia-lifetime version modified for the study of anxiety disorders: Rationale and conceptual development. *J. Psychiatr. Res.* 20: 317–325.

Mannuzza, S., Fyer, A. B., Martin, L. Y. et al. 1989. Reliability of anxiety assessment. *Arch. Gen. Psychiatry* 46: 1093–1101.

Marks, I. M., Marset, P., Boulougouris, J. et al. 1971. Physiological accompaniments of neutral and phobic imagery. *Psychol. Med.* 1: 299–307.

Marks, I. M. & Bebbington, P. 1976. Space phobia: Syndrome or agoraphobic variant? *Br. Med. J.* 2: 345–347.

Marks, I. M. 1981. Space 'phobia': a pseudo-agoraphobic syndrome. *J. Neurol. Neurosurg. Psychiatry* 44: 387–391.

Marks, I. M. 1987. *Fears, Phobias and Rituals.* Oxford University Press, New York.

Marks, I. M. 1988. Blood-injury phobia: A review. *Am. J. Psychiatry* 145: 1207–1214.

Marks, I. M., Viswanathan, R., Lipsedge, M. S. et al. 1972. Enhanced relief of phobias by flooding during waning diazepam effect. *Br. J. Psychiatry* 121: 493–505.

Marks, I. M. & Mathews, A. M. 1979. Brief standard self-rating for phobic patients. *Behav. Res. Ther.* 17: 263–267.

Mathews, A. M. 1971. Psychophysiological approaches to the investigation of desensitization and related procedures. *Psychol. Bull.* 76: 73–90.

Mathews, A. M., Gelder, M. G. & Johnston, G. W. 1981. *Agoraphobia: Nature and Treatment.* Tavistock, London.

McGlynn, F. D. & McNeil, D. W. 1990. Simple phobia in adulthood. In *Handbook of Child and Adult Psychopathology*, eds. M. Hersen, C. G. Last, Pergamon Press, New York.

McGlynn, F. D., Moore, P. M., Rose, M. P. et al. 1995. Effects of relaxation training on fear and arousal during in vivo exposure to a caged snake among DSM-III-R simple (snake) phobics. *J. Behav. Ther. Exper. Psychiatry* 26: 1–8.

McNally, R. J. 1994. Choking phobia: A review of the literature. *Compr. Psychiatry* 35: 83–89.

McNally, R. J. & Steketee, G. S. 1985. The etiology and maintenance of severe animal phobias. *Behav. Res. Ther.* 23: 431–435.

McNeil, D. W., Vrana, S. R., Melamed, B. G. et al. 1993. Emotional imagery in simple and social phobia: Fear versus anxiety. *J. Abnorm. Psychol.* 102: 212–225.

Melendez, J. C. & McCrank, E. 1993. Anxiety-related reactions associated with magnetic resonance imaging examinations. *JAMA* 270: 745–747.

Merckelbach, H., Arntz, A., De Jong, P. et al. 1993. Effects of endorphin blocking on conditioned SCR in humans. *Behav. Res. Ther.* 31: 775–779.

Miller, L. C., Barrett, C. L. & Hampe, E. 1974. Phobias of childhood in a prescientific era. In *Child Personality and Psychopathology: Current Topics*, ed. A. Davis, John Wiley, New York.

Mountz, J. M., Modell, J. G., Wilson, M. W. et al. 1989. Positron emission tomographic evaluation of cerebral blood flow during state anxiety in simple phobia. *Arch. Gen. Psychiatry* 46: 501–504.

Mower, O. H. 1960. *Learning Theory and Behavior*. John Wiley, New York.

Murris, P. & Herckelbach, H. 1996. Defense style and behaviour outcome in a specific phobia. *Psychol. Med.* 26: 635–639.

O'Carroll, R. E., Moffoot, A. P., Van Beck, M. et al. 1993. The effect of anxiety induction on the regional uptake of ^{99m}Tc-Exametazime in simple phobia as shown by single photon emission tomography (SPECT). *J. Affect. Disord.* 28: 203–210.

Öman, A. & Soares, J. F. 1994. 'Unconscious anxiety': Phobic responses to masked stimuli. *J. Abnorm. Psychol.* 103: 231–240.

Öst, L-G. & Hugdahl, K. 1981. Acquisition of phobias and anxiety response patterns in clinical patients. *Behav. Res. Ther.* 19: 439–447.

Öst, L-G. & Sterner, U. 1987. Applied tension: A specific behavioral method for treatment of blood phobia. *Behav. Res. Ther.* 25: 25–29.

Persson, G., Alstrom, J. E. & Nordlund, C. L. 1984. Prognostic factors with four treatment methods for phobic disorders. *Acta Psychiatr. Scand.* 69: 307–318.

Rachman, S. 1977. The conditioning theory of fear-acquisition: A critical examination. *Behav. Res. Ther.* 15: 375–387.

Rauch, L. S., Savage, C. R., Alpert, N. M. et al. 1995. A positron emission tomography study of simple phobic symptom provocation. *Arch. Gen. Psychiatry* 52: 20–28.

Regan, M. & Howard, R. 1995. Fear conditioning, preparedness, and contingent negative variation. *Psychophysiology* 32: 2208–2214.

Robins, L. N., Helzer, J. E., Weissman, M. M. et al. 1984. Lifetime prevalence of specific psychiatric disorders in three sites. *Arch. Gen. Psychiatry* 41: 949–958.

Rothbaum, B. O., Hodges, L., Watson, B. A. et al. 1996. Virtual reality exposure in the treatment of fear of flying: A case report. *Behav. Res. Ther.* 34: 477–481.

Roy-Byrne, P. P., Milgrom, P., Khoon-May, T. et al. 1994. Psychopathology and psychiatric diagnosis in subjects with dental phobia. *J. Anxiety Dis.* 8: 19–31.

Ruetz, P. P., Johnson, S. A., Callahan, R. et al. 1967. Fainting: A review of its mechanisms and a study in blood donors. *Medicine* 46: 363–384.

Schneier, F. R., Marshall, R. D., Street, L. et al. 1995. Social phobia and specific phobias. In *Treatments of Psychiatric Disorders*, ed. G. O. Gabbard, American Psychiatric Press, Washington, DC.

Seligman, M. E. P. 1971. Phobias and preparedness. *Behav. Ther.* 2: 307–320.

Silverman, W. K. & Nelles, W. B. 1990. Simple phobia in childhood. In *Handbook of Child and Adult Psychopathology*, eds. M. Hersen, C. G. Last, pp. 183–195, Pergamon Press, New York.

Spitzer, R. L., Williams, J. B. W., Gibbon, M. et al. 1992. The structured clinical interview for DSM-III-R (SCID) I: History, rationale, and description. *Arch. Gen. Psychiatry* 49: 624–629.

Steptoe, A. & Wardle. J. 1988. Emotional fainting and the psychophysiologic response to blood and injury: Autonomic mechanisms and coping strategies. *Psychosom. Med.* 50: 402–417.

Szymanski, J. & O'Donohue, W. 1995. Fear of spiders questionnaire. *J. Behav. Ther. Exper. Psychiatry* 26: 31–34.

Thyer, B. A. & Curtis, G. C. 1984. The effects of ethanol intoxication on phobic anxiety. *Behav. Res. Ther.* 22: 599–610.

Thyer, B. A., Himle, J. & Curtis, G. C. 1985. Blood-injury-illness phobia: A review. *J. Clin. Psychol.* 41: 451–456.

Torgersen, S. 1979. The nature and origin of common phobic fears. *Br. J. Psychiat.* 134: 343–351.

Tyrer, P. 1989. *Classification of Neurosis.* John Wiley, New York.

Verburg, C., Griez, E. & Meijer, J. 1994. A 35% carbon dioxide challenge in simple phobias. *Acta Psychiatr. Scand.* 90: 420–423.

Wallin, B. G. & Sundlof, G. 1982. Sympathetic outflow to muscles during vasovagal syncope. *J. Auton. Nerv. Sys.* 6: 287–291.

Warshaw, M. G., Keller, M. B. & Stout, R. L. 1994. Reliability and validity of the longitudinal interval follow-up evaluation for assessing outcome of anxiety disorders. *J. Psychiatr. Res.* 28: 531–545.

Watson, J. B. & Morgan, J. J. B. 1917. Emotional reactions and psychological experimentation. *Am. J. Psychol.* 28: 163–174.

Watson, J. P. 1973. Prolonged exposure in the therapy of phobias. *Curr. Psychiatric Ther.* 13: 83–89.

Windheuser, H. J. 1977. Anxious mothers as models for coping with anxiety. *Behav. Anal. Modif.* 2: 39–58.

Wolpe, J. 1958. *Psychotherapy by Reciprocal Inhibition.* Stanford University Press, Stanford, CA.

Wolpe, J. & Lang, P. 1964. Fear Survey Schedule for use in behavior therapy. *Behav. Res. Ther.* 2: 27–30.

World Health Organization. 1992. *The ICD-10 Classification of Mental and Behavioral Disorders.* pp. 91–101. World Health Organization, Geneva.

Zitrin, C. M., Klein, D. F. & Woerner, M. G. 1983. Treatment of phobias I. Comparison of imipramine and placebo. *Arch. Gen. Psychiatry* 40: 125–138.

6

Posttraumatic stress disorder

Definition

Posttraumatic stress disorder (PTSD) consists of a clearly defined syndrome that develops in the aftermath of a traumatic experience and that persists longer than 1 month. Shorter reactions to stressors or traumatic events are classified as acute stress reaction or, when milder, as adjustment disorders (American Psychiatric Association, 1994). While DSM-III and its subsequent modifications eliminated theoretical or aetiological explanations for psychiatric disorders and substituted a descriptive approach, an exception was made for these three disorders by linking them etiologically to specific adverse events (Brett et al., 1988). As PTSD is the more serious and usually more enduring disorder, most of this chapter deals with PTSD.

The impact of traumatic events on the psyche has been described by poets since antiquity. Vivid descriptions of traumatic reactions are provided by Shakespeare, whose Lady Macbeth cannot free her mind of Duncan's murder, and by Pushkin, whose Boris Godonov is plagued by memories of the murdered Zarevich. Samuel Peppy's diary records his reaction to the Great Fire of London in 1666, including anxiety, insomnia, nightmares and feelings of guilt for having saved himself and his property (Daly, 1983). In the nineteenth century, physicians became observant of the psychological and psychophysiological effects of massive trauma. They described physical and mental exhaustion and 'neurasthenia' in soldiers exposed to fighting in the American Civil War. A syndrome consisting of physical symptoms, phobias, nightmares and nervousness was named 'irritable heart' by DaCosta (Ramsay, 1990). During World War I similar symptoms in soldiers exposed to combat were called 'shell shock' and were attributed to brain injury. Greater awareness of the psychological impact of stress developed during World War II when Kardiner & Spiegel (1947) named the effect of trauma 'physioneurosis'. The classification of reactions to trauma was initiated in DSM-I with the category of 'gross stress reaction'. Subsequently this disorder's significance was reduced and relabeled 'transitory situational disturbance'. Influenced by increasing casualties from the Vietnam War, DSM-III defined posttraumatic stress disorder in 1980. The criteria for the disorders were subsequently modified in DSM-III-R and DSM-IV. In DSM-IV acute stress disorder, an earlier and more transitory reaction to traumas was added.

Acute stress disorder

Transitory reactions to trauma are common and may represent a healthy response. They may last hours, days or weeks, then fade in short time, or persist longer as an adjustment disorder, specific phobia, generalized anxiety disorder, or depression. Acute stress disorder is an acute reaction to trauma that is phenomenologically related to PTSD. Table 6.1 shows the DSM-IV criteria for this disorder. Its transitory nature makes it less well studied than PTSD. Acute stress disorder has been examined primarily in combat soldiers, hence the alternative label, acute combat stress reaction. It manifests itself in restlessness, psychomotor retardation, social withdrawal, sympathetic hyperactivity, increased startle response, confusion, dissociation, amnesia, reduction of awareness, derealization, nausea, vomiting, and paranoid thinking. In addition, overwhelming fear and reluctance to leave a secure setting have been described. Soldiers on the battlefield may become disorganized and act in ways that jeopardize their safety and that of their unit (Tomb, 1994).

By arbitrary rule, symptoms of acute stress disorder must occur within a month of the trauma, last for at least 2 days and resolve within 4 weeks; if symptoms last longer the disorder must be re-diagnosed. During the specified time, typical PTSD symptoms, including re-experiencing of traumatic events, avoidance of trauma-related stimuli, increased psychological arousal, and impaired functioning must occur (American Psychiatric Association, 1994; Spiegel & Classen, 1995). Thus, acute stress disorder resembles PTSD (Blank, 1993; Tomb, 1994); however, the disorder is more fluid than PTSD and can assume a multiplicity of forms. There is little evidence that individuals who develop adjustment disorders following traumatic events later develop PTSD (Rothbaum & Foa, 1993). On the other hand, acute stress disorder can be seen as a milder and briefer form or precursor of PTSD. In a sample of Israeli soldiers, 56% of those who developed combat-related acute stress disorder were subsequently diagnosed as having PTSD, whereas only 17% of combat soldiers without

Table 6.1. *DSM-IV Criteria for acute stress disorder*

A. The person has been exposed to a traumatic event in which both of the
    following were present:
    (1) the person experienced, witnessed, or was confronted with an event or
        events that involved actual or threatened death or serious injury, or a
        threat to the physical integrity of self or others
    (2) the person's response involved intense fear, helplessness, or horror
B. Either while experiencing or after experiencing the distressing event, the
    individual has three (or more) of the following dissociative symptoms:
    (1) a subjective sense of numbing, detachment, or absence of emotional
        responsiveness
    (2) a reduction in awareness of his or her surroundings (e.g., 'being in a daze')
    (3) derealization
    (4) depersonalization
    (5) dissociative amnesia (i.e., inability to recall an important aspect of the
        trauma)
C. The traumatic event is persistently reexperienced in at least one of the
    following ways: recurrent images, thoughts, dreams, illusions, flashback
    episodes, or a sense of reliving the experience; or distress on exposure to
    reminders of the traumatic event
D. Marked avoidance of stimuli that arouse recollections of the trauma (e.g.,
    thoughts, feelings, conversations, activities, places, people)
E. Marked symptoms of anxiety or increased arousal (e.g., difficulty sleeping,
    irritability, poor concentration, hypervigilance, exaggerated startle response,
    motor restlessness)
F. The disturbance causes clinically significant distress or impairment in social,
    occupational, or other important areas of functioning or impairs the
    individual's ability to pursue some necessary task, such as obtaining
    necessary assistance or mobilizing personal resources by telling family
    members about the traumatic experience
G. The disturbance lasts for a minimum of 2 days and a maximum of 4 weeks
    and occurs within 4 weeks of the traumatic event
H. The disturbance is not due to the direct physiological effects of a substance
    (e.g., a drug of abuse, a medication) or a general medical condition, is not
    better accounted for by brief psychotic disorder, and is not merely an
    exacerbation of a pre-existing axis I or axis II disorder

From American Psychiatric Association (1994). Reprinted with permission.

acute stress disorder later developed PTSD (Solomon, 1993a). Thus, acute
stress disorder indicates heightened vulnerability to PTSD.

Posttraumatic stress disorder

In DSM-IV requirements for the diagnosis of PTSD are contained in six
categories. The diagnostic criteria are shown in Table 6.2. Criterion A

Table 6.2. *DSM-IV Criteria for posttraumatic stress disorder*

A. The person has been exposed to a traumatic event in which both of the following were present:
   (1) the person experienced, witnessed, or was confronted with an event or events that involved actual or threatened death or serious injury, or a threat to the physical integrity of self or others
   (2) the person's response involved intense fear, helplessness, or horror. Note: In children, this may be expressed instead by disorganized or agitated behavior
B. The traumatic event is persistently reexperienced in one (or more) of the following ways:
   (1) recurrent and intrusive distressing recollections of the event, including images, thoughts, or perceptions. Note: In young children, repetitive play may occur in which themes or aspects of the trauma are expressed
   (2) recurrent distressing dreams of the event. Note: In children, there may be frightening dreams without recognizable content
   (3) acting or feeling as if the traumatic event were recurring (includes a sense of reliving the experience, illusions, hallucinations, and dissociative flashback episodes, including those that occur on awakening or when intoxicated). Note: In young children, trauma-specific reenactment may occur
   (4) intense psychological distress at exposure to internal or external cues that symbolize or resemble an aspect of the traumatic event
   (5) physiological reactivity on exposure to internal or external cues that symbolize or resemble an aspect of the traumatic event
C. Persistent avoidance of stimuli associated with the trauma and numbing of general responsiveness (not present before the trauma), as indicated by three (or more) of the following:
   (1) efforts to avoid thoughts, feelings, or conversations associated with the trauma
   (2) efforts to avoid activities, places, or people that arouse recollections of the trauma
   (3) inability to recall an important aspect of the trauma
   (4) markedly diminished interest or participation in significant activities
   (5) feeling of detachment or estrangement from others
   (6) restricted range of affect (e.g., unable to have loving feelings)
   (7) sense of a foreshortened future (e.g., does not expect to have a career, marriage, children, or a normal life span)
D. Persistent symptoms of increased arousal (not present before the trauma), as indicated by two (or more) of the following:
   (1) difficulty falling or staying asleep
   (2) irritability or outbursts of anger
   (3) difficulty concentrating
   (4) hypervigilance
   (5) exaggerated startle response
E. Duration of the disturbance (symptoms in criteria B, C, and D) is more than 1 month
F. The disturbance causes clinically significant distress or impairment in social, occupational, or other important areas of functioning.
   Specify:
      Acute (duration of symptoms is less than 3 months)
      Chronic (duration of symptoms is 3 months or more)
   Specify:
      With delayed onset (onset of symptoms is at least 6 months after the stressor)

From American Psychiatric Association (1994). Reprinted with permission.

describes the traumatic stressor as the direct personal experience of actual or threatened death or serious injury; witnessing the death or injury of another person; or learning about the unexpected or violent death or injury of a family member or close associate. The person must respond with intense fear, helplessness, or horror. Thus, DSM-IV provides considerable latitude in the definition of a stressor as long as it elicits a strong emotional response. Criteria B, C, and D specify the required symptoms. Criterion B requires persistent reexperiencing of the traumatic event and Criterion C describes persistent avoidance of stimuli associated with the trauma and numbing of general responsiveness. Criterion D describes symptoms of increased arousal and Criterion E requires that the full symptom picture be present for more than 1 month. As previously indicated, PTSD-like reactions of short duration are classified as acute stress disorder. Finally, Criterion F requires that the disturbance must cause clinically significant distress or impairment. PTSD is subdivided into an acute form lasting less than 3 months, a chronic form lasting longer than 3 months, and an infrequently seen delayed form that has its onset at least 6 months after the traumatic event.

DSM-IV differs from DSM-III-R in its definition of a traumatic event. In DSM-III-R the event had to be 'markedly distressing to almost everyone'; in DSM-IV the emphasis is placed on exposure to trauma coupled with the patient's reaction. Thus, DSM-IV takes into account the patient's vulnerability, and instead of insisting on an objectively-defined severe traumatic event, includes comparatively minor events as long as they elicit a strong emotional response. DSM-IV also requires that both persistent avoidance of stimuli associated with the trauma and numbing of general responsiveness be present for the diagnosis.

The International Classification of Diseases, 10th Revision (ICD-10) (Tyrer, 1989) guidelines are similar to those of DSM-III-R in emphasizing exposure to a traumatic event of exceptional severity within 6 months of symptom onset (Table 6.3). A 'probable' diagnosis can be given if typical PTSD symptoms emerge more than 6 months after the trauma. In addition to trauma, the patient must experience repetitive, intrusive recollections or re-enactments of the event in memories, daytime imagery, or dreams. In contrast to DSM-IV, frequent clinical features such as emotional detachment, numbing of feelings, and avoidance of stimuli that might prompt recall of the trauma, are not essential features. Autonomic disturbances, mood alternations and behavioral abnormalities contribute, but are not of prime importance to the diagnosis (De Silva, 1993).

Phenomenologically, PTSD is a composite of intrusive memories that

Table 6.3. *ICD-10 Criteria for posttraumatic stress disorder*

A. The patient must have been exposed to a stressful event or situation (either short- or long-lasting) of exceptionally threatening or catastrophic nature, which would be likely to cause pervasive distress in almost anyone
B. There must be persistent remembering or 'reliving' of the stressor in intrusive 'flashbacks', vivid memories, or recurring dreams, or in experiencing distress when exposed to circumstances resembling or associated with the stressor
C. The patient must exhibit an actual or preferred avoidance of circumstances resembling or associated with the stressor, which was not present before exposure to the stressor
D. Either of the following must be present:
   (1) inability to recall, either partially or completely, some important aspects of the period of exposure to the stressor
   (2) persistent symptoms of increased psychological sensitivity and arousal (not present before exposure to the stressor), shown by any two of the following:
      (a) difficulty in falling or staying asleep
      (b) irritability or outbursts of anger
      (c) difficulty in concentrating
      (d) hypervigilance
      (e) exaggerated startle response
E. Criteria B, C, and D must all be met within 6 months of the stressful event or of the end of a period of stress. (For some purposes, onset delayed more than 6 months may be included, but this should be clearly specified)

From WHO (1993). Reprinted with permission.

occur after traumatic experiences and of phobic reaction to these memories. Intrusive thoughts and images, even those that lead to transitory misinterpretation of sensory perceptions, are not unique to PTSD. They may be experienced during severe grief (Averill, 1968), longing for a loved one, or artistic creativity. In PTSD, intrusive memories are centered on the traumatic event and elicited by reminders of the trauma. In PTSD, recollections of the trauma provoke anxiety and, frequently, guilt feelings, so the individual develops phobic responses to and avoidance of provocative stimuli. The presence of hyperarousal, irritability, anxiety and depression further aggravates the condition in severely afflicted individuals.

Reliability and validity

Before accepting PTSD as a clearly defined syndrome one has to recognize that its conceptualization is still in flux. In contrast to most DSM-III and -IV diagnoses, PTSD is seen as having an etiological basis and this causes conceptual problems. If one assumes that trauma is the primary cause of

PTSD, then one must define or specify the types of trauma. Field studies, however, have shown that severe trauma fails to cause PTSD in some individuals, while in others apparently trivial events give rise to the syndrome. Moreover, similar traumas may not only precipitate PTSD but also phobias, general anxiety and depression as well.

The impact of a single trauma differs from that of a succession of insults. How much control one has over his or her environment also plays an important role in the development of PTSD. In captivity or after a disaster, starvation, physical illnesses, body injuries and uncertainty about the future may lower an individual's resistance. Some traumas hold consequences beyond the actual event. For instance, victims of disaster may have lost not only friends and family members but also homes and livelihood, and they may have to build a new life. Victims of the holocaust or refugees from war-torn countries may have to adjust to new cultures and may have to struggle with questions about the meaning of their suffering (Frankl, 1984).

It is not surprising that the impact of traumatic events and circumstances vary greatly. As Pugh & Trimble (1993) have stated: ' From the medical point of view, the crystallization of PTSD has been far from satisfactory. While it has defined some basic clinical features of a more generalized reaction to stress, it has also brought a concreteness to the concept, often with failure to think beyond it'.

Also, the diagnosis of PTSD is based primarily on self-report, and for this reason, its diagnosis and severity cannot always be assessed objectively. Symptoms of PTSD can easily be feigned. For instance, ratings on the Minnesota Multiphasic Personality Inventory (MMPI), a self-report questionnaire, could not distinguish Vietnam veterans with PTSD from healthy professionals who feigned symptoms of the disorder (Perconte & Goreczny, 1990). One study actually described cases of fictitious PTSD among veterans who had never seen combat (Lynn & Belza, 1984). In addition, memories of traumatic experiences change with time. In one study, individuals with symptoms recalled an event while many of those without symptoms had forgotten it (McFarlane, 1988b); however, the accuracy of recall has been shown to decay with time (McFarlane, 1990).

Thus PTSD, as defined in DSM-IV, is a condition characterized – but also limited – by specific symptoms that develop in the aftermath of a traumatic event that have caused strong emotion. Hence the validity is based on a somewhat circular definition. Its reliability depends on the quality of assessment instruments and, as always, the training and experience of the assessor.

Measurement

Several diagnostic and descriptive instruments for rating PTSD have been developed. As Allen (1994) has pointed out, the current diagnostic framework of PTSD calls for a categorical assessment, indicating the presence or absence of the condition. As our understanding of the disorder evolves, different subtypes may become evident, necessitating the development of new instruments. Instruments can be divided into self-report measures and structured interviews. The commonly used scales for adults are described below; scales applicable to children are described by Allen (1994).

Self-report measures

The Impact of Events Scale (IES) is one of the earliest and most frequently used scales. It was developed on a civilian population but has been tested on groups exposed to combat (Zilberg et al., 1982). The scale asks the respondent to describe a target event and then rate the frequency with which 15 symptoms have occurred during the past week. It measures, on a continuum, intrusion and avoidance. The IES was developed before DSM-III and, therefore, does not assess a wide range of important symptoms. The scale has good internal consistency and test-retest reliability. Its main drawback is that of all self-report scales, namely its vulnerability to false reporting.

The Mississippi Scale for Combat-related Post-traumatic Stress Disorder (M-PTSD) is a 35-item, Likeret scale questionnaire designed to assess PTSD symptoms in Vietnam veterans (Keane et al., 1988). A revised version was developed for use in female veterans. The M-PTSD correlates well with the Structured Clinical Interview for DSM-IV diagnosis of PTSD and provides a useful measure of change. The test-retest reliability and internal consistence are high, and the scale has a good diagnostic sensitivity and specificity.

Another self-report instrument is the Penn Inventory. This 26-item inventory assesses DSM-III-R symptoms and provides measures of the degree, frequency, and intensity (Hammarberg, 1992). It has been validated on civilian and combat-exposed populations and has good internal consistency, test-retest reliability, sensitivity, and specificity. It compares favorably with the M-PTSD.

A specific PTSD subscale has been developed from statements in the MMPI (Litz et al., 1991). The resulting 49 items have shown good psychometric properties, and the scale was able to distinguish veterans

Table 6.4. *Sample of items from the 17-item Davidson Self-rating PTSD Scale*

In the past week, how much trouble have you had with the following symptoms? Place a number in the box that best describes your answers.

Please identify the trauma which is most disturbing to you:	*Frequency*	*Severity*
	0 = Not At All	0 = Not At All Distressing
	1 = Once Only	1 = Minimally Distressing
	2 = 2–3 Times	2 = Moderately Distressing
	3 = 4–6 Times	3 = Markedly Distressing
	4 = Everyday	4 = Extremely Distressing
2. Have you had distressing dreams of the event?	☐	☐
4. Have you been upset by something which reminded you of the event?	☐	☐
6. Have you been avoiding any thoughts or feeling about the event?	☐	☐
10. Have you been unable to have sad or loving feelings, or have you generally felt numb?	☐	☐
13. Have you been irritable or had outbursts of anger?	☐	☐
17. Have you been physically upset by reminders of the event? (*This includes sweating, trembling, racing heart, shortness of breath, nausea, diarrhea*).	☐	☐

Source: Reproduced with permission from Multi-Health Systems Inc., 908 Niagara Falls Blvd, North Tonawanda, NY 14120-2060, (800) 456-3003.

with PTSD from veterans without PTSD but did less well in separating veterans with PTSD from other psychiatric patients.

The Davidson Self-rating PTSD Scale (Table 6.4) is a 17-item self-rated scale that covers reexperiencing of traumatic events, avoidance of stimuli associated with the trauma, and arousal induced by stimuli. Each item is rated for frequency and severity. This scale has a good test-retest reliability and is useful for assessing symptoms in the course of treatment (J. R. T. Davidson, personal communication).

Structured interviews

The Structured Clinical Interview for DSM-IV(SCID) is frequently used to provide a diagnostic evaluation of PTSD (First et al., 1996). As it also evaluates the presence of other psychiatric disorders, it is useful in assessing comorbidity. The SCID does not provide a measure of severity, and therefore, cannot be used as a measure of change.

The Post-traumatic Stress Disorder Interview (PTSD-I) was designed specifically for PTSD. It closely corresponds to DSM-III-R and provides dichotomous and continues data for each symptom (Watson et al., 1991). It has good test-retest reliability and internal consistency as well as high sensitivity and specificity. It can be used for diagnostic assessment as well as an outcome measure.

Another instrument for PTSD is the Structured Interview for PTSD (SI-PTSD). This 13-item instrument rates each item on a 5-point scale for severity at present and for the worst time ever (Davidson et al., 1990). The items fall into three categories: re-experiencing of traumatic events, avoidance of stimuli associated with the trauma, and increased arousal. The scale has good inter-rater and test-retest reliability and diagnostic sensitivity, and can be used to measure changes.

Epidemiology

Prevalence

As the development of PTSD depends on severity of the trauma, on social support during and after the trauma, and most importantly, on a person's vulnerability, it is not surprising that estimates of prevalence vary greatly. Moreover, epidemiological data depend on sampling methods. For instance, McFarlane found that the Diagnostic Interview Schedule performed well when administered by clinicians, but Kulak found it missed many cases of PTSD when administered by non-clinicians (Blank, 1993). In addition, investigator prejudice may color the interpretation of results; some investigators emphasize the scarcity of long-term effects in psychologically healthy individuals while others use data to support a variety of opinions and causes.

Data from various studies suggest that even the most devastating traumas seldom lead to PTSD in more than 50% of the population (McFarlane, 1990). In general, women appear more vulnerable than men. The National Comorbidity Survey estimated the lifetime prevalence at

7.8%, with combat exposure and witnessing the most frequent traumas in men and rape and sexual molestation the most frequent in women (Kessler et al., 1995). The National Vietnam Veterans Readjustment Study estimated that PTSD had occurred in 15% of all male veterans, including 2.5% of those who served outside the Vietnam theater (Friedman et al., 1994). The Epidemiological Catchment Area (ECA) study found that PTSD had occurred in 20% of wounded Vietnam veterans (Helzer et al., 1987) while those not wounded had a much lower prevalence.

Incarceration accompanied by torture and constant threats of death may have especially severe psychological consequences. Among holocaust victims living in Montreal, 46% met current criteria for PTSD, including 65% of those who survived concentration camps (Kuch & Cox, 1992). In a community survey of holocaust victims conducted in Jerusalem, 16% of male and 23% of female victims continued to experience emotional distress (Levav & Abramsom, 1984). Among Cambodian survivors of the Pol Pot War, 20% of adolescents, 50% of mothers and 33% of fathers had symptoms of PTSD (Sack et al., 1994). Also, in a 40-year follow-up of World War II prisoners of war, two-thirds had had PTSD at one time or another (Ramsay, 1990).

Among civilians, the ECA study estimated the lifetime prevalence of PTSD at 1% of the population (Helzer et al., 1987). Davidson et al. (1991) obtain a similar estimate that included 3.5% in civilians exposed to physical attack. Resnick et al. (1993), who interviewed more than 4000 women, reported a lifetime exposure to trauma in 69%, exposure to crime in 36%, and lifetime prevalence for PTSD of 12.3%. Exposure to rape led to a particularly high incidence, ranging from 57% to 80% (Davis et al., 1994). Breslau et al. (1991), who examined a high risk group of young adults belonging to an HMO in Detroit, reported a 39% exposure to traumatic events and a 9.2% lifetime prevalence of PTSD.

Accidents also cause PTSD. Sixteen percent of London underground drivers, who injured or killed persons who had jumped in front of trains, experienced PTSD (Farmer et al., 1992). Thirty-eight percent of survivors of motor vehicle accidents reported simple phobias, and approximately the same number experienced PTSD (Kuch et al., 1994). After an occupational exposure to toxic substances 14% developed PTSD, while a third developed somatoform disorders. Those with somatoform disorders had more often had chronic or repeated, but less severe, exposures, while those who developed PTSD had experienced single, life-threatening events (Schottenfeld et al., 1985).

The incidence of PTSD after disasters varies greatly. After the eruption of Mount St. Helens, 11% of highly exposed men and 21% of women developed anxiety, depression or PTSD. Similar findings were reported after mud slides and floods that killed many people in Puerto Rico. Other studies found PTSD in 5–22%, depending on the type of disaster (Green & Lindy, 1994).

In children, the prevalence of posttraumatic symptoms has varied – depending on the age, nature of traumatic event, and social support – from 27% to 100% (McNally, 1993). In the aftermath of hurricane Hugo only 5% of the children warranted a diagnosis of PTSD.

Risk factors

As only a fraction of those who are exposed to traumatic events subsequently develop PTSD, increased vulnerability plays a crucial role in the development of the disorder. Factors that predispose individuals to PTSD include past or present psychiatric illness and family history of psychiatric illness. Several studies have reported that a positive family history, particularly for depression, anxiety disorders or alcoholism, predisposes an individual to PTSD (Davidson et al., 1985, 1991; McFarlane, 1988a).

In the ECA study, almost 80% of persons with PTSD in St. Louis had a past or present psychiatric disorder, compared to about a third of those without PTSD (Davidson & Fairbank, 1993). In fact, McFarlane (1989) noted that a history of psychological treatment was a better predictor of PTSD than a traumatic event. Also, Beslau et al. (1991) found that pre-existing anxiety and depression made individuals more vulnerable to stressors.

Comorbidity

PTSD rarely occurs in the absence of other psychiatric disturbances. In some cases, a psychiatric disorder is already present when the trauma occurrs, thereby increasing the individual's vulnerability. In other cases, the trauma induces symptoms of other disorders, such as phobias, generalized anxiety or depression in addition to PTSD. PTSD may also activate latent psychiatric disorders in predisposed persons. Finally, PTSD may lead to alcohol or substance abuse and impulsive or violent behavior in personality-disordered individuals.

Major depressive disorder, generalized anxiety disorder, panic disorder and somatization disorder frequently coexist with PTSD (Davidson & Fairbank, 1993). After a disaster involving fire fighters, McFarlane &

Papay (1992) found that 77% of persons with PTSD had additional diagnoses, most often major depression. Comorbidity, especially with pre-existing anxiety and depression, may be an important predictor of chronic PTSD (Breslau et al., 1991). Fifty percent of Vietnam veterans with PTSD also met criteria for at least one concurrent, DSM-III-based disorder in the 6 months prior to assessment (Davidson & Fairbank, 1993). Substance abuse (Faustman & White, 1989), intermittent explosive disorder and antisocial behavior are also more commonly seen in combat veterans (Grady et al., 1989; Friedman et al., 1994).

Family and twin studies

While PTSD is regarded as a reaction to trauma, a genetic predisposition may also contribute to development of the disorder. Davidson et al. (1989) found a greater prevalence of anxiety disorders among the relatives of veterans with PTSD than among the relatives of controls veterans who had experienced combat. A large study of Vietnam veterans, who were mono-zygotic or dizygotic twins, found a significant genetic influence on symp-tom liability, even after adjusting for differences in combat exposure. Genetic factors accounted for 13–30% of the variance in reexperiencing the trauma, 30–34% in symptoms of avoidance, and 28–32% in symptoms of arousal (True et al., 1993). The importance of the trauma was demonstrated in a study of monozygotic twins who served in Southeast Asia. In that study, the prevalence of PTSD was 16% compared to only 5% in twins who did not serve (Goldberg et al., 1990).

Etiology and pathogenesis

Biological factors

Pathological learning and memory

As the principal symptoms of PTSD are intrusive thoughts, images and dreams, it is plausible that the disorder is caused by pathological implanta-tion of memories during extreme arousal. Research has demonstrated that learning and acquisition of memories requires change in synaptic trans-mission called long-term potentiation (LTP). In the presence of excitatory amino acids, LTP is induced by specific neuronal inputs to the limbic system. The hippocampus is thought to be necessary for the acquisition of declarative memory and the amygdala for acquisition of conditioned emo-tional responses (Hoehn-Saric et al., 1991; Charney et al., 1994; Davis et al.,

1994). Changes in noradrenaline, corticotropin-releasing hormone (CRH) and, indirectly, serotonin, that occur during heightened arousal enhance the formation of LTP. This may explain why intrusive memories and phobias, which represent pathological excess, are enhanced during heightened arousal (Davis et al., 1994). Once a learned response, including fear, has been established, drugs that are capable of blocking acquisition of the response may lose their effectiveness. Unlearning of a response, including habituation, again requires an active process and the same mechanisms that were involved in the acquisition (Davis, 1992).

Intrusive memories are triggered by minimal and harmless stimuli that remind a person of the trauma. Memories of this kind tend to become less strong and frequent if they occur in an environment where negative feelings are not reinforced and the individual learns they are harmless. When intrusions are accompanied by severe anxiety, pathological learning is reinforced and symptoms are maintained or strengthened; therefore, in some patients, intrusive memories do not extinguish and become relatively resistant to pharmacotherapy. To be extinguished, they require active relearning through emotional-cognitive techniques, such as flooding and stress inoculation. Non-directive, insight-oriented psychotherapy is less efficient in bringing about changes.

Neurotransmitter systems

As many PTSD patients exhibit heightened arousal and symptoms of sympathetic hyperactivity, it has been hypothesized that their noradrenergic system is overstimulated. The locus ceruleus-noradrenergic system modifies levels of arousal and heightens the effect of internal and external stimuli by increasing the signal-to-noise ratio (Aston-Jones et al., 1994). It also increases peripheral sympathetic tone. When this system is overstimulated, for instance with the administration yohimbine, the result is disorganization and heightened anxiety, including panic attacks (Charney et al., 1987). Provocation with yohimbine increases the startle response in veterans with PTSD but not in controls (Morgan, 1993). This, and increased urinary catecholamine levels (Mason et al., 1990), shows a heightened central noradrenergic and peripheral sympathetic tone in some PTSD patients. Not all such patients exhibit heightened sympathetic activity; this is limited to severe, possibly predisposed cases. A study examining plasma norepinephrine in patients with PTSD found no increase (Murburg et al., 1995). The authors concluded that previous reports of increased catecholamine levels reflected response to stimulation but not resting activity.

The serotonergic system, which is closely associated with the norad-renergic system, has also been implicated in the etiology of PTSD. In part this is because medications that cause serotonin uptake inhibition amelior-ate PTSD symptoms (Charney et al., 1993); however, little is known about how the complex serotonergic system functions. The fact that medications that alter it also improve PTSD cannot be taken to mean that the system is etiologically important. Changes in brain serotonin may alter the functions of other brain systems that are affected by the disorder. Based on studies in animals and in veterans that found increased urinary dopamine levels in response to stress, changes in the dopaminergic system also have been implicated in the pathogenesis of PTSD (Antelman & Yehuda, 1994).

CRH is another neurotransmitter that is likely to be involved in PTSD. CRH not only increases the output of ACTH and cortisol, but within the brain, activates areas associated with anxiety, including the locus ceruleus and the limbic system. Intrathecally injected CRH causes behavioral and endocrine changes in animals that are identical to responses seen during stress (Dunn & Berridge, 1990). Alterations in brain CRH are believed to be responsible for biological changes seen in anxiety as well as depression (Gold et al., 1988). The peripheral effects of CRH are increased ACTH and cortisol. Moderately increased cortisol levels have a protective effect on the brain; however, large increases may damage hippocampal neurons (McEwen, 1988). A recent MRI study that compared brain structures of Vietnam veterans with those of controls found that veterans had an 8% smaller right hippocampus associated with deficits in short-term verbal memory (Bremner et al., 1995). The authors hypothesized that stress-induced high cortisol levels had damaged the hippocampus. As interesting as this finding is, it is hard to reconcile it with findings by Yehuda et al. (1993, 1995) of lower cortical levels in war veterans and holocaust survivors than in controls.

Neuroanatomical localization

Two imaging studies, measuring cerebral blood flow, have been conducted on PTSD victims. Liberzon (1995) measured regional blood flow in vet-erans using SPECT, during stimulation with white noise or combat sounds. Combat sounds increased blood flow in the right and left parahip-pocampal gyrus, the left striatum, and certain upper brain stem structures. Rauch et al. (1996) measured cerebral blood flow with the help of a PET scanner while patients listened to script-driven descriptions of their trauma or neutral scripts. Activation normalized blood flow in right-sided limbic, paralimbic, and visual areas. Thus, both studies found that reexperiencing the trauma activated limbic and paralimbic systems. Stronger activation of the right hemisphere in the second study corresponds to findings of Davidson (1994) showing that greater activity in the right hemisphere is associated with increased vulnerability to anxiety and depression.

An electroencephalographic study of evoked potentials in persons who had been attacked a month earlier showed a significant decrease in the P300 amplitude. These changes were associated with disturbances in information processing (Charles et al., 1995).

Psychophysiological abnormalities

PTSD is frequently associated with hyperarousal and emotional overreaction to trauma-related cues. Subjective reports of somatic symptoms have been confirmed with psychophysiological measures; however, these reports should be interpreted cautiously because most studies were conducted with chronic PTSD war veterans. In such veterans, some studies have found higher heart rates than in controls, which suggests sympathetic arousal. Other studies have not found such differences (Orr, 1990; Hoehn-Saric & McLeod, 1993). When exposed to laboratory stimuli or stressors that were unrelated to the trauma – for example a neutral script, a videotape of a car accident, or mental arithmetic – veterans exhibited similar or even lower physiological responses than controls. This suggests that they do not respond to non-specific stressors with indiscriminate autonomic overreaction, but at times, underreaction, a phenomenon seen in other anxiety disorders. When exposed to trauma-related stressors, such as tape-recorded combat sounds or combat-related scripts, patients showed heightened physiological arousal including increased heart rate, blood pressure, skin conductance and muscle tension (Hoehn-Saric & McLeod, 1993). PTSD patients also recover physiologically more slowly after exposure (Hoehn-Saric & McLeod, 1993). This indicates they have been conditioned to stimuli that represent the trauma. Hyperaroused PTSD patients also startle easily (Butler et al., 1990). There are, however, a significant number of patients with PTSD who do not overreact to trauma-related cues (Orr, 1990). For instance, rape victims who were asked to imagine and visualize a standardized sexual assault had no heightening of heart rate or skin conductance (Kozak, quoted by Orr, 1990).

One of the most common complaints among persons with PTSD is disturbed sleep. Patients report difficulty falling asleep, frequent awakenings and excessive movement during sleep. Also, nightmares and nocturnal panic attacks frequently occur. In former prisoners of war with PTSD, van Kammen et al. (1990) found significantly less sleep, increased time to fall asleep, lower sleep maintenance, decreased stage 2 and delta sleep, but increased rapid eye movement (REM) sleep. In contrast to findings in depression, these investigations did not find REM latency shortened. Other studies have found shortened as well as prolonged REM latency, possibly because of the diversity of cases and frequent comorbidity with depression (Dreissig & Berger, 1991); however, some sleep disturbances may precede PTSD. For example, in one study, the tendency to have bad dreams and interrupted sleep before the trauma appeared to increase an individual's post-trauma morbidity (Mellman et al., 1995a).

Neuroendocrine abnormalities

Some, but not all, studies have found increased catecholamine levels in veterans with PTSD compared with normals and other psychiatric patients. (Hoehn-Saric & McLeod, 1993). A recent study shows that combat veterans with PTSD do not differ from controls on overall catecholamine excretion but that, during disturbed sleep, excretion decreases (Mellman et al., 1995b). The total number of platelet alpha-2-receptor binding sites, particularly those with high-affinity, were also reduced, suggesting a down regulation and desensitization of receptors (Giller et al., 1990). Increased levels of catecholamines were found in persons living close to the Three Mile Island reactor involved in a nuclear accident. Alterations in the dopaminergic system have also been suggested, based on studies in stressed animals and veterans (Antelman & Yehuda, 1994).

Both increased and decreased cortisol levels have been found in PTSD patients. Yehuda and colleagues (1993, 1995) reported lower cortisol levels in veterans and holocaust victims with PTSD compared with victims without PTSD and controls. Along these lines, suppression of steroids has been observed in chronically stressed animals (Mason et al., 1990). The findings suggest an inhibitory or suppressive mechanism acting on the pituitary–adrenal–cortical system, perhaps in response to initial, stress-induced hyperactivity. A psychological explanation of the phenomenon is also possible. Individuals, who under stress exhibit high levels of denial, may have low cortisol levels (Mason et al., 1990). Thus, avoidance and emotional numbness may contribute to hypoactivity of the hypothalamic–pituitary–adrenal system. Other studies have found no differences or even increased cortisol levels in veterans with PTSD (Southwick et al., 1994). Subjects living close to the Three Mile Island nuclear reactor had higher urinary cortisol levels than controls 17 months after the accident (Schaeffer & Baum, 1984). The reason for discrepant findings concerning steroid response is not known. It is possible that the extreme,

but temporary, stress experienced by soldiers and holocaust victims induces different adaptive mechanisms than the milder, but more persistent,
stress of living next to a nuclear reactor that might melt down.

Psychological factors

Freud, in 1921 (quoted from Ramsey 1990), believed that a 'traumatic
neurosis' develops when an individual's adaptive capabilities are exceeded
and the person reverts to earlier, more primitive forms of defense, otherwise
called repetition compulsion. By actively reexperiencing an event, an individual gradually masters it, or if he or she does not succeed, develops
numbing to avoid painful recollections.

Janet hypothesized that trauma results in a breaking up of mental
cohesion, such that behavioral, cognitive and emotional residues of past
experiences continue to govern current behavior (Choy & Bosset, 1992).
Horowitz (1985) developed a cognitive model of information processing,
according to which trauma disrupts an individual's information processing
system, and this results in intrusions. The distress caused by intrusions then
leads to numbing and avoidance.

Various psychological factors have been shown to be associated with
increased vulnerability to PTSD. They include unfavorable childhood
environment, parental poverty, childhood abuse, separation from a parent
before age 10 years, low education and early conduct problems (Breslau et
al., 1991). The children of parents with PTSD may also be more vulnerable.
This has been observed in children of holocaust victims who, as soldiers,
were more likely to develop PTSD (Solomon et al., 1988).

Personality

In adults, personality traits, particularly neuroticism, have predicted who
will develop PTSD (McFarlane, 1989). Fire fighters who developed PTSD
scored high on introversion and neuroticism, traits associated with anxiety
and depressive reactions to everyday stressors. In Israeli soldiers, poor
social adjustment was an important vulnerability factor. Among these
soldiers, vulnerability to combat stress increased inversely with personality
characteristics such as punctuality, sociability and intelligence. On the
other hand, Israeli officers, who had been highly selected, were five times
less susceptible to war stress than soldiers in the lower ranks (Levav et al.,
1979). Similarly, in Vietnam veterans with PTSD, borderline, obsessive-
compulsive, avoidant and paranoid personality disorders have frequently
been observed (Faustman et al., 1989). Among persons in a large city,

extroversion, antisocial and narcissistic personality, low intelligence and limited coping abilities predisposed individuals to PTSD. Extroverts may be more vulnerable by virtue of the fact that they expose themselves to potentially traumatic situations more often (Breslau et al., 1991). Premorbid factors become less important as the severity of the trauma increases (Davidson & Fairbank, 1993). For instance, soldiers with an external locus of control (i.e., unwilling to accept responsibility for their actions) were more prone to develop PTSD when battle intensity was low, but when battle intensity was high, the locus of control made little difference (Solomon et al., 1989).

Social environment

Poor social adjustment also heightens a person's vulnerability to stress. Among civilians, persons who develop PTSD have histories of job instability (Davidson et al., 1991). In the military, disciplined units have less PTSD than undisciplined ones (De Silva, 1993). PTSD is more frequent among individuals who abuse drugs, probably because they expose themselves to potentially traumatic situations (Cottler et al., 1992). During the Gulf War, lower class evacuees exhibited more extensive and severe psychopathological symptoms (Solomon et al., 1993).

Preparation for trauma

Preparation to deal with trauma has a protective effect. Expectation permits mental preparation. Traumatic experiences that were handled well in the past increase self-confidence and lessen the impact of later traumas. Individuals who are unprepared for situations – for instance, inexperienced body carriers during the Gulf War – are more affected by the task than those who are used to such trauma (McCarroll et al., 1993). Persons who expected torture were often less affected by it than those tortured unexpectedly.

Previous traumatic experiences

Previous traumatic experiences can strengthen or weaken a person. Individuals with strong personalities learn to cope with repeated traumas. A good example is the former Yugoslav politician, Milovan Djilas, who emerged strengthened from repeated imprisonments, torture, and horrors of the Partisan Wars (Djilas, 1973). In a recent survey, almost half the women who had been sexually abused as children, reported having received some benefit from their experience. They felt better equipped to protect their children from similar abuse, and some even viewed themselves stronger (McMillen et al., 1995). Vulnerable persons, however, become sensitized by traumas and are, subsequently, more likely to develop PTSD. For instance, train drivers, who had previously been involved in accidents, reacted more strongly to a new accident than those who had not (Karlehagen et al., 1993). Sensitization is particularly strong when the trauma is severe and occurs in an environment that limits coping, such as a concentration camp. For instance, during the Gulf War, even holocaust victims who were without PTSD were more vulnerable to the stress of that war (Solomon & Prager, 1992).

Cultural factors

Vulnerability to PTSD is not influenced by culture, but culture modifies the clinical picture. During World War II, British soldiers reported more anxiety and psychosomatic complaints, while Indian soldiers, for whom the expression of anxiety was culturally unacceptable, exhibited more hysterical symptoms (De Silva, 1993). Among Cambodians, who also lose face when they express strong emotion, somatization was the most common presentation; therefore, they were more responsive to medication than psychotherapy (Cheung, 1993).

Consequences of trauma

The consequences of the trauma are of great psychological importance. Some individuals are affected by the reception they receive after the trauma. For instance, a lack of attention to a soldier who expects to be treated as a hero, or a feeling among comrades that the victim may have betrayed them under torture, may be more important than the trauma itself.

As trauma frequently – and often justifiably – opens the way for compensation, secondary gains – financial or otherwise – influence the course of symptoms. Requests for financial compensation are commonplace in civilian accidents and symptoms frequently remain unresolved until compensation has been obtained or the injured party accepts the futility of further attempts. Among war veterans, only 4% of those who developed PTSD applied for compensation. Secondary gain need not be financial. Some combat veterans, who had become nearly free of symptoms, relapsed and became the center of sympathetic concern after they returned home. Often individuals of this kind had functioned marginally before their induction into the military. Through symptoms of PTSD, they could now attract the always-desired but never-attained attention from their families. Other persons with personality disorders use PTSD as an excuse for impulsive and antisocial behavior; however, the majority of PTSD patients are not seeking secondary gains or excuses for undisciplined behavior (Blank, 1993).

Clinical picture

Symptoms may develop during a traumatic experience or after some delay. While the severity of the trauma plays an important role (Bryant & Harvey, 1995), its subjective perception is also important. For instance, even the prediction of a possible disaster, such an earthquake, can induce mild PTSD symptoms (Kiser et al., 1993). PTSD can emerge under continuing traumatic circumstances, for instance, in an overburdened manager or a woman caring for a dying husband (Scott & Stradling, 1994), after childbirth (Ballard et al., 1995) or in cancer survivors (Alter et al., 1996); however, a traumatic event involving potential for personal injury generally has greater impact (Breslau & Davis, 1987). Continuous stress, such as confinement in a concentration camp, may induce protective emotional numbing with the development of trauma-related symptoms after liberation.

Immediately after an acute stress, individuals may become disorganized, dysfunctional and highly suggestible. The most prominent symptoms are intrusive memories and dreams. These may occur spontaneously but generally are triggered by what often seems like irrelevant stimuli that remind them of their experience. Even odors that have a link to the trauma may provoke flashbacks (Kline & Rausch, 1985). Intrusive thoughts cause various degrees of distress that may reach the intensity of panic attacks. Some flashbacks are exciting and involve heightened tension and a sense of control, followed by calm and relaxation (Solursh, 1988).

In addition, symptoms of excessive arousal, such as hypervigilance, increased startle, and disrupted sleep, are common. Persistent anxiety may contribute to fatigue and emotional instability. In less severe cases, such psychophysiological reactions may not occur (Malt et al., 1993). More severe cases experience increased muscle tension, palpitations, sweating, shortness of breath, and dissociative symptoms. Anxiety with the suddenness and intensity of a panic attack may occur whenever patients experience flashbacks. When the distress becomes overwhelming, patients avert it by employing emotional numbing and by avoiding stimuli that trigger memories. Such reactions lead to social withdrawal, irritability and explosive behavior when avoidance is not possible.

For a minority of patients PTSD becomes chronic. In those instances, symptoms may remain stationary or wax and wane, and symptoms that resolve may reemerge under stress or without apparent reason (Ramsay, 1990). The severity of the symptoms varies greatly. The majority of patients continue to function socially, although with some restrictions such as phobic avoidance or diminished social interactions. Patients often cannot return to their work place after a traumatic event has occurred. For instance, most of the sailors who were rescued after a marine explosion were unable to return to sea duty (Leopold & Dillon, 1963). Patients with severe anxiety and depression may become incapacitated. They may reexperience, but at the same time avoid, thoughts and feelings relating to the traumatic event. Hyperarousal is the most common symptom. Restricted affect, amnesia, and survival guilt are less common (Kilpatrick & Resnick, 1993). An increase in somatoform symptoms, including gastrointestinal and muscular distress, chronic fatigue and physical weakness, are frequently seen (Tomb, 1994). Vietnam veterans exhibit more soft neurological signs than veterans without PTSD, but do not show differences on electroencephalogram or neuropsychological testing (Gurvits et al., 1993).

Dissociative symptoms may include amnesia which tends to be selective (Bremner et al., 1993). Veterans with PTSD exhibit a bias for combat on memory tests; i.e., they show poor memory for everything but combat words (Zeitlin & McNally, 1991). PTSD victims also show higher hypnotizability scores than controls, but it is not clear if trauma makes individuals more hypnotizable or hypnotizable persons are more prone to PTSD (Stutman & Bliss, 1985). General cognitive impairment, including memory difficulty, reduced ability to learn, decreased motivation for tasks and impaired coping with stress or new situations, can complicate the clinical picture (Tomb, 1994).

Time can distort the recall of traumatic memories. Retrospectively retrieved memories, particularly those of early childhood, are easily distorted and can lead to a false memory syndrome (Tomb, 1994). Independent verification of an event should be obtained whenever possible.

PTSD symptoms may become complex, and when there is a history of multiple events, may include aspects of each trauma (Kilpatrick & Resnick, 1993). Patients who have recovered from the emotional effects of a trauma are often more vulnerable to new traumatic experiences (Solomon, 1993).

Guilt feelings about apparent cowardice, selfishness or atrocities committed may further complicate the picture and lead to chronic dysphoria. Persons with strong inner values or (conversely) with few moral scruples overcome trauma better than people who believe that under stress they betrayed their principles (Kral, 1951). A strong Weltanschauung, or belief in an orderly, purposeful world, can also be protective. Avery, a religious and non-political inmate of a concentration camp, described how prisoners with strong religious or political beliefs endured the hardships better than those who, like himself, could see no reason for their suffering (Hoehn-Saric, 1974).

Clinical subgroups

Combat-related PTSD

Symptoms of an acute stress disorder may occur during or soon after combat exposure. In some soldiers, symptoms develop days, weeks or, rarely, months later. Symptoms often take on a cultural flavor. For instance, during World War I, tremor was accepted as a trauma-induced symptom and was seen frequently. During World War II, trembling was not accepted and was rarely seen (Dreissig & Berger, 1991). In Eastern cultures, where excessive expression of emotions is frowned upon, somatic symptoms usually replace the psychic symptoms seen in Western soldiers (De Silva, 1993).

Stress in the military is often cumulative. The life of soldiers is disrupted by separation from their family, and ordinary social restraints are relaxed. Previously unacceptable habits, such as excessive alcohol and substance abuse, become commonplace, particularly when units are poorly led. Soldiers in combat also gain an opportunity to take out frustrations, anger, and aggression on helpless victims. Participation in atrocities, with subsequent feelings of guilt, then increases the risk of PTSD (Hendin et al., 1983; Breslau & Davis, 1987; Yehuda et al., 1992). Suicide among Vietnam veterans was associated with combat-related guilt (Hendin & Haas, 1991).

Guilt feelings, emotional withdrawal and aggression often make it difficult for veterans with PTSD to resume the former roles of father, husband and breadwinner. Wives and children of these veterans are often affected by their pathology and sometimes develop symptoms themselves (Carroll et al., 1985; Solomon, 1988). Even in less severe cases, the reentering of civilian life is a difficult period of readjustment. Wives, when left alone, may have developed greater independence and may no longer fit the often idealized picture the soldier had retained in his mind. Unsuccessful individuals, who in the military held positions of power, often return home to roles of lesser significance (Hobfoll et al., 1991). These factors, although unrelated to the trauma, may contribute greatly to the chronicity of PTSD.

Victims of the holocaust

Victims of prolonged, repeated exposure to trauma, under circumstances of powerlessness and uncertainty, exhibit a syndrome that differs from that seen in victims of isolated trauma. For some victims of persecution the experience results in loss of cultural past and continuity. Jews who survived the holocaust experienced an almost total loss of family and friends, and in addition, had no graves to symbolize their loss or continuity with the deceased. They lost their homes, countries, traditions, styles of living and culture. They suffered from the effects of discrimination, defamation, lawlessness, loss of individuality and social position. In the camps, they were under the constant threat of death, physical maltreatment, hunger and disease. Once liberated, they had to deal with the trauma of emigration and adjust to a new culture (Peters, 1989). Some victims were unable to tear themselves away from their past and integrate themselves into a new environment.

In many victims, the concentration camp caused an existential crisis with bitterness over having been forsaken by human beings and by God (Wiesel, 1960) and guilt feelings about having survived when others perished. While in the camp, belief in a personal future and in the meaning of life, was essential for survival. When it was lost, life was also lost. Such insights gave birth to existential thinking that became the foundation of 'logotherapy' (Frankl, 1946).

Blocking of feelings was a protective mechanism in concentration camps. After liberation this suppression loosened, allowing anxiety and depression to emerge (Peters, 1989). Along with intrusive thoughts and dreams as well as protracted depressions, survivors of concentration camps often became hypervigilant, anxious and agitated, and had numerous somatic complaints. They tended to be forgetful with disturbances of time sense, memory, and concentration. The rupture in continuity between the present and past often persisted long after release from confinement (Herman, 1993).

It is surprising that the majority of holocaust victims adjusted relatively well. A community survey in Jerusalem showed that only 38% of concentration camp survivors – 16% males and 23% females – were still emotionally distressed (Levav & Abramsom, 1984). Not surprisingly, the more brutal the holocaust experience, the greater was the demoralization (Fenig et al., 1991). Children who were in death camps suffer more 50 years later than those who went through other forms of persecution (Robinson et al., 1994). A survey of holocaust survivors in Montreal, showed that most had mild psychiatric symptoms regardless of the age at which they experienced the holocaust. Somatic complaints predominated, consisting of weakness, headache, sour stomach, anxiety, restlessness, excessive worry, depression and feelings of social isolation (Eaton et al., 1982). Even in apparently well-adjusted individuals, an increased vulnerability emerged with the experience of new stressors. For instance, non-clinical holocaust survivors were more vulnerable to stress caused by the Persian Gulf War than were persons in the general population (Solomon & Prager, 1992). PTSD may affect entire families; among holocaust victims, symptoms of distress were often transmitted to the second, but apparently not the third, generation (Allodi, 1994).

Victims of torture and political persecution

Torture involves pain, humiliation, exhaustion, physical injury, unpredictability, and uncertainty regarding one's future. Often prisoners are exposed to prolonged periods of sensory deprivation through blindfolding and isolation. In women, torture is more frequently sexual, and this, consequently, affects their subsequent sexual adaptation (Allodi & Stiasny, 1990). Unexpected torture generally has a greater impact than torture that is expected. In survivors of torture in Turkey, the perceived severity was related to PTSD symptoms, but subsequent anxiety and depressive symptoms were related to the lack of social support. Thus, PTSD is shaped by psychosocial stressors that follow captivity, such as loss of job, emigration, distancing of acquaintances, and suspicion of betrayal on the part of comrades. As in other PTSD subgroups, a family history of psychiatric illness has been shown to correlate highly with symptoms (Basoglu et al., 1994).

Victims of crime and violence

In spite of the frequency of physical violence, at least in North American cities, rape is the only assault condition studied extensively. Victims of other crimes frequently develop fears of further violence, phobic symptoms and PTSD. Predisposing factors include history of previous – especially childhood – violence, preexisting anxiety and depression, as well as poor coping mechanisms (Breslau et al., 1991). Lack of social support and self-blame both contribute to chronicity (Shepherd et al., 1990).

PTSD follows rape more frequently than exposure to other crimes (Kilpatrick & Resnick, 1993). Victims often experience, besides anxiety, feelings of humiliation, embarrassment, anger, desire for revenge, and self-blame. Rape represents for them a personal injury, a loss of control over situations that may not have been threatening before, and a loss of self-esteem that is not present in other victims of assault. The response of victims to such trauma is not uniform. Foa et al. (1995b) observed two patterns: one was characterized by PTSD symptoms and the other by phobic reactions. Phobic reactions reflected the circumstances of the trauma, namely a fear of indoor areas in women who were attacked while sleeping, and a fear of outdoor areas in women attacked on the street. Assaulted women often fear being alone as well as being in crowds or, when on the street, a fear of people behind them. Above all, they develop fears related to sex (Burgess & Holmstrom, 1974).

Major depression with sleep disturbance and dysphoria has been observed in 43% of victims. Older women are more often affected. Suicidal ideation and attempts were frequently observed among those assaulted (Kilpatrick et al., 1985). The depression tended to diminish after 3 months, and mood continued to stabilize over the next 6–12 months (Frank et al., 1984). In addition, rape victims more often reported poor perceived health, somatic symptoms and functional impairment (Golding, 1994), as well as symptoms of generalized anxiety and drug abuse (Frank & Anderson, 1987; Frank & Stewart, 1987). Nightmares occurred frequently. In early dreams, victims often tried to defend themselves but could not; later, when improving, they became able, in their dreams, to fight off or injure their assailant (Burgess & Holmstrom, 1974). Eventually, the trauma-related dreams faded.

Victims of accidents

PTSD caused by accidents varies greatly but is often complicated by expectations of compensation. Miller (1961) observed that after accidents with head injuries, psychological disturbances were more frequent in patients without radiological evidence of skull fractures than in patients with fractures. Those with psychological disturbances were more likely to have been unskilled workers who were dependent, insecure and craving sympathy, and who, at the same time, had paranoid personality traits. Symptoms were presented in exaggerated form. Patients displayed an attitude of martyred gloom and became defensive when told that their condition might improve. Their complaints of amnesia were at variance with the circumstantial detail with which they described events that led to the accident. The most consistent feature in these subjects was their unshakable conviction of unfitness for work and the equanimity with which they accepted the tedium of idleness. Often their symptoms improved after legal issues were resolved. Other patients are more concerned about the recognition of suffering rather than monetary rewards (Mayou, 1996).

Most victims of accidents develop only transitory symptoms. Sixty-one per cent of drivers of the London underground, who were involved in fatal accidents while operating trains, experienced no persistent consequences. These accidents involved injury or death of mostly suicidal persons who jumped before a moving train without injury to the driver. Twenty-three per cent of drivers experienced phobias and depression and some had to take time off work. Only 16% satisfied the criteria for PTSD and were absent from work for any substantial time after the accident (Farmer et al., 1992). Another study reported that most train drivers were able to overcome the effects of fatal accidents in a short time. Premorbid variables such as pre-accident worries influenced their stress response. Furthermore, involvement in previous accidents induced feelings of vulnerability and produced stronger acute responses in certain drivers (Malt et al., 1993). Only 10% of drivers reported being sick more than a week after the accident. On follow-up, symptoms of distress were significantly reduced 1 month after the accident. Premorbid factors and variables unrelated to the accident were more important for long-term outcome than the event itself (Karlehagen et al., 1993).

Fear of driving and of having panic attacks in cars is frequently seen in survivors of motor vehicle accidents (Kuch et al., 1994). In one study (Blanchard et al., 1996), the majority of patients whose PTSD followed a motor vehicle accident had had prior major depression, experienced a fear of dying during the accident, received extensive physical injuries or initiated litigation. Past anxiety disorders predispose one to fears but may not determine the content. 'Accident phobia' is particularly prevalent among patients with 'whiplash injury', combining phobic and chronic pain symptoms. Accident phobics complain of pain in more body locations than non-phobic accident victims and use health care more frequently. In some cases, pain improves when anxiety remits. In a study of road accident victims, half of those who meet the criteria for PTSD improved significantly within 6 months. Avoidance and numbing symptoms declined more than hyperarousal (Blanchard et al., 1995). Overprotection of victims by their families contributed substantially to chronicity (Tarsh & Royston, 1985).

One study showed that the effects of a marine explosion on people in the boat were more persistent. Surviving crew members exhibited nervousness, tension, anxiety and general upset. Some also reported depression, preoccupation with the details of the accident, and phobic reactions. A re-examination after 3 years showed considerable deterioration with more somatic complaints, particularly of a gastrointestinal and musculoskeletal nature. Only 39% of sailors went back to sea on a regular basis after this accident (Leopold & Dillon, 1963).

A different picture has been observed in burn victims, who not only have to manage memories of a traumatic event but also the serious physical injuries. A study of burn victims showed that a lack of perceived social support predicted PTSD better than the severity of the physical injury, indicating that the development of PTSD was more dependent on subjective factors than on the seriousness of the injury (Perry et al., 1992). Burn victims develop symptoms similar to other accident victims, but their emergence is often delayed until after discharge. In one study, only 7% of adults were symptomatic while they were on the burn unit, but 22% had psychological symptoms 4 months after discharge. Symptoms of emotional numbing and avoidance in response to the disfigurement tended to emerge after leaving the hospital (Roca et al., 1992). This study provides a good example of symptoms emerging when patients have to deal with the consequences of a trauma rather than the trauma itself.

Acquired blindness

Sudden accidental blindness is a severe trauma that necessitates adjustment to a permanent disability. Soldiers acutely blinded in combat are often disturbed by battle dreams from which they awaken in disbelief. Afterwards, they grow despondent. Gradually, they stabilize emotionally and learn to wash, feed themselves, walk and read Braille. Their perceptual thresholds shift gradually. They experience feelings of inferiority, jealousy, suspicion, envy, impatience, and irritability; they also may joke about their disability and become aggressive sexually. Somatic symptoms are frequently expressed. Nightmares gradually recede and alternate with pleasant dreams (Wittkower et al., 1946). Improvement and readjustment depend on personality and social support. Totally blinded individuals achieved an adequate emotional adjustment more quickly than partially blinded ones who retained false hopes for improvement. Some victims with unusual strong personalities may overcome the trauma within days and make goal-directed strides toward rehabilitation (Hoehn-Saric et al., 1981a). Among 150 blinded soldiers, Diamond & Ross (1945) reported that 60% adjusted well. Improving soldiers were free of preexisting neurotic and psychopathic traits and approached rehabilitation courageously and constructively.

Victims of inadequate surgical anesthesia

Modern surgical procedures are conducted under light anesthesia. In approximately one out of 3000 patients, the anesthesia is so light that patients become conscious during surgery, but because of profound muscle relaxation and tracheal intubation, are unable to communicate. During the operation, patients experience severe anxiety and some subsequently develop PTSD. Particularly distressing to the patients are tactless or derogatory remarks made by the staff who believed the patient was unconscious. Moreover, during their semiconscious state, patients may misunderstand remarks they overheard. Such misunderstanding may remain fixed in the patient's mind and cause further distress (MMW Report, 1996).

Victims of disaster

Disasters occur suddenly, often unexpectedly, and involve large numbers of people and, to varying degrees, loss of lives, homes, and livelihood. Outpourings of sympathy and help occur but are often insufficient for reducing prolonged hardship. Acute stress disorder occurs frequently after disasters but has been insufficiently studied.

Immediately after a disaster 12–25% of the victims remain 'coolheaded', another 75% are stunned but cooperative, and the remaining 12–25% will behave in grossly inappropriate ways (Logue et al., 1981). The prevalence of subsequent PTSD varies from 5% to 22% depending on the type of disaster. Artificially made disasters appear to cause more protracted reactions than natural disasters (Green & Lindy, 1994). Men and women differ in symptoms; women report more PTSD, anxiety and depression and men more somatic symptoms, alcohol abuse and hostile aggressive actions. Symptoms other than those of PTSD also occur. A year after a flash flood in Puerto Rico, a high prevalence of unexplained physical symptoms, including abdominal pain, vomiting, nausea and excessive gas, was noted (Escobar et al., 1992).

The incidence and duration of PTSD depend not only on the severity of a disaster but on the ability of a community to reorganize and normalize its life. While the majority recuperate, some individuals experience decreasing symptoms over the years but do not return to normal. A small number of victims remain disabled. Patients in whom PTSD resolves in a short time seldom have coexisting psychiatric disorders. The longer the symptoms persist, the greater is the role played by several vulnerability factors, such as neuroticism, a personal or family history of psychiatric illness, and a tendency not to confront conflict (McFarlane, 1990).

Trauma in children

Elbedour et al. (1993) stated that a child's capacity to cope with the stress of war depends on its emotional resources, the reaction of parents and care givers, and the cohesiveness of the community. In addition to the intensity and duration of war stress, cultural, historical and political factors influence the child's reaction. Similar statements can be made about other traumatic events in childhood.

Exposure to violence triggers PTSD in children more consistently than other stressors such as natural disasters; however, children exposed to long-lasting war and combat tend to be more sad and fearful (Zivcic, 1993). Family violence is especially destructive because the child sees itself threatened by those who should be its protectors; however, physical abuse in children and adolescents more frequently causes emotional, behavioral and social difficulties than it does PTSD (Parry-Jones & Barton, 1995). Research indicates that sexual abuse does not routinely produce PTSD in children. The impact depends on the type of abuse. For instance, abuse by siblings is usually less traumatic than abuse by a parent or another adult; seduction is less traumatic than the use of force, particularly when it is violent. Cultural values leading to guilt feelings also influence the outcome of abuse (McNally, 1993).

The response of a child to trauma depends on its age. Stressors traumatic to an adolescent – for instance, a devastating hurricane – may not be traumatic to a younger child who only responds to its mother's behavior and emotional state. In general, children manifest more pervasive hyperarousal and hyperreactivity, more global confusion, and fewer stimulus-specific PTSD symptoms than adults. Children respond differently according to their developmental level, ranging from nonspecific to focused responses. Children may react to stimuli that are not directly associated with the original trauma. They also may show regressive behavior. For the most part, adult criteria adequately capture the response to trauma in children but there are some differences: these include repetitive play involving aspects of the trauma, loss of recently acquired skills, regression to an earlier maturational level, and disturbance of future orientation. With the latter, a child does not anticipate achieving life goals of career, family or even adulthood and experiences fearfulness and separation anxiety (Brett et al., 1988). In younger children, distressing dreams of the event may change into generalized nightmares. Children often relive traumas through repetitive play of car crashes or combat. Somatization in the form of stomach aches and headaches is frequent.

Trait anxiety might be the single strongest risk factor for posttraumatic reactions in children exposed to disaster (Lonigan et al., 1994). In addition, parental anxiety modifies the impact of trauma. Children of parents with PTSD are more likely to develop the disorder themselves (Schwarz &

Perry, 1994). After a natural disaster, the risk of PTSD also depends on the time needed for the community to reorganize itself (Galante & Foa, 1986).

The assessment and treatment of children depends on their age. In young children, it may require play and art therapy; in older children, sympathetic conversations. One has to keep in mind that suggestible and eager-to-please youngsters can easily be led to believe and describe convincingly a version of events suggested by biased adults; therefore, mental health professionals need to exercise extreme caution not to induce false memories (Schwarz & Perry, 1994).

Recovery from PTSD depends on the type and severity of the trauma as well as its duration and subsequent support. Thus, recovery rates will vary. Children assessed 4 years after they had been kidnaped on a bus still showed pathology (Terr, 1983). On the other hand, children assessed 17 years after the Buffalo Creek Dam had collapsed showed a high recovery rate. The rate of PTSD in those children fell from 32% to 7% (Green & Lindy, 1994). Similarly, Krell (1993) reported that most children who survived the holocaust lived normal and creative adult lives in spite of symptoms. They had learned how to cope with bereavement and memories; however, heightened vulnerability often surfaced under stress (Solomon & Prager, 1992).

Natural history

Course and outcome

The course and outcome of PTSD depend on factors discussed earlier. The majority of victims recover completely or at least partially. In psychologically healthy individuals, who receive adequate support after the trauma, symptoms generally subside within a few days to weeks. Intrusions become less frequent and intense, and dreams become more benign in character. Emotional responses to stimuli also weaken. Some symptoms, such as intrusive thoughts or dreams, may remain but have little clinical importance. Recovery depends largely on a person's mental health and the social support obtained after the trauma.

Early posttraumatic symptoms resembling an adjustment disorder are unlikely to progress to PTSD. On the other hand, combat stress disorders, that correspond to the acute stress reaction in DSM-IV, signal a more severe disorder. In one study, combat stress disorder led to PTSD in 60% of the cases (Rothbaum & Foa, 1993).

Following motor vehicle accidents, 25% of the victims who originally met criteria for PTSD no longer did so after 4 months, and 50% no longer met criteria 6 months later (Blanchard et al., 1995). In the St. Louis ECA study, 49% of patients with PTSD experienced resolution of symptoms within 6 months, but 33% had symptoms that lasted beyond 26 months. Among prisoners of war seen 40 years later, 29% had fully recovered, 39% still reported mild symptoms, 24% moderate, and only 8% reported no improvement or worsening (Kluznik et al., 1986).

Chronic PTSD is more frequently found among persons who were attacked physically, were wounded in combat, or saw someone hurt or killed (Davidson & Fairbank, 1993). Several studies indicate that the presence of PTSD at approximately 3 months post-trauma predicts chronicity. The relative proportions of intrusion, avoidance, and hyperarousal symptoms may vary over time. Intrusion symptoms may be more prominent initially and avoidance symptoms later. In most cases, PTSD symptoms diminish over time, but in a small group of victims, they remain unchanged or worsen. In some instances, PTSD symptoms, such as nightmares, may be mild and isolated but persistent. Comorbidity may also change over time (Blank, 1993).

Studies indicate that severe PTSD has an adverse effect on functioning, and that over time, it may lead to difficulties in employment and marriage. Personality factors probably play an important role in social dysfunction because individuals who function well in the face of significant symptoms are common (Blank, 1993). For instance, veterans with PTSD who improved on treatment had a lower rate of alcohol consumption and a greater program participation than those who failed (Perconte & Griger, 1991).

Even after recovery, PTSD may leave a person more vulnerable to stress and susceptible to recurrences. Individuals may shed all or most of their symptoms for extended periods, but at times of stress, may experience them again. For instance, a patient who developed transitory PTSD during combat in Vietnam and who fully recovered within a few months, re-experienced trauma-related dreams 12 years later during the bankruptcy of his company and separation from his wife. In other instances, symptoms may reemerge for no obvious reason (Tomb, 1994).

Stressors of old age may also cause reemergence or worsening of PTSD. The aging process, when accompanied by diminished coping ability and increased social isolation, may increase the severity of PTSD. Depression is more frequently seen in older persons while anxiety is more common in younger victims (Dreissig & Berger, 1991). In a few soldiers, symptoms of traumatic stress, which had been latent since World War II, emerged in later years (Ramsay, 1990). Symptoms of holocaust victims often intensify after retirement, after children leave home, and illness occurs in old age. Being less distracted, elderly patients ruminate about their past and their experiences during persecution, particularly the loss of family members.

Predictors of outcome

Factors influencing the outcome of PTSD have been discussed in previous sections. Briefly, a family history of mental illness, pathological premorbid personality, previous traumatic experiences, mental illness at the time of the traumatic experience, the severity and repetition of trauma, development of anxiety disorders following the trauma, the presence of symptoms several months after the trauma, an inability to prevent or to control further traumas, a lack of support from family and friends and adverse social consequences of the trauma all are predictors for chronicity (Fontana & Rosenheck, 1994).

Complications

The clinical picture of PTSD can be complicated by alcoholism, substance abuse, major depression with suicidal ideation and attempts, and anxiety disorders. Frequent complications also are social withdrawal, violent outbursts, and personality changes, particularly in younger persons whose development may have been distorted by the trauma. Also, the infirmities of old age may make it difficult for patients' ability to cope with symptoms as they had previously. Secondary gains may exaggerate the clinical picture of PTSD. Some patients attribute other psychopathology to the traumatic experience thereby shifting responsibility for their actions away from themselves.

It is not clear whether PTSD can worsen a person's physical health. Tomb (1994) could find little evidence that PTSD increases the risk for medical disorders, such as hypertension, myocardial infarction or diabetes. Many patients exhibit a low effort tolerance without abnormalities on laboratory tests or physical examinations (Shalev et al., 1990). On the other hand, two studies show that the disorder may have an adverse effect on health. World War II Dutch resistance veterans with PTSD were at higher risk for cardiovascular diseases, particularly when they had type A personalities (Falger et al., 1992). Also, among fire fighters, the rate of cardiac disease, hypertension, respiratory diseases and diabetes increased significantly after a severe brush fire in Southern Australia (Clayer et al., 1985).

Adverse health practices, such as smoking, alcohol use, and poor dietary habits, may also contribute to physical deterioration (Shalev et al., 1990).

Differential diagnosis

The diagnosis and differential diagnosis of PTSD is easy when it follows a traumatic event and the patient exhibits classical PTSD symptoms. It is more difficult to decide to what extent coexisting general anxiety, phobias, panic, and depression are part of PTSD. Some of these symptoms may have preceded PTSD and others may have developed later and represent independent disorders. A preexisting disorder should be elicited by history, and if possible, verified by reliable sources. The preexistence of another disorder does not exclude PTSD but may mean that the symptoms are not the consequence of trauma alone.

On the other hand, trauma may give rise to an adjustment disorder, generalized anxiety disorder, somatization disorder, depression or phobias without classic PTSD symptoms. Even though such disorders are clearly trauma induced, they do not qualify for PTSD by present convention.

The most difficult differential diagnosis is malingering in an intelligent person. Evidence of ulterior motive and absence of PTSD symptoms when the patient feels unobserved are necessary to establish malingering. An exaggeration of mild PTSD symptoms should be considered when hope of financial gain through litigation is present (Blank, 1994).

Symptoms of PTSD may be mistaken for nightmare disorder, sleep terror or narcolepsy when vivid dreams emerge during a stressful period (Mellman et al., 1991).

Treatment

In the management of stress-induced disorders one has to consider symptoms, severity, duration and social ramification of the trauma. It is particularly important for treatment plannng to include co-occurring disorders. Psychological interventions are always required. Pharmacological treatments may be administered as adjuvants to psychological therapy or with the primary aim of suppressing stress-induced symptoms.

Pharmacological treatment

Acute stress disorder

No systematic studies have been conducted on the treatment of the newly described acute stress disorder. The therapeutic approach is symptomatic. Benzodiazepines are helpful to calm a person and induce sleep. Beta-blockers and clonidine have been used on the assumption that they reduce stress-induced noradrenergic hyperactivity. Clonidine also has anxiolytic and sedating effects that may be useful for reducing the intensity of anxiety (Hoehn-Saric et al., 1981b; Spiegel & Classen, 1995).

Posttraumatic stress disorder

In acute PTSD, benzodiazepines and possibly clonidine may be useful for reducing anxiety and hypervigilance. Sargent & Slater (1940) used medications such as ether to induce abreaction in soldiers with PTSD. Under the influence of the drug, and with guidance by the therapist, patients vividly relived their traumatic experience. This treatment was based on the assumption that uncovering of repressed or dissociated material through emotional abreaction might promote healing. In addition, reexperiencing the trauma in a controlled environment might lead to a perception of mastery over the experience. Abreaction studies in neurotic patients suggest that the healing effect lies primarily in an unfreezing of fixed response patterns that make patients temporarily more suggestible. The resulting altered state of mind permits the implantation of healthier attitudes. Abreaction alone is rarely helpful because newly gained attitudes must be reinforced through systematic therapy; however, it can act as catalyst that permits the initiation of change (Hoehn-Saric, 1977).

In chronic PTSD, pharmacotherapy is only modestly effective. Most controlled studies have been conducted on combat veterans. While benzodiazepines are helpful for brief, time-limited administration, antidepressants have gained a prominent role in chronic treatment. The tricyclic antidepressants, imipramine and amitriptyline, the monoamine oxidase inhibitor, phenelzine, and the selective serotonin reuptake inhibitor, fluoxetine, have proven superior to placebo in reducing PTSD symptoms (Foa et al., 1995a). The placebo response in controlled studies has been approximately 20%, which is lower than that for other anxiety disorders and depression. Antidepressants reduce intrusive, avoidance, and hyperarousal symptoms. In the treatment of chronic PTSD, it is important that sufficiently high doses be given and that the trials be of sufficient length. A minimum should be 5–8 weeks and preferably longer, because some patients improve only after several months of treatment. The antidepressants are generally only partially effective. Most patients continue to experience symptoms but to a lesser degree. Some may need lifelong pharmacotherapy, and for them, attempts to reduce the dose may lead to relapse even 20 or more years after combat exposure. Patients with severe symptoms often require a combination of pharmacotherapeutic agents combined with psychological interventions.

Carbamazepine, valproic acid, beta-blockers, and clonidine have been given to soldiers with PTSD, but no controlled studies have confirmed their effectiveness.

Psychological treatment

Acute stress disorder

There are no controlled treatment studies of acute stress disorder (Spiegel & Classen, 1995). Experience suggests that this disorder requires immediate attention. The value of debriefing alone – i.e., talking through the traumatic experience – has been questioned (Raphael et al., 1995). It is important to obtain detailed information about the trauma and its realistic consequences. Treatment should be given early, and it should be brief, problem-focused and simple. Patients should be placed in a safe area but preferably near the place where the trauma occurred. They should be told that they will recover quickly (Lundin, 1994), and if possible, returned in a short time to the environment in which the trauma occurred (Friedman et al., 1994).

Armstrong et al., (1991) developed a treatment program that consists of: (1) an introductory phase in which the therapist establishes contact and explains treatment procedures, (2) a fact-finding phase during which the patient retells personal experiences in relation to the traumatic event, (3) a cognitive phase during which reactions to the most stressful aspects of the event are explored, (4) an affective phase in which the patient is encouraged to discuss emotional reactions to the event, with emphasis on those that do not constitute weakness, and (5) a phase in which enquiries are made about physical and emotional symptoms since the event. At that point common features of the stress response syndromes and their normalization are brought up, and (6) a final phase that focuses on reentry and consolidation is completed. Obviously, individual psychological and social needs have to be considered, and treatment may have to be modified accordingly.

Posttraumatic stress disorder

Controlled studies concerning the efficacy of various therapeutic interventions have been conducted in combat veterans and rape victims but not other PTSD populations. There is considerable controversy about how effective psychological interventions may be. Andrews (1991) suggested that cognitive-behavioral techniques are more effective than psychoanalytically-oriented psychotherapy. A carefully conducted study in Israeli veterans, whose treatment was based on cognitive, behavioral and social theories, led to subjective improvement but objective worsening of symptoms (Solomon et al., 1992); however, other outcome studies have yielded more favorable results. Foa et al. (1995a) compared three treatment modalities, namely stress inoculation, prolonged imaginal exposure and supportive counseling with a wait-list control in rape victims. Initially, stress inoculation was superior; however, by the fourth month, imaginal exposure appeared more beneficial. Imaginal exposure appeared to induce major changes in memory representations, and therefore, produced more a profound change than stress inoculation. The technique was helpful when first applied but lost some of its impact when patients stopped practicing it. Other outcome studies have been less clear. In some studies, one technique was superior to others, but in others no differences were found. Desensitization appeared to have only a modest impact. Flooding was effective in some patients but led to worsening and complications in others. The effect of flooding depends upon whether the emotion that is elicited can be processed and brought to a satisfactory resolution, or whether it opens emotional wounds without providing relief.

Discrepant results are not surprising when one considers differences not only between but also within apparently homogeneous groups of PTSD patients. Thus, individualization of treatment is essential. Recommended methods, while good for learning, should not be followed rigidly but modified according to the needs of individual patients. Psychosocial treatment strategies are discussed extensively by Meichenbaum (1994) and by Lehrer & Woolfolk (1993).

The best results have been obtained with anxiety management training, a treatment program that includes biofeedback, relaxation, and cognitive restructuring with stress inoculation training. This approach includes an educational phase and some coping skills training with homework. Coping skills include muscle relaxation, breathing control, covert modeling, exposure, thought stopping and guided self-dialogue. Studies show that, while all treatments are of some use, a combination tends to be more effective than a single method. Psychological interventions are less effective in veterans than in rape victims, probably because of the greater chronicity and comorbidity in the former group.

In practice, the treatment plan must include the formation of positive rapport. Some patients avoid formal mental health services because they cue for distressing memories (Schwarz & Kowalski, 1992). Patients need to develop a realistic appraisal of the trauma and be educated regarding their symptoms. At the same time, the meaning of the trauma for the individual needs to be explored. Important also is the examination of perceived responsibility for having been traumatized. This includes reassurance about one's behavior and actions taken during the traumatic experience. The goal is the acceptance of one's behavior and the gradual mastery over one's feelings. Among holocaust survivors, intrusive thoughts about deceased relatives may become less distressing when they are viewed as cherished memories of loved ones rather than recollections of horror (Krell, 1993). The feeling of gaining control over one's life and over potential new traumas has a strengthening effect.

Relaxation techniques alone or combined with exposure to trauma-related stressors may lead to desensitization. Flooding, i.e., direct, often maximal, exposure to traumatic cues, leads at first to abreaction that is followed, under the proper guidance of a therapist, to a calmer view of the traumatic event. During exposure, it is important for victims to give not only a detailed description of the stimuli but also their reactions, appraisal, and threat-related thoughts. During exposure, trust in the therapist is of crucial importance because it is his or her influence that modifies the emotional tone of the distressing memories. Memories of the insult may never become neutral but become less painful. When exposure to a stressor is not possible, guided recollection of memories can be used. Its aim is to reduce the hyperarousal and excessive reactivity to traumatic memories. In addition, avoidance, when it is present, needs to be reduced and social interaction improved (McFarlane, 1994).

As stated above, treatment must begin with the establishment of rapport. A full exploration of the circumstances of the trauma and its psychological and social impact precedes actual treatment. Then, a treatment program is developed in collaboration with the patient who needs to realize that progress can only be made if he or she takes an active role. First, the increased arousal is treated with relaxation techniques. Then attempts are made to reduce intrusive thoughts and images for which several approaches are available. The choice of technique depends on the patient's psychopathology and ability to participate in treatment. With systematic desensitization, the therapist induces fearful images while the patient is in a relaxed state. It obviously is not effective if the patient cannot relax. Imaginary or in vivo exposure involves repeated reliving of the trauma with the aim of processing the experience and deriving a satisfactory

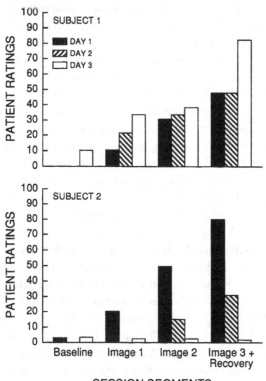

Figure 6.1 Ratings of fear on an analogue scale (0 to 100) before and after three subsequent imagings of a traumatic event during three different days of treatment. Subject 1 had chronic PTSD with poor prognosis; subject 2 had acute PTSD with good prognosis. For details see text.

closure. Cognitive working through of the traumatic experience under the guidance of a therapist is essential for bringing about change. Avoidance is treated with gradual exposure to the feared situations. The sequencing of exposures and demands for behavioral change need to be tailored individually. Realistic expectations for outcome should be set from the beginning. Patients need to realize that treatment will most likely reduce but not alleviate their symptoms. The goal of therapy should be better functioning in spite of the persistent symptoms.

Acute PTSD generally responds better than chronic PTSD. Figure 6.1 shows anxiety levels of an acute and a chronic patient during repeated imaginary exposures to a trauma. Each patient was asked to rate his or her anxiety on a scale ranging from 0 to 100 when not imagining, and then, while imagining the trauma repeatedly. This was done during the first week of treatment and repeated during a session 6–8 weeks later. Subject 1 had been involved in an industrial accident 2 years earlier in which he had almost lost his life. He had a history of alcohol abuse, his marriage was deteriorating, and he subsequently received little support from his employer. During imagining, the patient responded with increased fear to each exposure, and his fear became worse during 6 weeks of treatment. He needed prolonged therapy in addition to a monoamine oxidase inhibitor, and then he only partially recovered. Subject 2 was a prison guard who became involved in a shooting while transporting prisoners. He had no previous psychiatric problems, the incident was recent, and he had good social support. He experienced severe anxiety during the first session but was free of distress during a follow-up session 8 weeks later. Having received only behavior therapy with imaginary and in vivo exposure, he made a full recovery within 3 weeks.

The treatment plan needs to take into account the special needs of a patient. Disaster victims need to be resettled and helped to rebuild their lives. Victims of crime need help in dealing with stressful legal matters such as cross examination during the trial of a perpetrator. As noncompliance is frequent, the therapist needs to be patient and flexible in dealing with patent's anxieties and often changing feelings. Cultural aspects also have to be considered in the treatment of PTSD. For instance, Asians from far east regions are culturally prohibited from expressing strong or negative emotions, and, therefore, tend to somatize. Belief in the physical nature of their distress and 'karma', the idea that the disaster is a consequence of evil deeds done in previous lives, is a stumbling block to psychotherapy (Cheung, 1993). Such patients accept pharmacotherapy combined with reassurance and direct advice better than they do Western-style cognitive-emotional psychotherapies.

References

Allen, S. N. 1994. Psychological assessment of post-traumatic stress disorder: Psychometrics, current trends, and future dimensions. *Psychiatr. Clin. North Am.* 17: 327–349.

Allodi, F. & Stiasny, S. 1990. Women as torture victims. *Can. J. Psychiatry* 35: 144–148.

Allodi, F. A. 1994. Post-traumatic stress disorder in hostages and victims of torture. *Psychiatr. Clin. North Am.* 17: 279–288.

Alter, C. L., Pelcovitz, D., Axelrod, A. et al. 1996. Identification of PTSD in cancer survivors. *Psychosomatics* 37: 137–143.

American Psychiatric Association. 1994. *Diagnostic and Statistical Manual of Mental Disorders*, Fourth Edition, American Psychiatric Association, Washington, DC.

Andrews, G. 1991. The evaluation of psychotherapy. *Curr. Opin. Psychiatry* 4: 379–383.

Antelman, S. M. & Yehuda, R. 1994. Time-dependent change following acute stress: Relevance to the chronic and delayed aspects of PTSD. In *Catecholamine Function in Post-traumatic Stress Disorder*, ed. M. M. Murburg, pp. 87–98, American Psychiatric Press, Washington, DC.

Armstrong, K., O'Callaham, W. & Marmar, C. R. 1991. Debriefing Red Cross disaster personnel: The multiple stressor debriefing model. *J. Traum. Stress* 4: 481–491.

Aston-Jones, G., Valentino, R. J., Van Bockstaele, E. J. et al. 1994. Locus coeruleus, stress, and PTSD: Neurobiological and clinical parallels. In *Catecholamine Function in Post-traumatic Stress Disorder*, ed. M. M. Murburg, pp. 17–62, American Psychiatric Press, Washington, DC.

Averill, J. R. 1968. Grief: It's nature and significance. *Psychol. Bull.* 70: 721–748.

Ballard, C. G., Stanley, A. K. & Brockington, I. J. 1995. Post-traumatic stress disorder (PTSD) after childbirth. *Br. J. Psychiatry* 166: 525–528.

Basoglu, M., Paker, M., Ozmen, E. et al. 1994. Factors related to long-term traumatic stress responses in survivors of torture in Turkey. *JAMA* 272: 357–363.

Blanchard, E. B., Hickling, E. J., Vollmer, A. J. et al. 1995. Short-term follow-up of post-traumatic stress symptoms in motor vehicle accident victims. *Behav. Res. Ther.* 33: 369–377.

Blanchard, E. B., Hickling, E. J., Taylor, A. E. et al. 1996. Who develops PTSD from motor vehicle accidents? *Behav. Res. Ther.* 34: 1–10.

Blank, A. S. 1993. The longitudinal course of posttraumatic stress disorder. In *Posttraumatic Stress Disorder: DSM-IV and Beyond*, eds. J. R. T. Davidson, E. B. Foa, pp. 3–22, American Psychiatric Press, Washington, DC.

Blank, A. S. 1994. Clinical detection, diagnosis, and differential diagnosis of post-traumatic stress disorder. *Psychiatr. Clin. North Am.* 17: 351–383.

Bremner, J. D., Scott, T. M., Delaney, R. C. et al. 1993. Deficits in short-term memory in posttraumatic stress disorder. *Am. J. Psychiatry.* 150: 1015–1019.

Bremner, J. D., Randall, P., Scott, T. M. et al. 1995. MRI-based measurement of hippocampal volume in patients with combat-related posttraumatic stress disorder. *Am. J. Psychiatry* 152: 973–981.

Breslau, N. & Davis, G. C. 1987. Post-traumatic stress disorder: The etiologic specificity of wartime stressors. *Am. J. Psychiatry* 144: 578–583.

Breslau, N., Davis, G. C., Andreski, P. et al. 1991. Traumatic events and posttraumatic stress disorder in an urban population of young adults. *Arch. Gen. Psychiatry* 48: 216–222.

Brett, E. A., Spitzer, R. L. & Williams, J. B. W. 1988. DSM-III-R criteria for posttraumatic stress disorder. *Am. J. Psychiatry* 145: 1232–1236.

Bryant, R. A. & Harvey, A. G. 1995. Posttraumatic stress in volunteer firefighters: Predictors of distress. *J. Nerv. Ment. Dis.* 183: 267–271.

Burgess, A. W. & Holmstrom, L. L. 1974. Rape trauma syndrome. *Am. J. Psychiatry* 131: 981–985.

Butler, R. W., Braff, D. L., Rausch, J. L. et al. 1990. Physiological evidence of exaggerated startle response in a subgroup of Vietnam veterans with combat-related PTSD. *Am. J. Psychiatry* 147: 1308–1312.

Carroll, E. M., Rueger, D. B., Foy, D. W. et al. 1985. Vietnam combat veterans with post-traumatic stress disorder: Analysis of marital and cohabitating adjustment. *J. Abnorm. Psychol.* 94: 329–337.

Charles, G., Hansenne, M., Ansseau, M. et al. 1995. P300 in posttraumatic stress disorder. *Biol. Psychiatry.* 32: 72–74.

Charney, D. S., Woods, S. W., Goodman, W. K. et al. 1987. Neurobiological mechanisms of panic anxiety: Biochemical and behavioral correlates of yohimbine-induced panic attacks. *Am. J. Psychiatry* 144: 1030–1036.

Charney, D. S., Deutch, A. Y., Krystal, J. H. et al. 1993. Psychobiologic mechanisms of posttraumatic stress disorder. *Arch. Gen. Psychiatry* 50: 294–305.

Charney, D. S., Southwick, S. M., Krystal, J. H. et al. 1994. Neurobiological mechanisms of PTSD. In *Catecholamine Function in Post-traumatic Stress Disorder*, ed. M. M. Murburg, pp. 131–158, American Psychiatric Press, Washington, DC.

Cheung, P. 1993. Somatization as a presentation in depression and post-traumatic stress disorder among Cambodian refugees. *Aust. N. Z. J. Psychiatry* 27: 422–428.

Choy, T. & De Bosset, F. 1992. Post-traumatic stress disorder: An overview. *Can. J. Psychiatry* 37: 578–583.

Clayer, J. R., Brookless-Pratz, C. & Haris, R. L. 1985. Some health consequences of a natural disaster. *Med. J. Aust* 143: 182–184.

Cottler, L. B., Compton, W. M., III., Mager, D. et al. 1992. Posttraumatic stress disorder among substance users from the general population. *Am. J. Psychiatry* 149: 664–670.

Daly, R. J. 1983. Samuel Pepys and post-traumatic stress disorder. *Br. J. Psychiatry* 143: 64–68.

Davidson, J. R. T., Swartz, M., Storck, M. et al. 1985. A diagnostic and family study of posttraumatic stress disorder. *Am. J. Psychiatry* 142: 90–93.

Davidson, J. R. T., Smith, R. D.& Kudler, H. S. 1989. Familial psychiatric illness in chronic posttraumatic stress disorder. *Compr. Psychiatry* 4: 339–345.

Davidson, J. R. T., Kudler, H. S. & Smith, R. D. 1990. Assessment and pharmacotherapy of posttraumatic stress disorder. In *Biological Assessment and Treatment of Posttraumatic Stress Disorder*, ed. E. L. Giller, pp. 203–233, Psychiatric Press, Washington, DC.

Davidson, J. R. T. Hughes, D., Blazer, D. G. et al. 1991. Post-traumatic stress disorder in the community: An epidemiological study. *Psychol. Med.* 21: 713–721.

Davidson, J. R. T. & Fairbank, J. A. 1993. The epidemiology of posttraumatic stress disorder. In *Posttraumatic Stress Disorder. DSM-IV and Beyond*, eds. J. R. T. Davidson, E. B. Foa, pp. 147–169, American Psychiatric Press, Washington, DC.

Davidson, R. J. 1994. Asymmetric brain function, affective style, and psychopathology: The role of early experience and plasticity. *Dev. Psychopathol.* 6: 741–758.

Davis, G. C. & Breslau, N. 1994. Post-traumatic stress disorder in victims of civilian trauma and criminal violence. *Psychiatr. Clin. North Am.* 17: 289–299.

Davis, M. 1992. The role of the amygdala in fear-potentiated startle: Implications for animal models of anxiety. *TIPS* 13: 35–41.

Davis, M., Rainnie, D. & Cassell, M. 1994. Neurotransmission in the rat amygdala related to fear and anxiety. *TIPS* 17: 208–214.

De Silva, P. 1993. Post-traumatic stress disorder: Cross-cultural aspects. *Int. Rev. Psychiatry* 5: 217–229.

Diamond, B. L. & Ross, A. 1945. Emotional adjustment of newly blinded soldiers. *Am. J. Psychiatry* 102: 367–371.

Djilas, M. 1973. *Memoir of a revolutionary*. Harcourt Brace Jovanovich, New York.

Dreissig, H. & Berger, M. 199.1 Posttraumatische Stresserkrankungen: Zur Entwicklung des gegenwärtigen Krankheitskonzepts. *Nervenarzt*. 62: 16–26.

Dunn, A. J. & Berridge, C. W. 1990. Physiological and behavioral responses to corticotropin-releasing factor administration: Is CRF a mediator of anxiety or stress responses? *Brain Res. Rev.* 15: 71–100.

Eaton, W. W., Sigal, J. J. & Weinfeld, M. 1982. Impairment in Holocaust survivors after 33 years: Data from an unbiased community sample. *Am. J. Psychiatry* 139: 773–777.

Elbedour, S., Ten Bensel, R. & Bastien, D. T. 1993. Ecological integrated model of children of war: Individual and social psychology. *Child Abuse Negl.* 17: 795–803.

Escobar, J. I., Canino, G., Rubio-Stipec, M. et al. 1992. Somatic symptoms after a natural disaster: A prospective study. *Am. J. Psychiatry* 149: 965–967.

Falger, P. R. J., Op Den Velde, W., Hovens, J. E. et al. 1992. Current posttraumatic stress disorder and cardiovascular disease risk factors in Dutch resistance veterans from World War II. *Psychother. Psychosom.* 57: 164–171.

Farmer, R., Tranah, T., O'Donnell, I. et al. 1992. Railway suicide: The psychological effects on drivers. *Psychol. Med.* 22: 407–414.

Faustman, W. O. & White, P. A. 1989. Diagnostic and psychopharmacological treatment characteristics of 536 inpatients with posttraumatic stress disorder. *J. Nerv. Ment. Dis.* 177: 154–159.

Fenig, S. & Levav., I. 1991. Demoralization and social supports among Holocaust survivors. *J .Nerv. Ment. Dis.* 179: 167–172.

First, M. B., Spitzer, R. L., Gibbon, M. et al. 1996. *Structured Clinical Interview for DSM-IV Axis I Disorders* – Patient Edition (SCID-I/P, version 2.0). Biometrics Research Department, New York State Psychiatric Institute, New York, NY.

Foa, E. B., Davidson, J. & Rothbaum, B. O. 1995a. Posttraumatic stress disorder. In *Treatments of Psychiatric Disorders*, Second Edition, ed. G. O. Gabbard, pp. 1499–1519, American Psychiatric Press, Washington, DC.

Foa, E. B., Riggs, D. S. & Gershuny, B. S. 1995b. Arousal, numbing, and intrusion: Symptom structure of PTSD following assault. *Am. J. Psychiatry* 152: 116–120.

Fontana, A. & Rosenheck, R. 1994. Posttraumatic stress disorder among Vietnam theater veterans: A causal model of etiology in a community sample. *J. Nerv. Ment. Dis.* 182: 677–684.

Frank, E. & Stewart, B. D. 1984. Depressive symptoms in rape victims: A revisit. *J. Affect. Disord.* 7: 77–85.

Frank, E. & Anderson, B. P. 1987. Psychiatric disorders in rape victims: Past history and current symptomatology. *Compr. Psychiatry* 28: 77–82.

Frankl, V. E. 1946. *Ein Psycholog erlebt das Konzentrationslager*. Verlag für

Jugend und Volk, Wien.
Frankl, V. E. 1984. *Man's Search For Meaning: An Introduction to Logotherapy.* Simon and Schuster, New York, NY.
Friedman, M. J.,Schnurr, P. P. & McDonagh-Coyle, A. 1994. Post-traumatic stress disorder in military veterans. *Psychiatr. Clin. North Am.* 17: 265–277.
Galante, R. & Foa, D. 1986. An epidemiological study of psychic trauma and treatment effectiveness for children after a natural disaster. *J. Am. Acad. Child Adolesc. Psychiatry* 25: 357–363.
Giller, E. L., Perry, B. D., Southwick, S. et al. 1990. Psychoendocrinology of posttraumatic stress disorder. In *Posttraumatic Stress Disorder: Etiology, Phenomenology, and Treatment*, eds. M. E. Wolf, A. D. Mosnaim, pp. 158–167, American Psychiatric Press, Washington, DC.
Gold, P. W., Kling, M. A., Demitrack, M. A. et al. 1988. Clinical studies with corticotropin releasing hormone: Implications for hypothalamic-pituitary-adrenal dysfunction in depression and related disorders. *Curr. Top. Neuroendocrin* 8: 55–77.
Goldberg, J., True, W. R., Eisen, S. A. et al. 1990. A twin study of the effects of the Vietnam War on post-traumatic stress disorder. *JAMA* 263: 1227–1232.
Golding, J. M. 1994. Sexual assault history and physical health in random selected Los Angeles women. *Heal. Psych.* 13: 130–138.
Grady, D. A., Woolfolk, R. L. & Budney, A. J. 1989. Dimensions of war zone stress: An empirical analysis. *J. Nerv. Ment. Dis.* 177: 347–350.
Green, B. L. & Lindy, J. D. 1994. Post-traumatic stress disorder in victims of disaster. *Psychiatr. Clin. North Am.* 17: 301–309.
Gurvits, T. V., Lasko, N. B., Schachter, S. C. et al. 1993. Neurological status of Vietnam veterans with chronic posttraumatic stress disorder. *J. Neuropsychiatr.* 5: 183–188.
Hammarberg, M. 1992. Penn inventory for posttraumatic stress disorder: Psychometric properties. *Psychol Assess.* 4: 67–76.
Helzer, J. E., Robins, L. N. & McEvoy, L. 1987. Post-traumatic stress disorder in the general population: Findings of the Epidemiological Catchment Area Survey. *N. Eng. J. Med.* 317: 1630–1634.
Hendin, H., Haas, A. P., Singer, P. et al. 1983. The influence of precombat personality on posttraumatic stress disorder. *Compr. Psychiatry* 24: 530–534.
Hendin, H. & Haas, A. P. 1991. Suicide and guilt as manifestations of PTSD in Vietnam combat veterans. *Am. J. Psychiatry* 148: 586–591.
Herman, J. L. 1993. Sequelae of prolonged and repeated trauma: Evidence for a complex posttraumatic syndrome (DESNOS). In *Posttraumatic Stress Disorder DSM-IV and Beyond*, eds. J. R. T. Davidson, E. B. Foa, pp. 213–228, American Psychiatric Press, Washington, DC.
Hobfoll, S. E., Spielberger, C. D., Breznitz, S. et al. 1991. War-related stress: Addressing the stress of war and other traumatic events. *Am. Psychol.* 46: 848–855.
Hoehn-Saric, R. 1974. Transcendence in psychotherapy. *Am. J. Psychother.* 28: 252–264.
Hoehn-Saric, R. 1977. Emotions in psychotherapies. *Am. J. Psychother.* 31: 83–96.
Hoehn-Saric, R., Frank, E., Hirst, L. W. et al. 1981a. Coping with sudden blindness. *J. Nerv. Ment. Dis.* 169: 622–655.
Hoehn-Saric, R., Merchant, A. F., Keyser, M. L. et al. 1981b. Effects of clonidine on anxiety disorders. *Arch. Gen. Psychiatry* 38: 1278–1282.
Hoehn-Saric, R., McLeod, D. R. & Glowa, J. R. 1991. The effects of NMDA

receptor blockade on the acquisition of a conditioned emotional response. *Biol. Psychiatry* 30: 170–176.

Hoehn-Saric, R. & McLeod, D. R. 1993. Somatic manifestations of normal and pathological anxiety. In *Biology of Anxiety Disorders*, eds. R. Hoehn-Saric, D. R. McLeod, pp. 177–222, American Psychiatric Press, Washington, DC.

Horowitz, M. J. 1985. Disaster and psychological response to stress. *Psychiatr. Ann.* 15: 161–167.

Kardiner, A. & Spiegel, H. 1947. *War Stress and Neurotic Illness.* Paul B. Hoeber, New York.

Karlehagen, S., Malt, U. F., Hoff, H. et al. 1993. The effect of major railway accidents on the psychological health of train drivers: II. A longitudinal study of the one-year outcome after the accident. *J. Psychosom. Res.* 37: 807–817.

Keane, T. M., Caddell, J. M. & Taylor, K. L. 1988. Mississippi scale for combat-related posttraumatic stress disorder: Three studies in reliability and validity. *J. Consult. Clin. Psychol.* 56: 85–90.

Kessler, R. C., Sonnega, A., Bromet, E. et al. 1995. Posttraumatic stress disorder in the National Comorbidity Survey. *Arch. Gen. Psychiatry* 52: 1048–1060.

Kilpatrick, D. G., Best, C. L., Veronen, L. J. et al. 1985. Mental health correlates of criminal victimization: A random community survey. *J. Consult. Clin. Psychol.* 53: 866–873.

Kilpatrick, D. G. & Resnick, H. S. 1993. Posttraumatic stress disorder associated with exposure to criminal victimization in clinical and community populations. In *Posttraumatic Stress Disorder. DSM-IV and Beyond*, eds. J. R. T. Davidson, E. B. Foa, pp. 113–143, American Psychiatric Press, Washington, DC.

Kiser, L., Heston, J., Hickerson, S. et al. 1993. Anticipatory stress in children and adolescents. *Am. J. Psychiatry* 150: 87–92.

Kline, N. A. & Rausch, J. L. 1985. Olfactory precipitants of flashbacks in post-traumatic stress disorder: Case reports. *J. Clin. Psychiatry* 46: 383–384.

Kluznik, J. C., Speed, N., Van Valkenburg, C. et al. 1986. Forty-year follow-up of United States prisoners of war. *Am. J. Psychiatry* 143: 1443–1446.

Kral, V. A. 1951. Psychiatric observations under severe chronic stress. *Am. J. Psychiatry* 108: 185–192.

Krell, R. 1993. Child survivors of the Holocaust: Strategies of adaptation. *Can. J. Psychiatry* 38: 384–389.

Kuch, K. & Cox , M. A. 1992. Symptoms of PTSD in 124 survivors of the Holocaust. *Am. J. Psychiatry* 149: 337–340.

Kuch, K., Cox, B. J., Evans, R. et al. 1994. Phobias, panic, and pain in 55 survivors of road vehicle accidents. *J. Anxiety Dis.* 8: 181–187.

Lehrer, P. M. & Woolfolk, R. L. (eds.) 1993. *Principles and Practice of Stress Management*, Second Edition, Guilford Press, New York.

Leopold, R. L. & Dillon, H. 1963. Psycho-anatomy of a disaster: A long term study of post-traumatic neuroses in survivors of a marine explosion. *Am. J. Psychiatry* 119: 913–921.

Levav, I., Greenfeld, H. & Baruch, E. 1979. Psychiatric combat reactions during the Yom Kippur War. *Am. J. Psychiatry* 136: 637–641.

Levav, I. & Abramsom, J. H. 1984. Emotional distress among concentration camp survivors – a community study in Jerusalem. *Psychol. Med.* 14: 215–218.

Liberzon, I., Fig, L. M. & Jung, T. D. 1995. Brain blood flow in posttraumatic stress disorder: SPECT. *Biol. Psychiatry* 37: 622. (Abstract).

Litz, B. T., Penk, W. E., Walsh, S. et. al. 1991. Similarities and differences between MMPI and MMPI-2 applications to the assessment of posttraumatic stress disorder. *J. Pers. Assess.* 57: 238–253.

Logue, J. N., Melnick, M. E. & Hansen, H. 1981. Research issues and directions in the epidemiology of health effects of disaster. *Epidemiol. Rev.* 3: 140.

Lonigan, C. J., Shannon, M. P., Taylor, C. M., Jr. et al. 1994. Children exposed to disaster: II. Risk factors for the development of post-traumatic stress symptomatology. *J. Am. Acad. Child Adolesc. Psychiatry* 33: 94–105.

Lundin, T. 1994. The treatment of acute trauma: Post-traumatic stress disorder prevention. *Psychiatr. Clin. North. Am.* 17: 385–391.

Lynn, E. J. & Belza, M. 1984. Factitious post-traumatic stress disorder: The veteran who never got to Vietnam. *Hosp. Community Psychiatry* 35: 697–701.

Malt, U. F., Karlehagen, S., Hoff, H. et al. 1993. The effect of major railway accidents on the psychological health of train drivers: I. Acute psychological responses to accident. *J. Psychosom. Res.* 37: 793–805.

Mason, J. W., Giller, E. L., Jr., Kosten, T. R. et al. 1990. Psychoendocrine approaches to the diagnosis and pathogenesis of posttraumatic stress disorder. In *Biological Assessment and Treatment of Posttraumatic Stress Disorder*, ed. E. L. Giller, Jr, pp. 65–86, American Psychiatric Press, Washington, DC.

Mayou, R. 1996. Accident memories revisited. *Br. J. Psychiatry* 168: 399–403.

McCarroll, J. E., Ursano, R. J. & Fullerton, C. S. 1993. Symptoms of posttraumatic stress disorder following recovery of war dead. *Am. J. Psychiatry* 150: 1875–1880.

McEwen, B. S. 1988. Steroid hormones and the brain: Linking 'nature' and 'nurture'. *Neurochem. Res.* 13: 663–669.

McFarlane, A. C. 1988a. The aetiology of posttraumatic stress disorders following a natural disaster. *Br. J. Psychiatry* 152: 116–121.

McFarlane, A. C. 1988b. The longitudinal course of posttraumatic morbidity: The range of outcomes and their predictors. *J. Nerv. Ment Dis.* 176: 30–39.

McFarlane, A. C. 1989. The aetiology of post-traumatic morbidity: Predisposing, precipitating and perpetuating factors. *Br. J. Psychiatry* 154: 221–228.

McFarlane, A. C. 1990. Vulnerability to posttraumatic stress disorder. In *Posttraumatic Stress Disorder; Etiology, Phenomenology, and Treatment*, eds. M. E. Wolf, A. D. Mosnaim, pp. 2–20, American Psychiatric Press, Washington, DC.

McFarlane, A. C. & Papay, P. 1992. Multiple diagnoses in posttraumatic stress disorder in the victims of a natural disaster. *J. Nerv. Ment. Dis.* 180: 498–504.

McFarlane, A. C. 1994. Individual psychotherapy for post-traumatic stress disorder. *Psychiatr. Clin. North Am.* 17: 393–408.

McMillen, C., Zuravin, S. & Rideout, G. 1995. Perceived benefit from child sexual abuse. *J. Consult. Clin. Psychol.* 63: 1037–1043.

McNally, R. J. 1993. Stressors that produce posttraumatic stress disorder in children. In *Posttraumatic Stress Disorder: DSM-IV and Beyond*, eds. J. R. T. Davidson, E. B. Foa, pp. 57–74, American Psychiatric Press, Washington, DC.

Meichenbaum, D. 1994. *A Clinical Handbook/ Practical Therapist Manual for Assessing and Treating Adults with Post-traumatic Stress Disorder (PTSD)*. Institute Press, Waterloo, Ontario.

Mellman, T. A., Ramsay, R. E. & Fitzgerald, S. G. 1991. Divergence of PTSD and narcolepsy associated with military trauma. *J. Anxiety Dis.* 5: 267–272.

Mellman, T. A., David, D., Kulick-Bell, R. et al. 1995a. Sleep disturbance and its relationship to psychiatric morbidity after Hurricane Andrew. *Am. J. Psychiatry* 152: 1659–1663.

Mellman, T. A., Kumar, A., Kulick-Bell, R. et al. 1995b. Nocturnal/daytime urine noradrenergic measures and sleep in combat-related PTSD. *Biol. Psychiatry* 38: 174–179.

Miller, H. 1961. Accident neurosis. *Br. Med. J.* 266: 919–998.

MMW Report, 1996. 'Zeit des Erwachens'. *Munch. Med. Wschr.* 138: 16–18.

Morgan, C. A., III. 1993. Yohimbine-facilitated acoustic startle reflex in humans. *Psychopharmacology.* 110: 342–346.

Murburg, M. M., McFall, M. E., Lewis, N. et al. 1995. Plasma norepinephrine kinetics in patients with posttraumatic stress disorder. *Biol. Psychiatry* 38: 819–825.

Orr, S. P. 1990. Psychophysiologic studies of posttraumatic stress disorder. In *Biological Assessment and Treatment of Posttraumatic Stress Disorder*, ed. E. L. Giller, pp. 135–157, American Psychiatric Press, Washington, DC.

Parry-Jones, W. & Barton, J. 1995. Post-traumatic stress disorder in children and adolescents. *Curr. Opin. Psychiatry* 8: 227–230.

Perconte, S. T. & Goreczny, A. J. 1990. Failure to detect fabricated post-traumatic stress disorder with the use of the MMPI in a clinical population. *Am. J. Psychiatry* 147: 1057–1060.

Perconte, S. T. & Griger, M. L. 1991. Comparison of successful, unsuccessful, and relapsed Vietnam veterans treated for posttraumatic stress disorder. *J. Nerv. Ment. Dis.* 179: 558–562.

Perry, S., Difede, J., Musngi, G. et al. 1992. Predictors of posttraumatic stress disorder after burn injury. *Am. J. Psychiatry* 149: 931–935.

Peters, U. H. 1989. Das überlebenden-Syndrom. *Fortschritte in Neurologie und Psychatie* 57: 169–191.

Pugh, C. & Trimble, M. R. 1993. Psychiatric injury after Hillsborough. *Br. J. Psychiatry* 163: 425–429.

Ramsay, R. 1990. Invited review: Post-traumatic stress disorder; a new clinical entity? *J. Psychosom. Res.* 34: 355–365.

Raphael, B., Meldrum, L. & McFarlane, A. C. 1995. Does debriefing after psychological trauma work? *Br. Med. J.* 310: 1479–1480.

Rauch, S. L., van der Kolk, B. A., Fisler, R. E. et al. 1996. A symptom provocation study of posttraumatic stress disorder using positron emission tomography and script-driven imagery. *Arch. Gen. Psychiatry* 53: 380–387.

Resnick, H. S., Kilpatrick, D. G., Dansky, B. S. et al. 1993. Prevalence of civil trauma and posttraumatic stress disorder in a representative national sample of women. *J. Consult. Clin. Psychol.* 61: 984–991.

Robinson, S., Rapaport-Ben-Sever, M. & Rapaport, J. 1994. The present state of people who survived the holocaust as children. *Acta Psychiatr. Scand.* 89: 242–245.

Roca, R. P., Spence, R. J. & Munster, A. M. 1992. Posttraumatic adaptation and distress among adult burn survivors. *Am. J. Psychiatry* 149: 1234–1238.

Rothbaum, B. O. & Foa, E. B. 1993. Subtypes of posttraumatic stress disorder. In *Posttraumatic Stress Disorder; DSM-IV and Beyond*, eds. J. R. T. Davidson, E. B. Foa, pp. 23–35, American Psychiatric Press, Washington, DC.

Sack, W. H., McSharry, S., Clarke, G. N. et al. 1994. The Khmer adolescent project: I. Epidemiologic findings in two generations of Cambodian refugees. *J. Nerv. Ment. Dis.* 182: 387–395.

Sargent, W. W. & Slater, E. 1940. Acute war neuroses. *Lancet* 140: 1–2.

Schaeffer, M. A. & Baum, A. 1984. Adrenal cortical response to stress at Three Mile Island. *Psychosom. Med.* 46: 227–237.

Schottenfeld, R. S. & Cullen, M. R. 1985. Occupation-induced posttraumatic stress disorders. *Am. J. Psychiatry* 2: 198–202.

Schwarz, E. D. & Kowalski, J. M. 1992. Malignant memories: Reluctance to utilize mental health services after a disaster. *J Nerv. Ment Dis.* 180: 767–772.

Schwarz, E. D. & Perry, B. D. 1994. The post-traumatic stress response in children and adolescents. *Psychiatr. Clin. North Am.* 17: 311–326.

Scott, M. J. & Stradling, S. C. 1994. Post-traumatic stress disorder without the trauma. *Br. J. Clin. Psychol.* 33: 71–74.

Shalev, A., Bleich, A. & Ursano, R. J. 1990. Posttraumatic stress disorder: Somatic comorbidity and effort tolerance. *Psychosomatics* 2: 197–203.

Shepherd, J. P., Qureshi, R., Preston, M. S. et al. 1990. Psychological distress after assaults and accidents. *Br. Med. J.* 301: 849–850.

Solomon, Z. 1988. The effect of combat-related posttraumatic stress disorder on the family. *Psychiatry* 51: 323–329.

Solomon, Z., Kotler, M. & Mikulincer, M. 1988. Combat-related posttraumatic stress disorder among second-generation Holocaust survivors: Preliminary findings. *Am. J. Psychiatry* 145: 865–868.

Solomon, Z., Mikulincer, M. & Benbenishty, R. 1989. Locus of control and combat-related posttraumatic stress disorder: The intervening role of battle intensity, threat appraisal and coping. *Br. J. Clin. Psychol.* 28: 131–144.

Solomon, Z., Bleich, A., Shoham, S. et al. 1992. The Koach project for the treatment of combat related PTSD: Rationale, aims and methodology. *J. Traum Stress* 5: 175–194.

Solomon, Z. & Prager, E. 1992b. Elderly Israeli Holocaust survivors during the Persian Gulf War: A study of psychological distress. *Am. J. Psychiatry* 149: 1707–1710.

Solomon, Z. 1993. Immediate and long-term effects of traumatic combat stress among Israeli veterans of the Lebanon War. In *International Handbook of Traumatic Stress Syndromes*, eds. J. P. Wilson, R. Raphael, Plenum Press, New York.

Solomon, Z., Laor, N., Weiler, D. et al. 1993. The psychological impact of the Gulf War: A study of acute stress in Israeli evacuees. *Arch. Gen. Psychiatry* 50: 320–321.

Solursh, L. 1988. Combat addiction: Post-traumatic stress disorder re-explored. *Psychiatr. J. Univ. Ottawa* 13: 17–20.

Southwick, S. M., Bremner, D., Krystal, J. H. et al. 1994. Psychobiological research in post-traumatic stress disorder. *Psychiatr. Clin. North Am.* 17: 251–264.

Spiegel, D. & Classen, C. 1995. Acute stress disorder. In *Treatments of Psychiatric Disorders*, ed. G. O. Gabbard, pp. 1521–1535, American Psychiatric Press, Washington, DC.

Stutman, R. K. & Bliss, E. L. 1985. Posttraumatic stress disorder, hypnotizability, and imagery. *Am. J. Psychiatry* 6: 741–743.

Tarsh, M. J. & Royston, C. 1985. A follow-up study of accident neurosis. *Br. J. Psychiatry.* 146: 18–25.

Terr, L. C. 1983. Chowchilla revisited: The effects of psychic trauma four years after school bus kidnapping. *Am. J. Psychiatry* 12: 1543–1549.

Tomb, D. A. 1994. The phenomenology of post-traumatic stress disorder.

Psychiatr. Clin. North Am. 17: 237–250.
True, W. R., Rice, J., Eisen, S. A. et al. 1993. A twin study of genetic and environmental contributions to liability for posttraumatic stress symptoms. *Arch. Gen. Psychiatry* 50: 257–264.
Tyrer, P. 1989. *Classification of Neurosis.* John Wiley, New York.
van Kammen, W. B., Christiansen, C., van Kammen, D. P. et al. 1990. Sleep and the prisoner-of-war experience – 40 years later. In *Biological Assessment and Treatment of Posttraumatic Stress Disorder*, ed. E. L. Giller, pp. 159–172, American Psychiatric Press, Washington, DC.
Watson, C. G., Juba, M. P., Manifold, V. et al. 1991. The PTSD interview: Rationale, description, reliability, and concurrent validity of a DSM-III based technique. *J. Clin. Psychol.* 47: 179–187.
Wiesel, E. 1960. *Nacht.* Hill and Wang, New York.
Wittkower, M. E. & Davenport, R. C. 1946. The war blinded: Their emotional, social and occupational situation. *Psychosom. Med.* 8: 121–137.
Yehuda, R., Southwick, S. M. & Giller, E. L. 1992. Exposure to atrocities and severity of chronic posttraumatic stress disorder in Vietnam combat veterans. *Am. J. Psychiatry* 149: 333–336.
Yehuda, R., Southwick, S. M., Krystal, J. H. et al. 1993. Enhanced suppression of cortisol following dexamethasone administration in posttraumatic stress disorder. *Am. J. Psychiatry* 150: 83–86.
Yehuda, R., Kahana, B., Binder-Brynes, K. et al. 1995. Low urinary cortisol excretion in Holocaust survivors with post-traumatic stress disorder. *Am. J. Psychiatry* 152: 982–986.
Zeitlin, S. B. & McNally, R. J. 1991. Implicit and explicit memory bias for threat in post-traumatic stress disorder. *Behav. Res. Ther.* 29: 451–457.
Zilberg, N. J, Weiss, D. S. & Horowitz, M. J. 1982. Impact of Event Scale: A cross-validation study and some empirical evidence supporting a conceptual model of stress response syndromes. *J. Consult. Clin. Psychol.* 50: 407–414.
Zivcic, I. 1993. Emotional reactions of children to war stress in Croatia. *J. Am. Acad. Child Adolesc. Psychiatry* 32: 709–713.

7

Anxiety in the medically ill: disorders due to medical conditions and substances

Definition

Anxiety disorders are not only prevalent among medically ill persons but are associated with substantial morbidity. These disorders are heterogeneous and have varying relationships with coexisting physical illness. Most are reactions to the stress of developing or continuing illness and represent adjustment disorders. They also arise from biological disturbances that accompany physical illness or its treatment and are classified in DSM-IV as disorders due to medical conditions or substances (American Psychiatric Association, 1994). Others represent preexisting conditons, such as generalized anxiety or panic disorder, that persist following the development of physical illness.

Importance of anxiety in the medically ill

Much of the importance of these disorders derives from their varied interaction with physical illness. To begin with, anxiety and associated autonomic arousal may contribute to the development of disease or complicate the course of existing conditions. For example, anxiety symptoms appear to increase the risk of hypertension, coronary artery disease, and death following myocardial infarction (Hayward et al., 1990). The reverse is also true; physical illness may precipitate, exacerbate, or worsen the course of an anxiety disorder. For example, illness may be associated with the onset of panic disorder or cause the re-emergence of attacks in persons whose symptoms had been controlled (Roy-Byrne et al., 1986). Conditions or treatments that are associated with increased adrenergic activity, such as cardiac or respiratory failure, may increase anxiety symptoms (Katon, 1991). Regardless of the mechanism, coexisting anxiety disorders are associated with lower levels of functioning and well-being in patients with chronic medical conditions (Sherbourne et al., 1996).

Coexisting anxiety, like depression, has a substantial impact on diagnosis and treatment. Anxiety disorders complicate the assessment of patients with chronic physical conditions and vice versa. For example, many patients who present with chest pain, but have normal coronary arteries, have anxiety disorders (Beitman et al., 1989). Most patients with anxiety disorders present with somatic symptoms, and this presentation – one that mimics physical illness – often leads to fruitless evaluations and missed psychiatric diagnoses (Katon, 1986). Even though anxiety disorders are associated with increased utilization of health services, they tend to go undiagnosed (Hankin et al., 1982). For instance, in an health maintenance organization (HMO) population only 44% of persons with significant anxiety had received treatment for it (Fifer et al., 1994). The tendency for patients and their physicians to regard anxiety as an expected consequence of being ill is another reason that potentially treatable disorders are overlooked (Sensky et al., 1989).

Anxiety disorders also complicate the treatment of physical illness. Adherence and retention in treatment are often undermined by excessive worry about complications and by anxiety-related avoidant behaviors. Anxious patients tend to respond poorly to treatment for their physical condition, and this failure is often falsely attributed to the condition itself. For example, breathlessness in chronic lung disease patients is often made worse by anxiety, and increasing the dose of anxiogenic bronchodilating agents may only increase anxiety further. Exaggerated health worry and alarming physical symptoms (of anxiety) often interfere with the rehabilitation of medical patients, especially those with heart and lung diseases (Guiry et al., 1987). Finally, treatments for the two types of disorders may interact in a negative manner (Stoudemire & Moran, 1993).

Diagnosis of anxiety disorders in the medically ill

Pathological anxiety

Anxiety that is intense and causes impairment in physically ill persons is considered pathological. It is characterized by moderate to severe apprehension or worry together with vigilance and scanning, signs of central nervous system arousal. These psychological manifestations are accompanied by motor tension and autonomic hyperactivity (American Psychiatric Association, 1987). Paroxysms of severe anxiety (attacks) accompanied by sympathetic discharge may also occur. Such anxiety must have persisted for 2 weeks or more and been present for at least half the time (Maguire et al., 1993a). In the medically ill, severe anxiety may reduce the threshold for physical distress especially pain, and as just described, interfere with medical treatment.

Problems with diagnosis

The diagnosis of anxiety disorders in medically ill patients is problematic (Strain et al., 1981; Derogatis & Wise, 1989). Somatic symptoms involve many organ systems, especially the cardiovascular, neurological, and gastrointestinal, and these overlap with symptoms of physical disease and the side-effects of treatment (Katon, 1984). For example, symptoms such as poor concentration, fatigue, and trouble sleeping may be due to advanced disease, especially when pain is present. Consequently, somatic symptoms are of less value in making a diagnosis and greater reliance must be placed upon psychological symptoms.

It is also unclear how suitable the DSM-IV criteria are for the medically ill (Stoudemire et al., 1989; Rosenbaum & Pollack, 1991). Most medically ill patients have adjustment disorders, but symptom criteria for them have not been developed. Also, many meet criteria for generalized anxiety disorder but lack the required 6 month duration. The criteria for generalized anxiety disorder were refined to make them more discriminatory, but the overlap with symptoms of physical illness is considerable. Also, acute anxiety in physically ill patients is accompanied by greater autonomic hyperactivity than is seen in chronically anxious patients (e.g., generalized anxiety disorder). Finally, anxiety and depressive symptoms commonly coexist, and mixed states may be important in the medically ill (Liebowitz, 1993).

Diagnostic criteria

The DSM-IV criteria for adjustment disorders specify an onset within 3 months of an identified stressor (American Psychiatric Association, 1994). The categories of anxiety disorder due to a general medical condition and substance-induced anxiety disorder were new additions to DSM-IV and ICD-10 (World Health Organization, 1993). They replaced the category of organic anxiety disorder that had first appeared in DSM-III (American Psychiatric Association, 1980). The criteria for these disorders are shown in Tables 7.1a, b and 7.2. Both place reliance on the temporal relationship

Table 7.1a. *DSM-IV criteria for anxiety disorder due to a general medical condition*

A. Prominent anxiety, panic attacks, or obsessions or compulsions predominate in the clinical picture
B. There is evidence from the history, physical examination, or laboratory findings that the disturbance is the direct physiological consequence of a general medical condition
C. The disturbance is not better accounted for by another mental disorder (e.g., adjustment disorder with anxiety in which the stressor is a serious general medical condition)
D. The disturbance does not occur exclusively during the course of a delirium
E. The disturbance causes clinically significant distress or impairment in social, occupational or other important areas of functioning

Table 7.1b. *DSM-IV criteria for substance-induced anxiety disorder*

A. Prominent anxiety, panic attacks, or obsessions or compulsions predominate in the clinical picture
B. There is evidence from the history, physical examination, or laboratory findings of either:
   1. the symptoms developed during, or within 1 month of, substance intoxication or withdrawal, or
   2. medication use is etiologically related to the disturbance
C. The disturbance is not better accounted for by an anxiety disorder that is not substance-induced. Evidence that symptoms may not be substance-induced include: the symptoms precede the onset of the substance or medication use; the symptoms persist for a substantial period (e.g. a month) after the cessation of acute withdrawal or intoxication or are substantially in excess of what would be expected, given the type or amount of substance used or the duration of use; or there is other evidence which suggests the existence of an independent nonsubstance-induced anxiety disorder
D. The disturbance does not occur exclusively during the course of a delirium
E. The disturbance causes clinically significant distress or impairment in social, occupational or other important areas of functioning

From American Psychiatric Association (1994). Reprinted with permission.

between anxiety symptoms and the medical condition or substance (i.e., intoxication or withdrawal) known to produce them.

Measurement of anxiety in the medically ill

A variety of instruments are used to screen for psychiatric cases in medical populations and to measure change in symptomatic distress over time. Some, like the General Health Questionnaire (GHQ), were designed to screen for mental disorders regardless of type (Goldberg & Hillier, 1979).

Table 7.2. *ICD-10 criteria for organic anxiety disorder*

A. Criteria for mental disorder due to brain dysfunction or to physical disease
  1. There is objective evidence (from physical and neurological examination and laboratory tests) and/or history of cerebral dysfunction or of systemic physical disorder known to cause cerebral dysfunction, including hormonal disturbance and the effects of non-psychoactive drugs
  2. There is a presumed relationship between the development (or marked exacerbation) of the underlying dysfunction and the mental disorder, the symptoms of which may have immediate onset or may be delayed
  3. There is recovery from or significant improvement in the mental disorder following removal or improvement of the underlying presumed cause
  4. There is insufficient evidence for an alternative causation of the mental disorders (e.g., family history of a similar disorder)
B. The condition must meet criteria for generalized anxiety disorder or panic disorder

---

From WHO (1993). Reprinted with permission.

Others, like the State-Trait Anxiety Inventory (STAI), are made up entirely of anxiety symptoms or contain anxiety subscales that may be used for these purposes (Spielberger et al., 1970). Examples of the latter include the Symptom Checklist-90 and the Profile of Mood States (Derogatis, 1983; Cella et al., 1987). The State-Trait Anxiety Inventory is frequently administered to medically ill patients, and for them, a shortened version is available (van Knippenberg et al., 1990).

The Hospital Anxiety and Depression Scale (HADS) was developed specifically for the medically ill (Zigmond & Snaith, 1983). The HADS is a brief, self-assessment scale that has subscales for anxiety and depression, each containing seven items rated on 4-point linear scales (0 absent to 3 severe). It contains only psychological items likely to distinguish anxiety and depression. Zigmond & Snaith (1983) found the scale useful for screening (a score of 8–10 for doubtful cases and 11 or more for definite cases on either scale) and a valid measure of severity. In one study, the anxiety subscale showed a sensitivity of 75%, a specificity of 90%, and a misclassification rate of 12% (Hopwood et al, 1991a).

Epidemiology

Prevalence in the general population

Epidemiological studies have shown increased rates of anxiety disorders among persons with certain chronic medical conditions. This increase appears to be part of an overall association between mental and physical

Table 7.3. *Prevalence of anxiety disorders[a] among persons with chronic medical conditions in the general population*

Medical condition	Current anxiety (% SE)	Lifetime anxiety (% SE)
No medical condition	6.0 ± 0.6	12.4 ± 1.0
Arthritis	11.9 ± 2.6[b]	20.7 ± 3.3[b]
Diabetes	15.8 ± 6.1	27.1 ± 7.0[b]
Heart disease	21.0 ± 5.7[c]	28.3 ± 5.8[c]
Chronic lung disease	10.0 ± 2.5	21.0 ± 4.1[b]
High blood pressure	12.1 ± 3.0[b]	16.1 ± 2.9

[a]Generalized anxiety disorder, panic disorder, phobic disorders, and obsessive-compulsive disorders.
[b]$p < 0.05$, [c]$p < 0.01$. p values from t-tests comparing prevalence among persons with the medical condition compared to persons with no medical condition.
Source: Modified from Wells et al. (1989a). © Elsevier Science Inc. Reprinted with permission.

disorders in the general population (Eastwood & Trevelyan, 1972). For example, the Epidemiological Catchment Area (ECA) study found a 41% increase in the relative risk of having a recent mental disorder among persons with chronic physical disease (Wells et al., 1988). The lifetime prevalence of any recent anxiety disorder (i.e., panic disorder, phobic disorders, obsessive-compulsive disorder) among persons with medical conditions was 11.9% compared to 6.0% among those without such conditions (Wells et al., 1988). When the prevalence of anxiety disorders was examined in relation to individual conditions, it was high in persons with arthritis, diabetes, heart disease, high blood pressure, and chronic lung disease (see Table 7.3).

Although both anxiety and depressive disorders were associated with lifetime medical conditions, only anxiety disorders were associated with current medical conditions (Wells et al., 1989a). This suggests that an anxiety disorder may be an early reaction to the development of a major medical condition (Wells et al., 1989b). Specifically, persons with panic disorder showed a high likelihood of having cardiovascular disorders. They had a higher risk (odds ratio) of high blood pressure (1.9), heart attack (4.5), and stroke (12.0) than persons with no psychiatric disorder (Weissman et al., 1990). Among the elderly, anxiety disorders are more prevalent in those with serious physical illness (Lindesay, 1990). In fact, the onset of agoraphobia was attributed by most in this age group to an episode of physical illness (Lindesay, 1991).

Prevalence in general medical populations

Until recently, data concerning anxiety in general medical populations were quite limited (Rogers et al., 1994). According to the World Health Organization collaborative study, 10.5% of primary care patients have current anxiety disorders, the most common being generalized anxiety disorder (7.9%), agoraphobia (with and without panic attacks, 1.5%), and panic disorder (1.1%) (Sartorius et al., 1996). Nearly half of the cases of anxiety appeared in patients who also had current depression. Findings from the Medical Outcomes Study were similar (Sherbourne et al., 1996). Among primary care outpatients with common medical conditions (i.e., hypertension, diabetes, and heart disease), 15–18% had current anxiety disorders and 26–28% had lifetime anxiety disorders. Thus, anxiety disorders are among the most common psychiatric problems seen by primary care physicians, making up perhaps a third of patients with a psychiatric diagnoses.

Earlier studies of medical outpatients and inpatients rarely focused on anxiety and, therefore, yielded little information about such disorders (reviewed by Cavanaugh & Wettstein, 1984; Mayou & Hawton, 1986). The resulting prevalence figures vary greatly as do the populations studied and methods employed (Zung, 1986); however, several general conclusions may be drawn. Most estimates of current anxiety disorders fall between 4% and 16% (Table 7.4) (Glass et al., 1978; Hoeper et al., 1979; Harding, 1980; Dhadphale et al., 1983; Kessler et al., 1985; Schulberg et al., 1985; Katon et al., 1986; Goldberg & Bridges, 1987; von Korff et al., 1987; Barrett et al., 1988; Ormel et al., 1991; Fifer et al., 1994). In general, anxiety disorders are less prevalent than depressive disorders or mixed states (von Korff et al., 1987; Barrett et al., 1988; Ormel et al., 1991). Where individual disorders are identified, phobias are most prevalent followed by generalized anxiety disorder (Hoeper et al., 1979; Kessler et al., 1985; Schulberg et al., 1985; von Korff et al., 1987). Relatively low rates for panic are reported but one study, limited to this disorder, found a rate of 6.5% (Katon et al., 1986).

A recent study by Fifer et al. (1994) focused on untreated anxiety among patients in a health maintenance organization. They found a surprising 10% had unrecognized anxiety symptoms or disorders, representing 56% of the patients with significant anxiety. Among those with untreated anxiety, 17% had posttraumatic stress disorder, 15% simple phobia, 14%

Table 7.4. *Prevalence of anxiety disorders in primary care outpatients*

Reference	N	Sample	Assessment	Criteria	Prevalence (%)	Comment
Glass et al. (1978)	82	University hospital	HSCL; psychiatric interview	Feighner criteria	28.0	Anxiety neurosis
Hoeper et al. (1979)	247	Primary care (rural)	GHQ-30; SADS	RDC	7.4	5.8% phobic disorder, 1.6% GAD
Harding (1980)	1624	Primary care (developing countries)	SRQ; PSE	ICD-8	4.3	Anxiety neurosis
Dhadphale et al. (1983)	388	Hospital outpatients (Kenya)	SRO; Standardized Psychiatric Interview	ICD-9	9.0	
Kessler et al. (1985)	166	Primary care	GHQ; SADS-L	RDC		High phobia, low GAD and panic disorder
Schulberg et al. (1985)	294	Primary care	CES-D; DIS	DSM-III	6.8	Phobic disorders, panic disorder, 1.7%
Katon (1986)	195	Family medicine	ZAS, SCL-90; DIS	DSM-III	6.5	Current panic disorder only
von Korff et al. (1987)	809	Internal medicine	DIS	DSM-III	8.5	4.6% GAD, 1.4% panic disorder, 1.1% OCD
Goldberg & Bridges (1987)	590	Family practice	GHQ-28; PAS	DSM-III, Bedford College	15.8	GAD, additional 12.1% adjustment disorders
Barrett et al. (1988)	1055	Primary care	HSCL, CES-D	RDC	2.9	4.1% mixed anxiety/ depression
Ormel et al. (1991)	557	General practice (Netherlands)	GHQ	Bedford College	1.8	22.7% borderline anxiety, 12.7% mixed anxiety/ depression
Fifer et al. (1994)	6037	Primary care (HMO)	SCL-52; DIS	DSM-III-R	10.0	Untreated anxiety (symptoms/disorders)

social phobia, 14% agoraphobia, 9% generalized anxiety disorder, 5% panic disorder, and 4% obsessive-compulsive disorder. These untreated patients had reduced functioning and well-being comparable to that associated with chronic physical diseases, such as diabetes and congestive heart failure.

Few studies have examined the prevalence of anxiety disorders among general medical inpatients and even fewer have used structured interviews or diagnostic criteria. In the only study to focus exclusively on anxiety, Schwab et al. (1966) found that 20% had moderate to severe anxiety symptoms. Subsequent studies identified 6–11% as having anxiety disorders, a range similar to that for outpatients (Kaufman et al., 1959; Maguire et al., 1974; Feldman et al., 1987; Deshpande et al., 1989).

Prevalence in specific medical populations

Cardiology patients

A relationship between anxiety and cardiovascular disturbances has long been observed. According to early estimates, the prevalence of 'irritable heart', 'effort syndrome', or 'neurocirculatory asthenia' ranged from 10–14% of cardiology practice (Wood, 1941). Now labeled panic disorder, this disturbance with prominent cardiac symptoms (i.e., chest pain, palpitations, shortness of breath) continues to be prevalent among patients visiting cardiologists. One study found the disorder in 9.2% of cardiology outpatients (Goldberg et al., 1990). Recent attention has been focused on patients with chest pain and normal coronary arteries who make up 10–30% of those undergoing angiography (Lavey & Winkle, 1979).

A substantial portion of the morbidity experienced by these patients is due to panic disorder (Katon, 1990; Beitman et al., 1991). Bass et al. (1983) found that 61% of chest pain patients with normal coronary arteries had psychiatric disorders compared to 23% of those with abnormal arteries. Also, Katon et al. (1988) found that 43% of such patients had panic disorder compared to 7% of patients with coronary stenosis, and others have reported similar findings (Beitman et al., 1989). In most studies, patients who proved not to have cardiac disease were younger, were more likely to be female, reported more autonomic symptoms, and were more likely to have atypical chest pain, all characteristics of patients with panic disorder (Cormier et al., 1988).

The prevalence of panic disorder is also high among patients with chest pain seen in acute care settings. For instance, 17.5% of such patients seen in an emergency department had panic disorder and 23.1% had major depressive disorder (Yingling et al., 1993). The prevalence of panic was similar in those with and without acute cardiac ischemia, indicating that the presence of anxiety does not rule out organic disease. Likewise, Carter et al. (1992) identified panic disorder in 55.5% of patients with negative cardiac findings admitted to a coronary care unit.

Thus, between 16% and 58% of patients with unexplained chest pain suffer from panic disorder. Patients with this disorder typically present with somatic symptoms suggestive of disease in the cardiovascular and other systems. In one series, 40% had consulted a cardiologist (Logue et al., 1993). This type of presentation often results in costly workups and repeated medical consultations (Clancy & Noyes, 1976). Many patients see numerous physicians without having their psychiatric disorder diagnosed. The fact that some patients report no fear during attacks only adds to the likelihood of a missed diagnosis (Beitman et al., 1990).

When panic disorder and coronary artery disease coexist, they may complicate one another. Panic attacks may provoke ischemic pain by increasing heart rate and blood pressure, and the resulting angina may provoke increased anxiety. Similarly, altered cardiac functioning may cause increased sympathetic activity that may, in turn, cause increased anxiety, setting up a vicious cycle of anxiety and pain. Angina may, under these circumstances, be resistant to antianginal agents yet respond to the treatment of panic disorder (Mendels et al., 1986).

Clinical studies have demonstrated mitral valve prolapse in 30–50% of patients with panic disorder, a higher rate than that found in controls (Crowe, 1985; Gorman et al., 1988a); however, failure to find an association in the community has suggested that treatment-seeking bias might explain the high rate in clinical populations (Crowe, 1985). If prolapse occurs in panic patients, it appears to be a mild variety that involves histologically normal leaflets (Gorman et al., 1988a). Consistent with this view, Matuzas et al. (1989) found that patients with prolapse were younger and more often female. They also weighed less and were more ectomorphic, which suggests that body habitus might be an intervening variable. Treatment of panic may cause echocardiograms to revert to normal (Gorman et al., 1988a). Regardless, the mitral valve prolapse observed in panic patients appears to have little clinical significance.

Pulmonary disease patients

Any compromise of respiratory function, as in suffocation or choking, may be perceived as a threat to life and evoke a panic response. Conversely, the fight or flight reaction includes increased ventilatory exchange. Not surprisingly then, pulmonary diseases are associated with anxiety disorders (Oswald et al., 1970). For instance, Yellowless et al. (1987) reported a 34% current prevalence of anxiety disorders, including 24% with panic disorder, among patients with chronic airflow obstruction admitted to a respiratory unit. Other studies have found high rates among patients referred for pulmonary function tests (41% panic attacks, 11% panic disorder), patients with chronic obstructive lung disease (16% anxiety disorders, 8% panic disorder), and lung transplant applicants (14% anxiety disorders, 7% panic disorder) (Craven, 1990; Pollack et al., 1996). Another study found a higher lifetime prevalence of respiratory diseases in patients with panic disorder than with other psychiatric disorders (Zandbergen et al., 1991).

Bronchial asthma appears to have an especially close link to anxiety (Thompson & Thompson, 1985). The disease is associated with frightening, even life-threatening, attacks that cause many children and adults to panic. The prevalence of anxiety disorders in clinical populations appears high. Shavitt et al. (1992) found that 19.6% of asthmatic outpatients had current anxiety disorders (panic disorder 6.5% and agoraphobia 13.1%). Similarly, Yellowless et al. (1988) observed these disorders in 28.6% (panic disorder 12.2%, phobic disorders 8.2%, post-traumatic stress disorder 8.2%) of patients with severe disease. One study found a higher rate among asthmatics with more severe disease (Garden & Ayres, 1993).

The observed relationships have prompted speculation about the interaction between lung disease and anxiety disorders (Karajgi et al., 1990). Severe asthma attacks or obstructive disease may elicit a phobic reaction (Agle & Baum, 1977). This reaction resembles panic disorder with agoraphobia (fear of leaving home or being alone) but is more properly regarded as a specific phobia of illness (Shavitt et al., 1992). Panic attacks are provoked by dyspnea or fear of suffocation, and situations that evoke such fear are avoided. Altered respiratory physiology may also precipitate panic. According to Gorman et al. (1988b), panic attacks in healthy persons result from hypersensitivity of medullary carbon dioxide chemoreceptors. In patients with lung disease, increased carbon dioxide may stimulate these receptors, triggering hyperventilation and, with it, the frightening sensation of dyspnea.

Regardless of the mechanism, anxiety contributes to the morbidity of asthma and chronic obstructive disease. By increasing dyspnea, it causes patients to work harder and less efficiently for breath. When this breathlessness is attributed to respiratory disease, they may unnecessarily restrict activities and use excess medication in an effort to control symptoms. A vicious cycle of increasing anxiety and dyspnea may interfere with rehabilitation and contribute to disability. Treatment of the anxiety disorder may result in substantial benefit (Agle & Baum, 1977).

Cancer patients

Studies of anxiety disorders in cancer patients have yielded variable estimates of prevalence (reviewed by Noyes et al., in press). The most widely quoted study by Derogatis et al. (1983) used DSM-III criteria and examined a large sample of both inpatients and outpatients. Based on clinical assessment, 44% were identified as having psychiatric disorders, two-thirds of which were adjustment disorders. Twenty-one per cent had prominent anxiety symptoms including 2% anxiety disorders, 6% adjustment disorder with anxious mood, and 13% adjustment disorder with mixed emotional features. Most studies have estimated the current prevalence in a range of 10–28%. Using a conservative cutoff on the Hospital Anxiety and Depression Scale (i.e., ≥ 11 anxiety scale), five studies identified between 9% and 19% as cases of anxiety. Thus, anxiety disorders are prevalent, and adjustment disorder with anxious mood is the most common.

Anxiety disorders are more common in persons with cancer than they are in persons without chronic illness in the general population. In the ECA study, cancer was one of the conditions that had an especially strong association with anxiety and other psychiatric disorders (Wells et al., 1988). Also, clinical studies have found a higher prevalence of anxiety among cancer patients than controls (Maguire et al., 1978; Dean, 1987; Brandenberg et al., 1992); however, anxiety disorders may or may not be more prevalent among cancer patients than patients with other medical illnesses. Cassileth et al. (1984), reported that the distress associated with chronic disease is similar for major illness groups including cancer, but there have been few other studies.

Neurological patients

As some anxious patients present with neurological symptoms (e.g., paresthesias, tremor), it is not surprising that anxiety disorders are prevalent among neurological outpatients and inpatients (Bridges & Goldberg, 1984; Katon & Roy-Byrne, 1989). Recent interest has focused on patients with Parkinson's disease who have an especially high prevalence. Current anxiety disorders have been found in 19–38% of Parkinson's patients

(Stein et al., 1990; Menza et al., 1993). These disorders fall into varied diagnostic categories and usually coexist with depression (Schiffer et al., 1988; Lauterbach & Duvoisin, 1991; Menza et al., 1993).

The relationship between Parkinson's disease and anxiety disorders has not been clarified. Stein et al. (1990) suggested that the dopaminergic deficit responsible for Parkinson's might also give rise to anxiety disorders. Jimenez-Jimenez et al. (1993) observed panic symptoms during the off phase of levodopa therapy and suggested that attacks might, in some patients, represent an abstinence syndrome. A study of patients taking levodopa/carbidopa that used symptom diaries supported this observation by demonstrating higher anxiety during off periods (Siemers et al., 1993). Regardless of the cause, anxiety disorders contribute to overall disability but are responsive to antianxiety drugs (Stein et al., 1990).

An association between migraine and anxiety is well established. Studies of patients with migraine have identified current anxiety disorders in 20–40% and depressive disorders in 10–15% (Devlen, 1994). Migraine and anxiety disorders are not only associated with one another in patient populations, but community studies have also shown a strong association (Merikangas et al., 1993). Among persons with migraine, odds ratios of 1.9–2.7 for all anxiety disorders and 3.5–6.0 for panic disorder have been found (Stewart et al., 1989, 1994; Merikangas et al., 1990; Breslau et al., 1991).

The nature of the association between migraine, anxiety, and depression has been explored in several studies. In them, anxiety generally came before the onset of migraine and depression came afterwards (Merikangas et al., 1990; Breslau et al., 1991). Anxiety disorders are unrelated to the frequency of migraine attacks, so they are not likely to be a reaction to migraine (Breslau & Davis, 1993). In a family history study, Merikangas et al. (1993) found a significant association between anxiety/depression and migraine among the relatives (i.e., odds ratio 2.3). They observed that rates of anxiety/depression were elevated only among relatives with migraine and concluded that migraine and anxiety/depression share a syndromatic relationship.

This research makes clear the importance of assessing patients with migraine for anxiety and depression and of treating the entire syndrome (Merikangas et al., 1993). The depression is associated with anergia, hypersomnia and irritability, so prophylactic medications that cause fatigue should be avoided. Antidepressants that are energizing or that are effective for anxious depression (e.g., monamine oxidase inhibitors) should be considered (Quitkin et al., 1991).

Otolaryngology patients

Dizziness is a common and disabling symptom that often goes unexplained. Surveys of patients presenting with this symptom have found a
high prevalence of psychiatric disorders, especially anxiety (Yardley et al.,
1994). In primary care patients who presented with dizziness, Sullivan et al.
(1993) found the highest rates of psychiatric disorders among patients
without vestibular disease; however, rates were also high among patients
with such disease. Specialty clinic patients have high rates of panic disorder. Clark et al. (1994) found that 20% had panic disorder compared to
none of a comparison group with hearing loss. Similarly, Stein et al. (1994)
found panic disorder and/or agoraphobia in 15% of vestibular clinic
patients. It is clear that the diagnosis of an anxiety disorder does not
exclude vestibular pathology; on the other hand, anxiety disorders contribute to the problem of dizziness.

Psychiatric morbidity often results from vestibular disease (Pratt &
McKenzie, 1958; Lilienfeld et al., 1989). In fact, specific syndromes, such as
space phobia and motorists' disorientation syndrome, have been described
in patients with vestibular abnormalities (Marks, 1981; Page & Gresty,
1985). Eagger et al. (1992) found a specific association between peripheral
vestibular disease and panic. In most patients, psychiatric disorders developed after the onset of vestibular symptoms. Over a quarter experienced
symptoms resembling agoraphobia, but some avoided activities that increased their sense of disequilibrium, such as entering car washes, looking
up at monuments, or putting garments on over their heads. In some
instances, feared consequences, such as appearing intoxicated in public, led
to avoidance (Eagger et al., 1992).

These observations have prompted a search for vestibular abnormalities
in panic disorder (Jacob et al., in press). Although studies have found
abnormalities in 71–88%, the rate in normal controls has been high as well
(42%) (Yardley et al., 1994; Jacob et al., in press). In a recent study, Jacob et
al. (1996) found test abnormalities in most panic patients who also had
agoraphobia (93%). Their vestibular dysfunction was associated with
space and motion discomfort (i.e., sense of imbalance, anxiety in situations
lacking adequate visual or proprioceptive cues) and with vestibular symptoms. Thus, subclinical vestibular dysfunction may contribute to the development of agoraphobia in patients with panic disorder (Jacob et al., 1996).

Gastroenterology patients

Interest has developed in the relationship between functional bowel disturbances, especially irritable bowel syndrome, and anxiety disorders. In his review, Clouse (1988) emphasized the importance of autonomic and neurohumoral regulation of gastrointestinal function, especially motility. A variety of experiments have demonstrated the influence of acute stress on gastrointestinal function, and similar pathways may be involved in the interaction between psychiatric disorders and irritable bowel syndrome. Clinical studies have found mental disorders including anxiety disorders in 54–100% of patients with this disturbance, a rate much higher than controls (reviewed by Walker et al., 1990); however, an association has not been clearly established in the community. Preliminary surveys show that the relationship in clinical samples may be the result of treatment-seeking bias (Smith et al., 1990).

Nevertheless, using available data from the ECA study, Walker et al. (1992) found a higher prevalence of psychiatric disorders in persons with irritable bowel symptoms than in those without such symptoms. Also, Lydiard et al. (1993) found increased reporting of irritable bowel symptoms in persons with panic disorder (7.2%) compared to those with no psychiatric disorder (0.7%). Among panic patients seeking treatment, Lydiard et al. (1991) found 42% who met the criteria for irritable bowel syndrome, some of whom listed gastrointestinal symptoms among their chief complaints.

Patients with human immunodeficiency virus infection

The prevalence of anxiety disorders is high in patients with AIDS (Atkinson et al., 1988; Williams et al., 1991). For instance, Atkinson et al. (1988) reported higher rates of anxiety in men with HIV infection than control men. Thirty-nine per cent of infected men had generalized anxiety disorder and 30% had other anxiety disorders (lifetime). In most instances, generalized anxiety symptoms began around the time of diagnosis, but other anxiety disorders began earlier in life, long before the HIV infection.

Studies have not found increases in psychiatric symptoms or disorders in seropositive compared to seronegative men (Ostrow et al., 1989; Williams et al., 1991). Men with AIDS have more psychiatric symptoms, but within this group, little relationship to stage of illness, immune status, complications, or even cognitive dysfunction has been found (Dew et al., 1990; Williams et al., 1991; Perdices et al., 1992). On the other hand, psychosocial factors appear to have an important relationship to psychiatric distress.

Anxiety as a risk factor for disease

Hypertension

There is increasing evidence of associations between anxiety and both hypertension and increased mortality from coronary artery disease (reviewed by Hayward et al., 1990). Although two studies showed an increased prevalence of hypertension among patients with anxiety disorders (Noyes et al., 1978; Katon, 1984), studies comparing blood pressure measurements have shown relatively few differences (Charney & Heninger, 1986). As described earlier, a relationship between anxiety disorders and high blood pressure was observed in the ECA study (Wells et al., 1989a, b).

Although an extensive literature shows the importance of psychosocial factors in hypertension (reviewed by Sommers-Flanagan & Greenberg, 1989), recent prospective studies have found trait anxiety a consistent predictor of later blood pressure (Haynes et al., 1978; Jenkins et al., 1983; Markovitz et al., 1991). In a 3-year follow-up of middle-aged normotensive women, those with high scores on the Framingham Tension Scale had greater increases in systolic blood pressure (Markovitz et al., 1991). This finding remained significant after controlling for biological and behavioral variables. Another study showed anxiety levels predictive of later hypertension in middle-aged men (Markovitz et al., 1993). Men with very high anxiety had a 2.2 relative risk of developing hypertension. Not all studies have yielded consistent results of the kind described (Sparrow et al., 1982).

Coronary artery disease

Evidence of a link between anxiety and cardiovascular death has come from a series of studies (reviewed by Hayward et al., 1990). In a 35-year follow-up of patients with panic disorder, Coryell et al. (1982) found excess cardiovascular mortality among men. Some later follow-up studies have found similar increased mortality while others have not (reviewed by Allgulander, 1994). Three prospective studies have found a relationship between phobic anxiety and subsequent ischemic heart disease (Haines et al., 1987; Kawachi et al., 1994a, b). As part of the Northwick Park Heart Study, Haines et al. (1987) followed up nearly 1500 men who had completed the Crown-Crisp Experimental Index 10 years earlier. The relative risk of death due to coronary disease was 3.8 times greater for men who scored above 5 on the phobic anxiety subscale compared to those who scored 1 or less. Findings from the Health Professionals Follow-up Study and the Normative Aging Study were very similar (Kawachi et al., 1994a, b). In both, anxiety or phobic symptoms were associated with an increase in subsequent death due to coronary disease or sudden death.

Possible causes of death include ventricular arrhythmia and coronary artery spasm (Kawachi et al., 1994a). Lown (1982) showed that psychological events may trigger ventricular arrhythmia and sudden death; also, hyperventilation – often associated with anxiety – is a well-known precipitant of coronary spasm (Reich et al., 1981; Freeman & Nixon 1985). Diminished heart rate variability contributes to sudden death after myocardial infarction and may cause arrhythmias (Bigger et al., 1992). Recent studies have demonstrated decreased heart rate variability in patients with panic disorder compared to patients with depression and normal controls (Yeragani et al., 1990a, 1993; Klein et al., 1995). In these patients, heart rate variability correlated with severity of panic symptoms and returned to normal with treatment (Klein et al., 1995).

Coronary risk factors

In their review of research, Hayward et al. (1990) noted that anxiety affects behaviors such as cigarette smoking, alcohol consumption, and overeating that may alter cardiovascular risk. Recent work focusing on panic disorder has demonstrated higher rates of hypertension, hyperlipidemia, lack of physical fitness, smoking, and alcohol abuse (Hayward et al., 1990). Findings of hypertension and hyperlipidemia have been inconsistent (Charney & Heninger, 1986; Taylor et al., 1987; Hayward et al., 1989; Yeragani et al., 1990b; Bajwa et al., 1992). Panic patients are not physically fit, perhaps due to exercise intolerance (Taylor et al., 1987; Gaffney et al., 1988). Thus, panic disorder is associated with risk factors for cardiovascular disease.

Etiology and pathogenesis

Demographic factors

In the general population, anxiety disorders are associated with female gender, younger age, and lower socioeconomic status. In medically ill populations these demographic variables appear less important. For instance, in studies of cancer populations, four found greater anxiety in women and five found no difference related to gender (reviewed by Noyes et al., in press). Concerning age, three studies found greater anxiety in younger patients and five found no difference. Three studies found no relationship to marital status and three found no relationship to social class or education. These differences suggest that, as illness variables become more important, demographic factors become less so.

Psychological factors

Premorbid adjustment

In his study of terminally ill patients, Hinton (1972) noted that mood changes, including anxiety, were usually consistent with previous patterns of reaction. Among patients who became anxious in the face of advanced disease, he identified premorbid anxious tendencies and obsessional personality traits. Prospective studies have tended to confirm these observations. For example, Fallowfield et al. (1990) reported that breast cancer patients with high trait anxiety were more likely to have clinically significant anxiety in the year after mastectomy. Likewise, high neuroticism predicted psychological morbidity after mastectomy (Morris, 1979). Such findings are in accord with epidemiological studies showing premorbid neurotic traits in persons who develop anxiety disorders (Angst & Vollrath, 1991).

Other factors that may contribute to anxiety include psychiatric history, low sense of control, and low social support. In his review, Greer (1994) noted that these factors influence the psychosocial adjustment of cancer patients. Most research in this area deals with psychological distress without looking specifically at anxiety. For example, emotional support reduced the psychological distress of women with breast cancer and improved their self-esteem and sense of control (Bloom, 1986). Among hemophilic men with AIDS, Dew et al. (1990) found that positive psychiatric history, family psychiatric history, low education, low social support, low sense of mastery, and recent life events were associated with high levels of anxiety and depressive symptoms. Others have also found psychiatric history and social support to be important in patients with HIV infection (Fell et al., 1993).

Severity of illness

In general, research has shown that mental health declines along with physical status (Cassileth et al., 1984; Noyes et al., 1990). In studies that examined stage of cancer, for example, six found greater anxiety among patients with more advanced disease and four found no difference (Noyes et al., in press). In cancer outpatients, Cassileth et al. (1986) observed an

Table 7.5. *Percent of patients with clinically significant anxiety in breast cancer patients and controls*

Time of assessment	Mastectomy (%)	Controls (%)	χ^2
Before discovery	10	10	NS
After discovery	23	26	NS
Before surgery	27	14	0.05
After surgery (4 months)	21	8	0.01
After surgery (1 year)	19	8	0.01

Source: Adapted from Maguire et al. (1978). Printed with permission of the BMJ Publishing Group. Reprinted with permission.

association between anxiety and treatment status. State anxiety rose sequentially in patients receiving follow-up care, active treatment, and palliative treatment. Patients receiving active treatment faced inconvenience, toxicity, and uncertainty but those receiving follow-up care had been freed from such stress.

Medical treatment

Treatments of medical illness, including surgery, chemotherapy, and radiotherapy are anxiety-provoking and may contribute to psychological morbidity (Schag & Heinrich, 1989). The psychological reaction to mastectomy has received considerable attention, and high levels of anxiety as well as depression have consistently been reported (Morris, 1979). These symptoms are not only a response to the loss of a breast but also to cancer, factors that are difficult to separate. As shown in Table 7.5, anxiety increases with the discovery of the tumor, peaks prior to surgery, remains high immediately afterward, then declines in the first postoperative year (Maguire et al., 1978).

Chemotherapy is a major cause of emotional distress including anxiety (Cella et al., 1987). Awareness of toxicity may cause anxiety before treatment begins, but repeated post-infusion nausea and vomiting often produces subsequent pre-infusion distress (Holland, 1989; Massie, 1989). Anticipatory nausea and vomiting, that affects a quarter to a half of patients, is a classically conditioned response to chemotherapy (Olafsdottir et al., 1986). Also, recent studies indicate that anticipatory anxiety, which may be similarly conditioned, develops in many patients and interacts with anticipatory nausea, each increasing the other (Andrykowski & Gregg, 1992; Jacobsen et al., 1993).

Patients undergoing radiotherapy may experience significant psychological distress including apprehension, anxiety, restlessness, feelings of helplessness, nightmares, and insomnia (Forester et al., 1978). Peck & Boland (1977), who observed moderate anxiety in 26% of patients, noted that many believed radiation might damage their bodies. This psychological distress may exceed the physical distress caused by radiation and remain high as therapy progresses (Andersen et al., 1984; Munro et al., 1989). This may be because of accumulating side-effects and the anticipation of treatment's end (Holland et al., 1979).

Organic factors

A variety of organic factors may also give rise to anxiety disorders in medically ill patients. As with psychological factors, these may involve the physical disease, its treatment, or factors unrelated to either. Most disturbances represent anxiety disorders due to general medical conditions or substance-induced anxiety disorders (American Psychiatric Association, 1994).

Pain

Poorly controlled pain is a common cause of anxiety (Massie, 1989). An association between psychiatric disorders and pain in cancer patients was demonstrated by Derogatis et al. (1983). Among patients with a psychiatric diagnosis, 39% had significant pain, whereas only 19% of those without a diagnosis had pain. It is estimated that 30% of patients with intractable pain have anxiety disorders, although more than half have comorbid depressive or substance use disorders as well (Bouckoms & Hackett, 1991). Anxiety may be both a consequence and a contributor to pain (Sternbach, 1974). Many patients believe that pain is indicative of disease progression, and this not only increases their pain but their apprehension.

Altered metabolic states

Altered metabolic states are often a cause of anxiety in medically ill patients (Lishman, 1987). Anxiety in seriously ill patients may be due to hypoxia. Hypoxic patients sense that something is wrong with their breathing and grow fearful. Sudden anxiety with chest pain may be the result of a pulmonary embolus (Dietch, 1981). Sepsis, that is accompanied by chills and fever, may also be associated with anxiety. In addition, anxiety and

Table 7.6. *Medical conditions associated with anxiety*

Cardiovascular conditions	Neurological conditions
Angina pectoris	Akathisia
Arrhythmia	Encephalopathy
Congestive heart failure	Mass lesion
Hypovolemia	Postconcussion syndrome
Myocardial infarction	Seizure disorder
Valvular disease	Vertigo
Endocrine conditions	Peptic ulcer disease
Carcinoid	Respiratory conditions
Hyperadrenalism	Asthma
Hypercalcemia	Chronic obstructive pulmonary
Hyperthyroidism	disease
Hypocalcemia	Pneumothorax
Hypothyroidism	Pulmonary edema
Pheochromocytoma	Pulmonary embolism
Metabolic conditions	Immunological conditions
Hyperkalemia	Anaphylaxis
Hyperthermia	Systemic lupus erythematosus
Hypoglycemia	
Hyponatremia	
Hypoxia	
Porphyria	

Source: Goldberg & Posner (1993). © 1993, Oxford University Press. Reprinted with permission.

restlessness may be early signs of delirium, regardless of the cause (Massie et al., 1983).

A variety of endocrine abnormalities are also associated with anxiety (Dietch, 1981; MacKenzie & Popkin, 1983; Raj & Sheehan, 1987). Table 7.6 lists these and other medical conditions often accompanied by anxiety (Goldberg & Posner, 1993). Hyperthyroidism is associated with anxiety that resembles generalized anxiety disorder (Kathol et al., 1986; Trzepacz et al., 1988). Kathol et al. (1986) and Trzepacz et al. (1988) found that three-quarters of such patients had anxiety symptoms beginning with the onset of the hyperthyroid state. Pheochromocytoma may also be associated with anxiety symptoms, although one study found them to be surprisingly infrequent (Starkman et al., 1985). Certain tumors, for instance pancreatic and lung cancer, may produce paraneoplastic syndromes that cause psychiatric disturbances including anxiety (Holland et al., 1986).

Central nervous system abnormalities

Anxiety syndromes may occur with cerebral lesions and abnormalities (reviewed by Strain & Ploog, 1988). Tumors of the central nervous system, especially those affecting the temporal lobes, may give rise to anxiety and panic attacks (Strain & Ploog, 1988). Likewise, viral encephalitis may be associated with anxiety. Anxiety and depression may develop following head injuries, but they are especially frequent in association with the postcontusional syndrome (Brooks, 1984). Tyerman & Humphrey (1984) found anxiety in 44% of head trauma patients 6 months after injury. This anxiety appeared to be related to difficulties in adjusting to the impairment in brain functioning. The postconcussion syndrome is often associated with anxiety symptoms as well.

Anxiety disorders, often in combination with depressive disorders, have been observed in 3–27% of stroke patients (Starkstein et al., 1990; Castillo et al., 1993; Burvill et al., 1995). Such disorders may represent reactions to life-threatening illness or its consequences (Storey, 1985; Burvill et al., 1995). According to Castillo et al. (1993), post-stroke anxiety is not associated with background characteristics or impairment but with the brain structures affected (right hemispheric lesions).

Anxiety associated with epilepsy was first described by Jackson (1881). He observed that anxiety and fear may occur as part of the aura of psychomotor seizures (Harper & Roth, 1962). Later, Williams (1956) reported that 37% of patients with partial complex seizures have ictal anxiety. Anxiety and anxiety attacks can be induced by stereotactic stimulation of the temporal lobes and other limbic structures, indicating that these structures are important in generating such symptoms (Gloor et al., 1982).

Substance-induced disturbances

Substance-induced anxiety disorders are common in medically ill patients. Corticosteroids cause major psychiatric disturbances in 5 and 10% of patients receiving high doses (Ling et al., 1981); however, minor mood disturbances, including anxiety symptoms, are common (Stiefel et al., 1989). These include anxiety, restlessness, emotional lability, insomnia, and agitation. Other medications that may cause anxiety symptoms are shown in Table 7.7.

Antiemetic drugs, such as metoclopramide and prochlorperazine, may cause anxiety-like symptoms. These neuroleptic drugs are given in high doses to control chemotherapy-related nausea and vomiting. Akathisia or

Table 7.7. *Medications associated with anxiety*

Anesthetics/analgesics
Antidepressants (tricyclics, SSRIs, bupropion)
Antihistamines
Antihypertensives
Antimicrobials
Bronchodilators
Caffeine preparations
Calcium-blocking agents
Cholinergic-blocking agents
Digitalis
Estrogen
Ethosuximide
Heavy metals and toxins
Hydralazine
Insulin
Levodopa
Muscle relaxants
Neuroleptics
Non-steroidal anti-inflammatories
Procaine
Procarbazine
Sedatives
Steroids
Sympathomimetics
Theophylline
Thyroid preparations

Source: Colon & Popkin (1996). © American Psychiatric Press. Reprinted with permission.

motor restlessness typically develops several hours to days after treatment. Uncontrollable movements involving the legs, hands and jaws are accompanied by anxiety. According to Fleishman et al. (1994), 50% of cancer patients receiving one of these drugs experience this side-effect.

A variety of other drugs are capable of producing anxiety symptoms especially in high doses (reviewed by Abramowicz, 1989). Thyroid replacement, when excessive, may cause anxiety symptoms (Hall, 1983). Also, bronchodilators and beta-adrenergic agonists can produce anxiety symptoms (Jacobs et al., 1976; Wiener, 1980). Stimulant drugs, such as methylphenidate and dextroamphetamine, may cause anxiety and insomnia in high dose. Likewise, excessive use of, or withdrawal from, caffeine may produce anxiety symptoms (Victor et al., 1981). Drugs of abuse, especially cocaine and marijuana, may cause panic attacks (Aronson & Craig, 1986). Exposure to organic solvents may also precipitate anxiety (Duger et al., 1987).

Discontinuation of certain drugs may also be associated with anxiety symptoms. If alcohol is abruptly stopped, withdrawal symptoms, including severe anxiety, may appear within the first day (Lerner & Fallon, 1985). Patients dependent upon narcotics, such as heroin, may also experience anxiety as part of a withdrawal syndrome. Also, benzodiazepines, especially short-acting drugs, are an increasing cause of withdrawal symptoms (Noyes et al., 1988). Similarly, discontinuation of sedative-hypnotics and narcotic analgesics may precipitate withdrawal syndromes.

Clinical picture

Acute anxiety symptoms

Although most anxiety disorders represent acute reactions to medical illness or its treatment, some are long-standing disturbances that have been exacerbated by illness or challenged by the treatment setting (Sharer et al., 1993). Regardless of cause, the symptoms experienced by most patients are similar. Their mood is anxious, and they are troubled by uneasiness, apprehension or, in more severe cases, a sense of impending doom. This mood is accompanied by an unpleasant feeling of arousal; patients feel keyed up, are irritable, and have a tendency to startle. They are unable to relax and have difficulty falling asleep.

Patients with acute anxiety find their minds filled with recurring, intrusive thoughts and images of illness or accident (Kaasa et al., 1993). They are beset by fears of bodily injury or death and dwell upon obtaining help or avoiding such threats (Stefanek et al., 1989). The thinking of anxious patients is often catastrophic and overgeneralized; they see unlikely dangers as probable and unfortunate consequences as overwhelming. Typically they view their situation as uncontrollable and see themselves as helpless victims.

Symptoms of autonomic arousal include rapid or forceful heartbeat, sweating, and a sinking sensation in the stomach. Many patients experience tightness in the chest, shortness of breath, feelings of dizziness and paresthesias, sympathetically-mediated symptoms. Some patients experience anxiety or panic attacks that leave them emotionally drained and fearful of future attacks. Parasympathetically-mediated symptoms such as abdominal distress, nausea and diarrhea, are common. Vegetative disturbances, such as loss of appetite and sexual interest, may also be part of the clinical picture.

Acutely anxious patients show physiological signs and behavioral manifestations. They appear worried and drawn. Many are distractible, perplexed, and emotionally labile. Others are fidgety, restless, and have trouble sitting still. They are often tremulous or diaphoretic. Trouble sleeping contributes to fatigue and a low tolerance for frustration. In response to anxious preoccupation about illness, many repeatedly check their bodies for signs of recurrence or progression. Acutely anxious patients feel an urge to avoid or escape from surroundings they see as threatening, prompting them to refuse treatment or to sign out of the hospital (Greenberg, 1991). Anxiety symptoms may contribute to physical morbidity as well. Loss of appetite, poor sleep, shortness of breath, fatigue, and pain are all symptoms that may worsen with anxiety.

Phobic symptoms

Phobic symptoms sometimes develop in reaction to illness or its treatment. Persons exposed to life-threatening medical events may become fearful of the circumstances or activities they regard as dangerous (Lloyd, 1991). Following a heart attack or stroke, for example, a patient may find him or herself preoccupied with thoughts or images of a recurrence (Burvill et al., 1995). Such patients are vigilant, unable to sleep, and have difficulty being away from a safe person in case something catastrophic were to happen. They may be afraid to leave home or be without ready access to emergency medical care (Bishay et al., 1995). Also, they may view activities involving physical exertion or emotional arousal (e.g., sexual activity) as dangerous and avoid them.

Patients with chronic lung disease often show a similar phobic response (Agle & Baum, 1977). In addition to tension, jumpiness, and tremulousness, they have overanxious concern about breathing and fears of suffocation. They hyperventilate, are fearful and avoid situations that they perceive as a threat to their breathing. Situations of this kind include taking a shower, going to the toilet, eating alone, and being without an inhaler or companion (Yellowless et al., 1987).

Posttraumatic stress symptoms

Posttraumatic stress symptoms may follow life-threatening accidents or injuries. For instance, up to 40% of hospitalized burn victims report symptoms of posttraumatic stress disorder (Perry et al., 1992; Roca et al., 1992; Powers et al., 1994). Other precipitants include accidents, assaults, and disasters which expose patients to the threat of death or serious injury.

Also, survivors of life-threatening illnesses, such as myocardial infarction and cancer, sometimes experience posttraumatic stress symptoms (Doerfler et al., 1994; Kutz et al., 1994; Alter et al., 1996). Patients exposed to such threats often experience painful and intrusive recollections of the traumatic event and find their sleep interrupted by frightening dreams (Noyes et al., 1971). They are overwhelmed by a sense of vulnerability, are preoccupied with the circumstances of the accident, and experience other symptoms typical of posttraumatic stress disorder (see Chapter 6).

Some persons develop unreasonable fears of illness in the absence of physical disease (Marks, 1987). They have illness phobia originally described by Ryle (1948). Fears of illness are relatively common in the general population and persons with illness phobia make up 15–34% of phobic outpatients (Agras et al., 1969; Marks, 1987). Illness phobics worry excessively that they might have one or another disease, and their fear persists despite reassurance (Noyes et al., 1992). They constantly search their bodies for signs and interpret benign bodily sensations as evidence of serious disease. Somatic symptoms of anxiety (e.g., palpitations) may themselves cause alarm. Fears of heart disease, cancer and, more recently, AIDS are commonly seen (Logsdail et al., 1991; Eifert, 1992).

Chronic anxiety symptoms

Many patients with chronic disturbances, such as generalized anxiety disorder and panic disorder, experience the re-emergence or intensification of symptoms with the development of physical illness. Persons whose panic and agoraphobic symptoms had been controlled may experience them again upon learning their diagnosis or being exposed to painful procedures, toxic medications, or crowded treatment facilities. Of course, fear of crowded or confined places (agoraphobia) may interfere with medical treatment, and panic attacks occasionally prompt patients to abruptly terminate procedures. Posttraumatic stress disorder may also be reactivated by medical illness (Hamner, 1994).

Specific phobias, especially blood/needle phobia and claustrophobia (fear of closed places), may also interfere with medical treatment. Patients with blood/needle phobia may be unable to tolerate injections, blood draws, or treatment procedures, and experience persistent anxiety in anticipation of such procedures (see Chapter 5). They show a characteristic vasovagal response to the feared object (i.e., bradycardia and fall in blood pressure). Claustrophobic patients are unable to tolerate procedures that require confinement in small spaces. These may include imaging studies, radiotherapy, administration of anesthetic agents, etc. According to Melendez & McCrank (1993), 5–10% of persons undergoing magnetic resonance imaging (MRI) scans experience severe panic or claustrophobic reactions.

Natural history

There is some evidence that new anxiety disorders among medical patients follow a favorable course, and that most remit without treatment. For instance, Kathol & Wenzel (1992) followed patients who, at the time of hospitalization, were identified as having anxiety or depressive disorders associated with their medical condition. These patients showed a significant decrease in psychiatric symptoms within days of admission, and roughly two-thirds showed resolution of their disorder without specific intervention. The authors concluded that patients improve as their medical condition improves and respond to support and reassurance (Kathol & Wenzel, 1992). Similarly, Kessler et al. (1985) observed that most anxiety and depressive disorders in primary care outpatients follow an episodic course.

Anxiety disorders that develop in patients with physical illness sometimes disappear with resolution of the crisis that precipitated them. In a study of adjustment disorders among inpatients referred for psychiatric consultation, Popkin et al. (1990) observed that two-thirds resolved, usually within 30 days. Longitudinal studies of cancer patients, beginning at the time of diagnosis or initiation of treatment, show a gradual decline in the number of patients with anxiety disorders. For instance, Maguire et al., (1978) reported that, of patients who suffered moderate to severe anxiety before surgery, 12% had symptoms that lasted 2–8 months, 17% had symptoms more than 8 months, and 4% still had symptoms after 1 year. Others have observed a similar decline in symptoms over 6 months to 1 year.

The same studies show that progression of disease and/or treatment influences psychological morbidity and that new cases of anxiety often develop along the way. For instance, Bergman et al. (1991) reported that anxiety declined in lung cancer patients who completed chemotherapy, but that this anxiety covaried with the tumor's response to therapy. Hopwood et al. (1991b) observed that 13 of 24 advanced breast cancer patients who had been cases of anxiety initially were borderline or well 1–3 months later, but that 11 more had become cases. Similarly, Devlen et al. (1987) found anxiety in lymphoma patients highest before treatment, but new episodes developed subsequently that, in many instances, were associated with treatment toxicity.

Anxiety disorders due to medical conditions or substances usually remit when the organic disturbance is corrected. According to Hall (1980), disorders due to medical conditions follow the course of the condition and resolve when it is treated. As an example, Kathol et al. (1986) observed that anxiety disorders associated with hyperthyroidism remit when the altered metabolic state is corrected. They concluded that treatment should be directed toward the organic disturbance and that additional treatment for anxiety may not be needed.

Differential diagnosis

Anxiety disorders that are associated with medical illness (or its treatment) fall into several diagnostic categories. When an illness serves as a stressful life event, an adjustment disorder may be diagnosed providing the disorder began within 3 months of the event, the symptoms do not meet the criteria for another anxiety disorder, and the symptoms do not persist for more than 6 months after termination of the stressor (American Psychiatric Association, 1994). The mere existence of a powerful stressor (e.g., heart attack, diagnosis of cancer) is not sufficient reason to identify an adjustment disorder. On the one hand, other anxiety disorders are frequently associated with life events, and on the other hand, many persons exposed to such events do not develop anxiety symptoms (Blazer et al., 1987). Acute life-threatening illness may also result in persistent re-experiencing of the event, persistent avoidance of stimuli associated with the trauma, and symptoms of increased arousal. In that case, a diagnosis of acute stress disorder or post-traumatic stress disorder may be warranted.

Anxiety disorders due to general medical conditions must be distinguished from disorders in which the medical condition serves as a psychological stressor (American Psychiatric Association, 1994). The former are caused by physiological disturbances that accompany the conditions, such as a hyperthyroid state. In such cases there is usually evidence from the literature that the condition can produce anxiety, and a temporal relationship between anxiety symptoms and the onset, exacerbation or remission of the condition usually exists. Also, clinical features that are atypical for primary anxiety disorders (e.g., late age of onset, remitting course, absent family history) are often present.

Anxiety disorders due to general medical conditions must also be distinguished from substance-induced anxiety disorders (American Psychiatric Association, 1994). Symptoms that develop during or shortly after (i.e., within 4 weeks) intoxication or withdrawal from a substance may be substance-related, depending upon the substance and the amount used. Substance-induced anxiety disorders occur only during drug intoxication or withdrawal; other anxiety disorders often precede the onset of substance use and persist during sustained abstinence. A history of exposure and laboratory evidence (i.e., drug screen) may be important in establishing this diagnosis. A substance-induced anxiety disorder should be diagnosed instead of substance intoxication or withdrawal only when the anxiety symptoms exceed those usually associated with the intoxication or withdrawal and are sufficient to warrant independent clinical attention. If anxiety symptoms persist more than 4 weeks after a substance or medication is stopped, the cause may be other than the substance.

In medically ill patients, anxiety symptoms are commonly caused by delirium. The presence of delirium precludes the diagnosis of an anxiety disorder due to a medical condition.

The differential diagnosis of anxiety disorders due to medical conditions includes a great variety of conditions which may present with anxiety or anxiety-like symptoms (Cameron, 1985). According to Hall et al. (1978, 1981), 2% of psychiatric outpatients and inpatients have medical disorders that present with anxiety. There are a number of reviews of such conditions (Hall, 1980; Dietch, 1981; Jefferson & Marshall, 1981; Mackenzie & Popkin, 1983; Raj & Sheehan, 1987; Goldberg, 1988). Most provide a list of illnesses and substances (including medications) commonly associated with anxiety. Any such lists, like those shown in Tables 7.6 and 7.7 are arbitrary. Many of the conditions included produce symptom patterns like those of generalized anxiety (e.g., hyperthyroidism) or panic disorder (e.g., paroxysmal atrial tachycardia), while others produce symptoms that only resemble anxiety syndromes (e.g., angina pectoris) (Hall, 1980).

The diagnosis of an anxiety disorder due to a general medical condition or substance requires evidence from medical history, physical examination, and laboratory testing of the condition. Routine screening for specific disorders is usually not called for when assessing anxious patients unless the basic evaluation points in that direction. As endocrine disorders, especially hyperthyroidism and pheochromocytoma, are commonly considered in the differential diagnosis, alertness to such disorders should remain high, but routine testing for them is likely to have a low yield. The commonest drug-related anxiety disturbances include intoxication with stimulants (e.g., cocaine) and withdrawal from alcohol. Here again, the history and physical examination, plus laboratory screening, should provide clues to the diagnosis.

Treatment

Treatment of anxiety disorders in the medically ill depends upon the relationship between anxiety symptoms and physical disease. Some patients have persisting symptoms or exacerbations of anxiety disorders that existed before the onset of physical disease. In that case, treatment should be similar to that given to patients without comorbid illness. Other patients, perhaps the majority, have disorders the onset of which coincides with illness-related events. In these instances, treatment needs to take the emotional reaction to events into account. Still other patients will have disorders caused by the altered biology of a disease or its treatment. These are disorders due to medical conditions or substances, and their treatment should begin with the medical conditions, many of which are reversible.

The pharmacological treatment of anxiety disorders in the medically ill is complicated by physical disease and its treatment. Sometimes medications used for anxiety adversely affect the underlying medical problems or interact negatively with the drugs used to treat these problems. For example, a benzodiazepine may suppress respiration if given to an anxious patient with chronic pulmonary disease, or a serotonin reuptake inhibitor may alter the metabolism of drugs used to control cardiac rhythm in a patient with heart disease. Of course, the reverse is also true; physical disease and its treatment may contribute to anxiety in ways that are sometimes difficult to modify. In the face of progressive and life-threatening disease, anxiety-generating treatment (e.g., chemotherapy) may be necessary. When factors that are contributing to anxiety symptoms are recognized, they can be taken into account in weighing treatment options.

The psychological treatment of anxiety in the medically ill employs a number of management techniques. These techniques are usually not time-consuming nor do they call for special training, yet they are surprisingly effective (Burton et al., 1991). For example, anxiety is best managed initially by providing emotional support and adequate information (Massie & Shakin, 1993). To do this, physicians should elicit and deal with the thoughts and feelings that are causing distress. Anxiety about procedures or treatments may be reduced by adequate preparation. Although the value of such simple measures is well documented, they are too often neglected (Egbert et al., 1964). Causes of anxiety to be explored include worry about practical matters such as finances, physical suffering, uncertainty about the future, loss of independence, loss of social role, fear of becoming a burden, fear of the manner of death, and spiritual concerns (Craig & Abeloff, 1974; Maguire et al., 1993b). Many patients can be helped by an opportunity to share their concerns and to feel understood (Maguire et al., 1993b).

In addition to supportive psychotherapy, anxiety management techniques (e.g., muscle relaxation), and cognitive behavioral interventions (e.g., modifying dysfunctional thoughts about illness) are often helpful.

Pharmacological treatment

Benzodiazepines

Benzodiazepines not only reduce anxiety but also induce sleep, promote muscle relaxation, control nausea and vomiting associated with chemotherapy, and bring about relaxation if not amnesia during procedures. There have been few controlled trials so that efficacy has not been established for most indications. In a controlled trial of patients with anxiety associated with cardiovascular disease, lorazepam in a dose of 3 mg daily proved superior to placebo (Samet & Geller, 1979). Tollefson et al. (1991) reported that, in an open trial of alprazolam, patients with coexisting generalized anxiety disorder and irritable bowel syndrome showed a reduction in both anxiety and bowel symptoms. Similarly, Holland et al. (1991) found that both alprazolam and progressive muscle relaxation resulted in a significant reduction in anxiety and depressive symptoms among cancer patients.

Benzodiazepines have also been shown to significantly reduce the anticipatory anxiety as well as the nausea and vomiting that accompanies chemotherapy (reviewed by Triozzi et al., 1988; Greenberg, 1991). Patients who receive lorazepam experience less anxiety and more sedation as well as less nausea and vomiting. When the drug is given intravenously (2–4 mg), many patients do not remember the treatment. Patients receiving benzodiazepines have been pleased with their effects, and in some instances, have been willing to continue otherwise intolerable treatments (Triozzi et al., 1988).

The choice of a benzodiazepine and its administration may be influenced by a patient's age and physical status. The metabolism of drugs that undergo microsomal oxidation is slowed in the elderly. This prolongs the half-life of long-acting drugs and increases the risk of toxicity from accumulation (reviewed by Stoudemire & Moran, 1993). The metabolism of drugs that undergo glucuronide conjugation, such as lorazepam, oxazepam, and temazepam, are little affected by age. Liver disease may also slow the metabolism and increase the risk of toxicity. In elderly patients, the starting dose of a benzodiazepine should be about half the usual dose.

Drugs that influence the activity of liver enzymes may alter the metabolism of benzodiazepines. Chronic sedative-hypnotic use can, by increasing enzymatic activity, increase the breakdown of benzodiazepines. Consequently, patients taking drugs like phenobarbital or phenytoin may require high doses. On the other hand, patients taking drugs that compete for metabolizing enzymes, such as cimetidine, disulfiram, isoniazid, erythromycin or estrogens, may require smaller doses. Elderly patients are more sensitive to the central effects of benzodiazepines including memory disturbance, drowsiness, depressed mood, ataxia, and falls.

Benzodiazepines may inhibit respiratory drive in patients with chronic pulmonary disease. This inhibition is usually only a problem in patients with chronic carbon dioxide retention. According to Stoudemire & Moran (1993), most asthmatic and chronic emphysematous patients are able to tolerate small doses of benzodiazepines. Use of a benzodiazepine is dangerous in patients suffering from sleep apnea because of respiratory suppression. Buspirone, because it is a mild respiratory stimulant, may be useful in patients with chronic obstructive lung disease. Open trials have indicated efficacy (Craven & Sutherland, 1991; Singh et al., 1993).

Lorazepam, alprazolam, and clonazepam are the benzodiazepines most frequently prescribed for medically ill patients. Lorazepam has no active metabolites and is unlikely to accumulate. Unlike most other drugs in this class, it may be administered by the oral, intramuscular, and intravenous routes, making it versatile. Control of anxiety is rapid, often occurring within the first few days. Drowsiness and fatigue, the most common side-effects, usually respond to dose adjustment or the passage of time. Alprazolam has antidepressant properties and may be tried where depressive symptoms coexist. Clonazepam is a longer-acting drug that has little interdose rebound that may be a problem with shorter-acting drugs (Tesar, 1990). Midazolam, a short-acting benzodiazepine that is available only in injectable form, is also used to control procedure-related anxiety.

Other antianxiety drugs

Several other classes of drugs are used to control generalized anxiety symptoms in the medically ill. These include azapirones, beta-blockers, and antihistamines. Buspirone, an azapirone, is a partial serotonin agonist that is free of sedation and effects on cognition (Kiev & Domantay, 1988). It does not appear to interact with drugs used in the medically ill. In addition to its value in pulmonary disease, it may control anxiety and agitation in patients with dementia and brain trauma (Tiller et al., 1988). The dose for elderly patients is similar to that for younger ones (i.e., 40–60 mg) (Robinson et al., 1988; Rickels et al., 1991).

Propranolol and other beta-adrenergic blocking agents relieve anxiety by blocking the peripheral autonomic response (Noyes, 1988). As with buspirone, they are useful for milder forms of anxiety but have little effect on panic disorder. Non-selective beta-blockers, such as propranolol, should not be used in patients with a history of asthma or obstructive pulmonary disease. Cardioselective agents, such as atenolol, may be used cautiously in such patients and may be best for patients with diabetes as they do not interfere with glycogenesis. Less lipophilic drugs, such as atenolol, have fewer central nervous system side-effects. Hydroxyzine and diphenhydramine, H1-histaminic blocking agents, are commonly used to treat mild anxiety and insomnia. Although considered safe, they may cause drowsiness and cognitive impairment in the elderly and medically ill. Also, they have anticholinergic and other side-effects to which elderly persons are particularly sensitive.

Although benzodiazepines are useful for the rapid control of more severe anxiety, other drugs, including the serotonin uptake inhibitors, tricyclic antidepressants, and monoamine oxidase inhibitors are also used to treat anxiety in the medically ill. The efficacy of these classes of drugs for various anxiety disorders has been reviewed elsewhere (see Chapters 2 and 3). The relative absence of cardiovascular effects has made the serotonin uptake inhibitors popular for treating anxiety and depression in the medically ill (Papp et al., 1995; Stoudemire & Fogel, 1995). They may alter the metabolism of a number of drugs used to treat medical illness because of their inhibition of cytochrome P_{450} liver enzymes. Consequently, possible interactions must be taken into account when they are prescribed. Drugs with mild stimulant properties, such as fluoxetine, may be more difficult for anxious patients to tolerate initially than drugs such as paroxetine or sertraline. In higher doses these agents may produce akasthisia that may be mistaken for worsening anxiety.

Cyclic antidepressants are well established antipanic agents and their efficacy for generalized anxiety has also been demonstrated (Hoehn-Saric et al., 1988); however, in the medically ill they have a number of potentially serious effects. These include orthostatic hypotension, anticholinergic effects, quinidine-like effects, and sedation. Nortriptyline has less potential for hypotension, and established blood levels are a useful guide to dosing. It is wise to begin with low doses (e.g., 10–25 mg) and increase gradually using electrocardiographic monitoring. Monoamine oxidase inhibitors may also be used in medically ill or elderly patients. Their superior efficacy for anxious depression and their energizing effects make them especially valuable for some patients. If no harmful drug interactions are anticipated, orthostatic hypotension is the chief concern with drugs such as phenelzine or tranylcypromine. Patients using these drugs must adhere to a tyramine-free diet and avoid indirect-acting sympathomimetic agents, some of which are available in over-the-counter cold preparations. Hypertensive crises resulting from such interactions are, fortunately, rare.

Psychological treatment

Medically ill patients may benefit from a variety of psychosocial interventions designed to reduce general distress, procedure-related discomfort, and acute anxiety. Few controlled trials have examined the effectiveness of such therapies for anxiety (reviewed by Derogatis & Wise, 1989). A review of controlled studies of psychological therapies in medically ill patients in 1981 found only 13 methodologically adequate trials, and a similar review in 1996 found just 14 (Guthrie,1996). In their review of controlled studies in cancer patients, Fawzy et al. (1995) identified several types of relatively brief interventions that have demonstrated efficacy. These included education, behavioral interventions, cognitive therapy, individual psychotherapy, and group therapy. Few of the studies specifically examined change in anxiety but included it among measures of psychological distress. Also, most interventions were compared to ineffective procedures which showed they were better than no treatment but not how they compared with other approaches.

Behavioral methods have been used in conjunction with many medical interventions to reduce physical as well as psychological distress, and these methods have, in general, proved beneficial. Techniques have included progressive muscle relaxation, hypnosis, deep breathing, meditation, biofeedback, and guided imagery (Fawzy et al., 1995). As reviewed by Goldberg (1982), these self-regulatory techniques reduce anxiety by evoking the relaxation response (Benson et al., 1974). Most are easily taught and quickly learned. Efficacy in medical populations has been demonstrated (Raskin et al., 1980). For instance, Davis (1986) reported significant improvement in anxiety among breast cancer patients receiving biofeedback and cognitive therapy, and other investigators observed reduced anxiety among cancer patients who received muscle relaxation and guided imagery (Gruber et al., 1993; Baider et al., 1994). Similar methods have been applied to patients with lung disease (Renfroe, 1988).

Behavioral techniques may also be useful for managing anxiety related to investigations or procedures (Wilson-Barnett, 1992). Relaxation training, systematic desensitization, and positive reinforcement have been used to reduce anxious and phobic reactions to medical treatments (Melamed & Seigal, 1980). Behavioral approaches, especially those for children undergoing painful procedures, usually involve a combination of positive motivation, emotive imagery, and hypnosis. Patients with claustrophobia or needle/blood phobia may be rapidly and successfully treated with behavioral methods (Öst et al., 1984). For needle/blood phobia, Öst et al. (1989) developed a technique called applied tension that may produce results quickly (see Chapter 5).

Cognitive therapy, an effective treatment for anxiety, is increasingly being used in the medically ill (reviewed by Sensky, 1993). This therapy focuses upon dysfunctional beliefs, especially those involving the illness itself, interaction with health care professionals, and the perceived impact on the patient's life (Bishay et al., 1995). The onset of physical illness often involves life-threatening events to which some patients, by virtue of their cognitive style, are vulnerable. Cognitive therapy begins with an exploration of a patient's understanding of his or her illness. The approach is educational and leads to the acquisition of skills that can be applied to present and future problems. Specific techniques have been developed for patients with such problems as cancer and chronic pain. Sensky (1993) has reviewed the efficacy of cognitive therapy in a variety of patient populations.

Individual psychotherapy has, in some controlled trials, resulted in reduced psychological distress and better coping in patients with neoplastic and other diseases (Fawzy et al., 1995). In a study that attempted to reduce psychological morbidity including anxiety, Greer et al. (1992) examined the effect of adjuvant psychological therapy. At 4 months and again at 12 months, patients who had received the therapy had significantly lower scores on anxiety than did controls (Moorey et al., 1994). Also, fewer therapy patients fell in the clinical range for anxiety than did controls. The study – one of the few to address anxiety specifically – demonstrated that a brief psychological intervention can not only reduce distress but also the rate of caseness a year afterward. Controlled studies have also shown psychotherapeutic interventions useful in reducing the distress following myocardial infarction (reviewed by Guthrie, 1996). In one such trial, patients who received counseling from coronary care nurses reported significantly lower levels of anxiety than controls immediately after admission as well as 6 months later (Thompson & Meddis, 1990).

Psychotherapy with medically ill persons is based on an understanding of the illness dynamics or factors affecting an individual's response to a specific disease at a particular time in his or her life (reviewed by Green, 1985, Rosenbaum & Pollack, 1991). Illness is experienced as both a threat and a loss and typically precipitates a grief reaction accompanied by anxiety (Green, 1993). Supportive rather than intensive psychotherapy is usually appropriate for anxiety resulting from illness (Derogatis & Wise, 1989). Winston et al. (1986) and Green (1993) have outlined the goals and techniques to be employed with this form of therapy. Blacher (1991) and Groves & Kucharski (1991) describe a series of brief intervention strategies that may be used by psychiatric consultants.

Group intervention may also be beneficial in medically ill patients (Fawzy et al., 1995). Group techniques include education, emotional support, stress management, coping strategies, behavioral training, and others. In an important study by Spiegel et al. (1981), patients who participated in psychological support groups for a year reported less tension and fewer phobias than did controls.

References

Abramowicz, M. 1989. Drugs that cause psychiatric symptoms. *Med. Lett.* 31: 113–118.
Agle, D. P. & Baum, G. L. 1977. Psychological aspects of chronic obstructive pulmonary disease. *Med. Clin. North Am.* 61: 749–758.
Agras, S., Sylvester, D. & Oliveau, D. 1969. The epidemiology of common fears and phobias. *Compr. Psychiatry* 10: 151–156.
Allgulander, C. 1994. Suicide and mortality patterns in anxiety neurosis and depressive neurosis. *Arch. Gen. Psychiatry* 51: 708–712.
Alter, C. L., Pelcoritz, D., Axelrod, A. et al. 1996. Identification of PTSD in cancer survivors. *Psychosomatics* 37: 137–143.
American Psychiatric Association 1980. *Diagnostic and Statistical Manual of Mental Disorders*, Third Edition, American Psychiatric Association, Washington, DC.
American Psychiatric Association 1987. *Diagnostic and Statistical Manual of Mental Disorders*, Third Edition-Revised, American Psychiatric Association, Washington, DC.
American Psychiatric Association 1994. *Diagnostic and Statistical Manual of Mental Disorders*, Fourth Edition, American Psychiatric Association, Washingon, DC.
Andersen, B. L., Karlson, J. A., Anderson, B. et al. 1984. Anxiety and cancer treatment: Response to stressful radiotherapy. *Health Psychol.* 3: 535–551.
Andrykowski, M. A. & Gregg, M. E. 1992. The role of psychological variables in post chemotherapy nausea: anxiety and expectation. *Psychosom. Med.* 54: 48–58.
Angst, J. & Vollrath, M. 1991. The natural history of anxiety disorders. *Acta Psychiatr. Scand.* 84: 446–452.

Aronson, T. A. & Craig, T. J. 1986. Cocaine precipitation of panic disorder. *Am. J. Psychiatry* 143: 643–645.

Atkinson, J. H., Grant, I., Kennedy, C. J. et al. 1988. Prevalence of psychiatric disorders among men infected with human immunodeficiency virus: A controlled study. *Arch. Gen. Psychiatry* 45: 859–864.

Baider, L., Uziely, B. & De-Nour, A. K. 1994. Progressive muscle relaxation and guided imagery in cancer patients. *Gen. Hosp. Psychiatry* 16: 340–347.

Bajwa, W. K., Asnis, G. M., Sanderson, W. C. et al. 1992. High cholesterol levels in patients with panic disorder. *Am. J. Psychiatry* 149: 376–378.

Barrett, J. E., Barrett, J. A., Oxman, T. E. et al. 1988. The prevalence of psychiatric disorders in a primary care practice. *Arch. Gen. Psychiatry* 45: 1100–1106.

Bass, C., Wade, C., Gardner, W. N. et al. 1983. Unexplained breathlessness and psychiatric morbidity in patients with normal and abnormal coronary arteries. *Lancet* 1: 605–609.

Beitman, B. D., Kushner, M. G., Lamberti, J. W. et al. 1990. Panic disorder without fear in patients with angiographically normal coronary arteries. *J. Nerv. Ment. Dis.* 178: 307–312.

Beitman, B. D., Kushner, M. G., Busha, I. et al. 1991. Follow-up status of patients with angiographically normal coronary arteries and panic disorder. *JAMA* 265: 1545–1549.

Beitman, B. D., Mukerii, J., Lamberti, J. W. et al. 1989. Panic disorder in patients with chest pain and angiographically normal coronary arteries. *Am. J. Cardiol.* 63: 1399–1403.

Benson, H., Beary, J. F. & Carol, M. P. 1974. The relaxation response. *Psychiatry* 37: 37–46.

Bergman, B., Sullivan, M. & Sorenson, S. 1991. Quality of life during chemotherapy for small cell lung cancer. I. An evaluation of generic health measures. *Acta Oncol.* 30: 947–957.

Bigger, J. T., Fleiss, J. L., Steinman, R. C. et al. 1992. Frequency domain measures of heart rate period variability and mortality after myocardial infarction. *Circulation* 85: 164–171.

Bishay, N. R., Tarrier, N. & Roberts, A. P. 1995. Cognitive therapy of agoraphobia in reaction to physical illness: An uncontrolled study. *Irish J. Psychol. Med.* 12: 135–138.

Blacher, R. 1991. Brief psychotherapy for medical and surgical patients. In *Handbook of Studies on General Hospital Psychiatry*, eds. F. K. Judd, G. D. Burrows, D. R. Lipsitt, pp. 143–152, Elsevier, Amsterdam.

Blazer, D., Hughes, D. & George, L. K. 1987. Stressful life events and the onset of generalized anxiety syndrome. *Am. J. Psychiatry* 144: 1178–1183.

Bloom, J. R. 1986. Social support and adjustment to breast cancer. In *Women and Cancer*, ed. B. Anderson, pp. 204–229, Springer, New York.

Bouckoms, A. & Hackett. T. P. 1991. The pain patient: Evaluation and treatment. In *Massachusetts General Hospital Handbook of General Hospital Psychiatry*, Third Edition, ed. N. Cassem, Mosby Year Book, St. Louis.

Brandenberg, Y., Bolund, C. & Sigurdardottir, J. J. 1992. Anxiety and depressive symptoms at different stages of malignant melanoma. *Psychooncology* 1: 71–78.

Breslau, N. & Davis, G. C. 1993. Migraine, physical health and psychiatric disorder: A prospective epidemiologic study in young adults. *J. Psychiatr. Res.* 27: 211–221.

Breslau, N., Davis, G. C. & Andreske, P. 1991. Migraine, psychiatric disorders, and suicide attempts: An epidemiologic study of young adults. *Psychiatry Res.* 37: 11–23.

Bridges, K. W. & Goldberg, D. P. 1984. Psychiatric illness in patients with neurological disorders: Patients' views on discussion of emotional problems with neurologists. *Br. Med. J.* 289: 656–658.

Brooks, N. 1984. *Closed Head Injury: Psychological, Social, and Family Consequences.* Oxford University Press, Oxford.

Burton, M. J., Parker, R. W. & Wollner, J. M. 1991. The psychotherapeutic value of a 'chat': A verbal response modes study of a placebo attention control with breast cancer patients. *Psychother. Res.* 1: 39–61.

Burvill, P. W., Johnson, G. A., Vamrozik, K. D. et al. 1995. Anxiety disorders after stroke: Results from the Perth Community Stroke Study, *Br. J. Psychiatry* 166: 328–332.

Cameron, O. G. 1985. The differential diagnosis of anxiety: Psychiatric and medical disorders. *Psychiatr. Clin. North Am.* 8: 3–24.

Carter, C., Maddock, R., Amsterdam, E. et al. 1992. Panic disorder and chest pain in the coronary care unit. *Psychosomatics* 33: 302–309.

Cassileth, B. R., Lusk, E. G. & Walsh, W. P. 1986. Anxiety levels in patients with malignant disease. *Hospice Journal* 2: 57–69.

Cassileth, B. R., Lusk, E. J., Strouse, T. B. et al. 1984. Psychosocial status in chronic illness: A comparative analysis of six diagnostic groups. *N. Engl. J. Med.* 311: 506–511.

Castillo, C. S., Starkstein, S. E., Fedoroff, J. P. et al. 1993. Generalized anxiety disorder after stroke. *J. Nerv. Ment. Dis.* 181: 100–106.

Cavanaugh, S. & Wettstein, R. M. 1984. Prevalence of psychiatric morbidity in medical populations. In *Psychiatric Update*, Vol. 3, ed. L. Grinspoon, pp. 187–215, American Psychiatric Press, Inc., Washington, DC.

Cella, D., Orofiamma, B., Holland, J. et al. 1987. The relationship of psychological distress, extent of disease and performance status in patients with lung cancer. *Cancer* 60: 1661–1667.

Charney, D. S. & Heninger, G. R. 1986. Abnormal regulation of noradrenergic function in panic disorders. *Arch. Gen. Psychiatry* 43: 1042–1054.

Clancy, J. & Noyes, R. 1976. Anxiety neurosis: A disease for the medical model. *Psychosomatics* 17: 90–93.

Clark, D. B., Hirsch, B. E., Smith, M. G. et al. 1994. Panic in otolaryngology patients presenting with dizziness or hearing loss. *Am. J. Psychiatry* 151: 1223–1225.

Clouse, R. E. 1988. Anxiety and gastrointestinal illness. *Psychiatr. Clin. N. Am.* 11: 399–418.

Colon, E. A. & Popkin, M. K. 1996. Anxiety and panic. In *Textbook of Consultation-Liaison Psychiatry*, eds. J. R. Randell, M. G. Wise, pp. 402–425, American Psychiatric Press, Washington, DC.

Cormier, L. E., Katon, W., Russo, J. et al. 1988. Chest pain with negative cardiac diagnostic studies: Relationship to psychiatric illness. *J. Nerv. Ment. Dis.* 176: 351–358.

Coryell, W., Noyes, R. & Clancy, J. 1982. Excess mortality in panic disorder: A comparison with primary unipolar depression. *Arch. Gen. Psychiatry* 39: 701–706.

Craig, T. J. & Abeloff, M. D. 1974. Psychiatric symptomatology among hospitalized cancer patients. *Am. J. Psychiatry* 131: 1323–1327.

Craven, J. and the Toronto Lung Transplant Group 1990. Psychiatric aspects of lung transplant. *Can. J. Psychiatry* 35: 759–764.

Craven, J. & Sutherland, A. 1991. Buspirone for anxiety disorder in patients with severe lung disease. *Lancet* 338: 249.

Crowe, R. R. 1985. Mitral valve prolapse and panic disorder. *Psychiatr. Clin. N. Am.* 8: 63–71.

Davis, H. IV. 1986. Effects of biofeedback and cognitive therapy on stress in patients with breast cancer. *Psychol. Rep.* 59: 967–974.

Dean, C. 1987. Psychiatric morbidity following mastectomy: Preoperative predictors and type of illness. *J. Psychosom. Res.* 31: 385–392.

Derogatis, L. R., Morrow, G., Fetting, J. et al. 1983. The prevalence of psychiatric disorders among cancer patients. *JAMA* 249: 751–757.

Derogatis, L. R. 1983. *SCL-90-R Administration, Scoring and Procedures Manual*, Second Edition. Procedures Psychometric Research. Baltimore.

Derogatis, L. R. & Wise, T. N. 1989. *Anxiety and Depressive Disorders in the Medical Patient*. American Psychiatric Press, Washington, DC.

Deshpande, S. N., Sundaram, K. R. & Wig, N. N. 1989. Psychiatric disorders among medical inpatients in an Indian hospital. *Br. .J Psychiatry* 154: 504–509.

Devlen, J. 1994. Anxiety and depression in migraine. *J. Roy. Soc. Med.* 87: 338–341.

Devlen, J., Maguire, P., Phillipos, P. et al. 1987. Psychological problems associated with diagnosis and treatment of lymphomas. II. Prospective study. *Br. Med. J. Clin. Res. Ed.* 295: 955–957.

Dew, M. A., Ragni, M. V. & Nimorwicz, P. 1990. Infection in the human immunodeficiency virus and vulnerability to psychiatric distress: A study of men with hemophilia. *Arch. Gen. Psychiatry* 47: 737–744.

Dhadphale, M., Ellison, R. H. & Griffin, L. 1983. The frequency of psychiatric disorders among patients attending semi–urban and rural general outpatient clinics in Kenya. *Br. J. Psychiatry* 142: 379–383.

Dietch, J. T. 1981. Diagnosis of organic anxiety disorders. *Psychosomatics* 22: 661–669.

Doerfler, L. A., Pbert, L. & DeCosimo, D. 1994. Symptom of posttraumtic stress disorder following myocardial infarction and coronary artery bypass surgery. *Gen. Hosp. Psychiatry* 16: 193–199.

Duger, S. R., Holland, J. P., Cowley, D. S. et al. 1987. Panic disorder precipitated by exposure to organic solvents in the work place. *Am. J. Psychiatry* 144: 1056–1058.

Eagger, S., Luxon, L. M., Davies, R. A. et al. 1992. Psychiatric morbidity in patients with peripheral vestibular disorder: A clinical neuro-otologic study. *J. Neurol. Neurosurg. Psychiatry* 55: 363–387.

Eastwood, M. & Trevelyan, M. 1972. Relationship between physical and psychiatric disorder. *Psychol. Med.* 2: 363–372.

Egbert, L. D., Battit, G. E., Welch, C. E. et al. 1964. Reduction of postoperative pain by encouragement and instruction of patients. *N. Engl. J. Med.* 170: 825–827.

Eifert, G. H. 1992. Cardiophobia: A paradigmatic behavioral model of heart-focused anxiety and non-anginal chest pain. *Behav. Res. Ther.* 30: 329–345.

Fallowfield, L. J., Hall, A., Maguire, G. P. et al. 1990. Psychological outcomes of different treatment policies in women with early breast cancer outside a clinical trial. *Br. Med. J.* 301: 575–580.

Fawzy, F. I., Fawzy, W. W., Arndt, L. A. et al. 1995. Critical review of psychosocial interventions in cancer care. *Arch. Gen. Psychaitry* 52: 100–113.

Feldman, E., Mayou, R., Hawton, K. et al. 1987. Psychiatric disorder in medical inpatients. *Quart. J. Med.* 63: 405–412.

Fell, M., Newman, S., Herns, M. et al. 1993. Mood and psychiatric disturbance in HIV and AIDS: Changes over time. *Br. J. Psychiatry* 162: 604–610.

Fifer, S. K., Mathias, S. D., Patrick, D. L. et al. 1994. Untreated anxiety among adult primary care patients in a health maintenance organization. *Arch. Gen. Psychiatry* 51: 740–750.

Fleishman, S. B., Lavin, M. R., Sattler, M. et al. 1994. Antiemetic-induced akathisia in cancer patients. *Am. J. Psychiatry* 15: 763–765.

Forester, B. M., Kornfeld, D. S. & Fleiss, J. 1978. Psychiatric aspects of radiotherapy. *Am. J. Psychiatry* 135: 960–963.

Freeman, L. J. & Nixon, P. G. F. 1985. Are coronary artery spasm and progressive damage to the heart associated with hyperventilation syndrome? *Br. Med. J.* 291: 851–852.

Gaffney, F. A., Fenton, B. J., Lane, L. D. et al. 1988. Hemodynamic, ventilation, and biochemical responses of panic patients and normal controls with sodium lactate infusion and spontaneous panic attacks. *Arch. Gen. Psychiatry* 45: 53–60.

Garden, G. M. F. & Ayres, J. G. 1993. Psychiatric and social aspects of brittle asthma. *Thorax* 48: 501–505.

Glass, R. M., Allan, A. T., Uhlenhuth, E. H. et al. 1978. Psychiatric screening in a medical clinic: An evaluation of a self–report inventory. *Arch. Gen. Psychiatry* 35: 1189–1195.

Gloor, P., Olivier, A., Quesney, L. F. et al. 1982. The role of the limbic system in experimental phenomena of temporal lobe epilepsy. *Ann. Neurology* 12: 129–144.

Goldberg, D. & Bridges, K. 1987. Screening for psychiatric illness in general practice: The general practitioner versus the screening questionnaire. *J. Roy. Coll. Gen. Pract.* 37: 5–18.

Goldberg, D. P. & Hillier, J. F. 1979. A scaled version of the General Health Questionnaire. *Psychol. Med.* 9: 139–145.

Goldberg, R., Morris, P., Christian, F. et al. 1990. Panic disorder in cardiac outpatients. *Psychosomatics* 31: 168–173.

Goldberg, R. J. 1982. Anxiety reduction by self-regulation: Theory, practice and evaluation. *Ann. Intern. Med.* 96: 483–487.

Goldberg, R. J. 1988. Clinical presentations of panic-related disorders. *J. Anx. Dis.* 2: 61–75.

Goldberg, R. J. & Posner, D. A. 1993. Anxiety in the medically ill. In *Psychiatric Care of the Medical Patient*, eds. A. Stoudemire, B. S. Fogel, pp. 87–103, Oxford University Press, New York.

Gorman, J. M., Fuer, M. R., Goetz, R. et al. 1988b. Ventilatory physiology of subjects with panic disorder. *Arch. Gen Psychiatry* 45: 31–39.

Gorman, J. M., Goetz, R. R., Fyer, M. et al. 1988a. The mitral valve prolapse – panic disorder connection. *Psychosom. Med.* 50: 114–122.

Green, S. 1985. *Mind and Body: The Psychology of Physical Illness.* American Psychiatric Press, Washington, DC.

Green, S. 1993. Principles of medical psychotherapy. In *Psychiatric Care of the Medical Patient*, eds. A. Stoudemire, B. Fogel, pp. 3–18, Oxford University Press, New York.

Greenberg, D. B. 1991. Strategic use of benzodiazepines in cancer patients. *Oncology* 5: 83–95.

Greer, S. 1994. Psycho-oncology: Its aims, achievements, and future tasks. *Psycho-oncology* 3: 87–101.

Greer, S., Moorey, S., Baruch, J. et al. 1992. Adjuvant psychological therapy for patients with cancer: A prospective randomized trial. *Br. Med. J.* 304: 675–680.

Groves, J. E. & Kacharski, A. 1991. Brief psychotherapy. In *Handbook of General Hospital Psychiatry*, ed. N. Cassem, pp. 321–341, St. Louis.

Gruber, B. L., Hersh, S. P., Hall, N. R. S. et al. 1993. Immunological responses of breast cancer patients to behavioral interventions. *Biofeedback Self Regulation* 18: 1–21.

Guiry, E., Conroy, R. M., Hickey, N. et al. 1987. Psychological response to an acute coronary event and its effect on subsequent rehabilitation and lifestyle change. *Clin. Cardiol.* 10: 256–260.

Guthrie, E. 1996. Emotional disorder in chornic illness: Psychotherapeutic interventions. *Br. J. Psychiatry* 168: 165–173.

Haines, A. P., Imeson, J. R., Meade, T. W. 1987. Phobic anxiety and ischemic heart disease. *Br. Med. J.* 295: 297–299.

Hall, R. C. W. 1980. *Psychiatric Manifestations of Medical Illness*. Spectrum Publications, New York.

Hall, R. C. W. 1983. Psychiatric effects of thyroid hormone disturbance. *Psychosomatics* 24: 7–18.

Hall, R. C. W., Popkin, M. K., Devaul, R. A. et al. 1978. Physical illness presenting as psychiatric disease. *Arch. Gen. Psychiatry* 35: 1315–1320.

Hall,. R. C. W., Gardner, E. R. & Popkin, M. K. 1981. Unrecognized physical illness prompting psychiatric admission: A prospective study. *Am. J. Psychiatry* 138: 629–635.

Hamner, M. B. 1994. Exacerbation of posttraumatic stress disorder symptoms with medical illness. *Gen. Hosp. Psychiatry* 16: 135–137.

Hankin, J. R., Steinwachs, D. M., Regier, D. A. et al. 1982. Use of general medical care services by persons with mental disorders. *Arch. Gen. Psychiatry* 39: 225–231.

Harding, T. W., De Arango, M. J., Batlazar, J. et al. 1980. Mental disorders in primary health care: A study of their frequency and diagnosis in four developing countries. *Psychol. Med.* 10: 213–241.

Harper, M. & Roth, M. 1962. Temporal lobe epilepsy and the phobic anxiety-depersonalization syndrome. Part I: A comparative study. *Compr. Psychiatry* 3: 129–151.

Haynes, S. G., Levine, S., Scotch, N. et al. 1978. The relationship of psychosocial factors to coronary heart disease in the Framingham Study. I: Methods and risk factors. *Am. J. Epidemiol.* 107: 362–383.

Hayward, C., Clark, D. B. & Taylor, C. B. 1990. Panic disorder, anxiety, and cardiovascular risk. In *Clinical Aspects of Panic Disorder*, ed. J. C. Ballenger, pp. 99–110, Wiley-Liss, New York.

Hayward, C., Taylor, C. B., Roth, W. T. et al. 1989. Plasma lipid levels in patients with panic disorder or agoraphobia. *Am. J. Psychiatry* 146: 917–919.

Hinton, J. 1972. Psychiatric consultation in fatal illness. *Proc. R. Soc. Med* 65: 1035–1038.

Hoehn-Saric, R., McLeod, D. R. & Zimmerli, W. D. 1988. Differential effects of alprazolam and imipramine in generalized anxiety disorder: Somatic versus psychic symptoms. *J. Clin. Psychiatry* 49: 293–301.

Hoeper, E., Nycz, G. R., Cleary, P. D. et al. 1979. Estimated prevalence of RDC mental disorders in primary medical care. *Int. J. Ment. Health* 8: 6–15.

Holland, J. C. 1989. Anxiety and cancer: The patient and the family. *J. Clin. Psychiatry* 50: 20–25.

Holland, J. C., Hughes, A., Korzan, A. H. et al. 1986. Comparative psychological disturbance in patients with pancreatic and gastric cancer. *Am. J. Psychiatry* 143: 982–986.

Holland, J. C., Morrow, G., Schmale, A. et al. 1991. A randomized clinical trial of alprazolam versus progressive muscle relaxation in cancer patients with anxiety and depressive symptoms. *J. Clin. Oncol.* 9: 1004–1011.

Holland, J. C., Rowland, J., Lebovits, A. et al. 1979. Reactions to cancer treatment: Assessment of emotional response to adjuvant radiotherapy as a guide to planned intervention. *Psychiatr. Clin. North Am.* 2: 347–358.

Hopwood, P., Howell, A. & Maguire, P. 1991a. Screening for psychiatric morbidity in patients with advanced breast cancer: Validation of two self-report questionnaires. *Br. J. Cancer* 64: 353–356.

Hopwood, P., Howell, A. & Maguire, P. 1991b. Psychiatric morbidity in patients with advanced cancer of the breast: Prevalence measured by two self-rating questionnaires. *Br. J. Cancer* 64: 349–352.

Jackson, J. H. 1881. On right- or left-sided spasms at the onset of epileptic paroxysms, and on crude sensation warnings and elaborate mental states. *Brain* 3: 192–206.

Jacob, R. G., Furman, J. M., Durrant, J. D. et al. 1996. Panic, agoraphobia, and vestibular dysfunction. *Am. J. Psychiatry* 153: 503–512.

Jacob, R. G., Furman, J. M. & Perel, J. M. In Press. Panic phobia and vestibular dysfunction. In *Vestibular Autonomic Regulation*, eds. B. Yates, A. Miller, CRC Press, New York.

Jacobs, M. A., Senior, R. M. & Kessler, G. 1976. Clinical experience with theophylline: Relationship between dosage, serum concentration, and toxicity. *JAMA* 235: 1983–1986.

Jacobsen, P. B., Bovberg, D. H. & Redd, W. H. 1993. Anticipatory anxiety in women receiving chemotherapy for breast cancer. *Health Psychology* 12: 469–475.

Jefferson, J. W. & Marshall, J. R. 1981. *Neuropsychiatric Features of Medical Disorders*. Plenum Medical Books, New York.

Jenkins, C. D., Sooervell, P. D. & Hames, O. G. 1983. Does blood pressure rise with age? . . . or with stress? *J. Hum. Stress* 9: 4–12.

Jimenez-Jimenez, J. A., Garcia-Ruiz, P. & Garcia-Urra, D. 1993. 'Panic attacks' in Parkinson's disease. *Acta Neurol. Scand.* 87: 14–18.

Kaasa, S., Malt, U., Jagen S. et al. 1993. Psychological distress in cancer patients with advanced disease. *Radiotherp. Oncol.* 27: 192–197.

Karajgi, B., Rifkin, A., Doddi, S. et al. 1990. The prevalence of anxiety disorders in patients with chronic obstructive pulmonary disease. *Am. J. Psychiatry* 147: 200–201.

Kathol, R. G., Turner, R. & Delahunt, J. 1986. Depression and anxiety associated with hyperthyroidism: Response to antithyroid therapy. *Psychosomatics* 27: 501–505.

Kathol, R. G. & Wenzel, R. P. 1992. Natural history of symptoms of depression and anxiety during inpatient treatment on general medicine wards. *J. Gen. Int. Med.* 7: 287–293.

Katon, W. J. 1984. Panic disorder and somatization: A review of 55 cases. *Am. J. Med.* 77: 101–106.

Katon, W. J. 1986. Panic disorder: Epidemiology, diagnosis, and treatment in primary care. *J. Clin. Psychiatry* 47 (Suppl. 10): 21–27.

Katon, W. J. , Hall, M., Russo, J. et al. 1988. Chest pain: Relationship to psychiatric illness to coronary angiographic results. *Am. J. Med.* 84: 1–9.

Katon, W. J. & Roy-Byrne, P. P. 1989. Panic disorder in the medically ill. *J. Clin. Psychiatry* 50: 299–302.

Katon, W. J. , Vitaliano, P., Russo, J. et al. 1986. Panic disorder: Epidemiology in primary care. *J. Family Practice* 23: 233–239.

Katon, W. J. 1990. Chest pain, cardiac disease, and panic disorder. *J. Clin. Psychiatry* 51: 27–30.

Katon, W. J. 1991. *Panic Disorder in the Medical Setting.* American Psychiatric Press, Washington, DC.

Kaufman, M. R., Lehrman, S., Franzblau, A. W. et al. 1959. Psychiatric findings in admissions to a medical service in a general hospital. *J. Mt. Sinai Hosp. N.Y.* 26: 160–170.

Kawachi, I., Colditz, G. A., Ascherio, A. et al. 1994a. Prospectrive study of phobic anxiety and risk of coronary heart disease in men. *Circulation* 89: 1992–1997.

Kawachi, I., Sparrow, D., Vokonas, P. S. et al. 1994b. Symptoms of anxiety and risk of coronary heart disease: The Normative Aging Study. *Circulation* 90: 2225–2229.

Kessler, L. G., Cleary, P. D. & Burke, J. D. 1985. Psychiatric disorders in primary care: Results of a follow-up study. *Arch. Gen. Psychiatry* 42: 583–587.

Kiev, A. & Domantay, A. G. 1988. A study of buspirone coprescribed with bronchodilators in 82 anxious ambulatory patients. *J. Asthma* 25: 281–284.

Klein, E., Cnaani, E., Harel, T. et al. 1995. Altered heart rate variability in panic disorder patients. *Biol. Psychiatry* 37: 18–24.

Kutz, I., Shabtai, H., Solomon, Z. et al. 1994. Posttraumatic stress disorder in myocardial infarction patients. *Israel J. Psychiatry Related Sci.* 31: 48–56.

Lauterbach, E. C. & Duvoisin, R. 1991. Anxiety disorders in familial parkinsonism. *Am. J. Psychiatry* 148: 274.

Lavey, E. D. & Winkle, R. A. 1979. Continuing disability of patients with chest pain and normal coronary arteriograms. *J. Chron. Dis.* 32: 191–196.

Lerner, W. D. & Fallon, H. J. 1985. The alcohol withdrawal syndrome. *N. Engl. J. Med.* 313: 951–952.

Liebowtiz, M. R. 1993. Mixed anxiety and depression: Should it be included in DSM-IV? *J. Clin. Psychiatry* 54 (Suppl. 5): 4–7.

Lilienfeld, S. O., Jacob, R. G. & Furman, J. M. R. 1989. Vestibular dysfunction followed by panic disorder with agoraphobia. *J. Nerv. Ment. Dis.* 177: 700–701.

Lindesay, J. 1990. The Guy's/Age Concern Survey: Physical health and psychiatric disorder in an urban elderly community. *Intern. J. Ger. Psychiatry* 5: 171–178.

Lindesay, J. 1991. Phobic disorders in the elderly. *Br. J. Psychiatry* 159: 531–541.

Ling, M. H., Perry, P. J. & Tsuang, M. T. 1981. Side effects of corticosteroid therapy: psychiatric aspects. *Arch. Gen. Psychiatry* 38: 471–477.

Lishman, W. A. 1987. *Organic Psychiatry*, pp. 428–485, Blackwell, London.

Lloyd, G. G. 1991. Psychological reactions in physically ill patients. In *Handbook of Studies in General Hospital Psychiatry*, eds. F. Judd, G. D. Burrows, D. Lipsitt, Elsevier, Amsterdam.

Logsdail, S., Lovell, K., Warwick, A. et al. 1991. Behavioral treatment of AIDS-focused illness phobia. *Br. J. Psychiatry* 159: 422–425.

Logue, M. B., Thomas, A. M., Barbee, J. G. et al. 1993. Generalized anxiety disorder patients seek evaluation for cardiological symptoms at the same frequency as patients with panic disorder. *J. Psychiat. Res.* 27: 55–59.

Lown, B. 1982. Mental stress, arrhythmia, and sudden death. *Am. J. Med.* 72: 177–180.

Lydiard, R. B., Fossey, M. D., Marsh, W. et al. 1993. Prevalence of psychiatric disorders in patients with irritable bowel syndrome. *Psychosomatics* 34: 229–234.

Lydiard, R. B., Greenwald, S., Weissman, M. M. et al. 1994. Panic disorder and gastrointestinal symptoms: Findings from the NIMH epidemiologic catchment area project. *Am. J. Psychiatry* 151: 64–70.

Mackenzie, T. B. & Popkin, M. K 1983. Organic anxiety syndrome. *Am. J. Psychiatry* 140: 342–344.

Maguire, G. P., Julier, D. L., Hawton, K. E. et al. 1974. Psychiatric morbidity and referral on two general medical wards. *Br. Med. J.* 1: 268–270.

Maguire, G. P., Lee, E. G., Bevington, D. J. et al. 1978. Psychiatric problems in the first year after mastectomy. *Br. Med. J.* 1: 963–965.

Maguire, P., Faulkner, A. & Regnard, C. 1993a. Managing the anxious patient with advancing disease – a flow diagram. *Palliative Med.* 7: 239–244.

Maguire, P., Faulkner, A. & Regnard, C. 1993b. Eliciting the current problems of the patient with cancer. *Palliative Med.* 7: 63–68.

Markovitz, J. H., Matthews, K. A., Kannel, W. B. et al. 1993. Psychological predictors of hypertension in the Framingham Study. *JAMA* 270: 2439–2443.

Markovitz, J. H., Matthews, K. A., Wing, R. R. et al. 1991. Psychological, health behavior, and biological predictors of blood pressure change in middle-aged women. *J. Hypertension* 9: 399–406.

Marks, I. M. 1981. Space phobia: Syndrome or agoraphobic variant. *J. Neurol. Neurosurg. Psychiatry* 44: 387–391.

Marks, I. M. 1987. *Fears, Phobias, and Rituals*, pp. 410–415, Oxford University Press, Oxford.

Massie, M. J. 1989. Anxiety, panic and phobias. In *Handbook of Psychooncology: Psychological Care of the Patient with Cancer*, eds. J. C. Holland, J. J. Rowland, pp. 300–309, Oxford University Press, New York.

Massie, M. J., Holland, J. C. & Glass, E. 1983. Delirium in terminally ill cancer patients. *Am. J. Psychiatry* 140: 1049–1050.

Massie, M. J. & Shakin, E. J. 1993. Management of depression and anxiety in cancer patients. In *Psychiatric Aspects of Symptom Management in Cancer Patients*, eds. W. Breitbart, J. C. Holland, pp. 1–21, American Psychiatric Press, Washington, DC.

Matuzas, W., Al-Sadir, J., Uhlenhuth, E. H. et al. 1989. Correlates of mitral valve prolapse among patients with panic disorder. *Psychiatry Res.* 28: 161–170.

Mayou, R. & Hawton, K. 1986. Psychiatric disorder in the general hospital. *Br. J. Psychiatry* 149: 172–190.

Melamed, B. G. & Seigal, L. J. 1980. *Behavioral Medicine*. Spring Publishing Company, New York.

Melendez, J. C. & McCrank, E. 1993. Anxiety-related reactions associated with magnetic resonance imaging. *JAMA* 270: 745–747.

Mendels, J., Chernoff, R. W. & Blatt, M. 1986. Alprazolam as an adjunct to propranolol in anxious outpatients with stable angina pectoris. *J. Clin. Psychiatry* 47: 8–11.

Menza, M. A., Robertson-Hoffman, D. E. & Bonapace, A. S. 1993. Parkinson's disease and anxiety: Comorbidity with depression. *Biol. Psychiatry* 34: 465–470.

Merikangas, K. R., Angst, J. & Isler, H. 1990. Migraine and psychopathology. Results of the Zurich cohort study of young adults. *Arch. Gen. Psychiatry* 47: 849–853.

Merikangas, K. R., Merikangas, J. R. & Angst, J. 1993. Headache syndromes and psychiatric disorders: Association and familial transmission. *J. Psychiatr. Res.* 27: 197–210.

Moorey, S., Greer, S., Watson, M. et al. 1994. Adjuvant psychological therapy for patients with cancer: Outcome at one year. *Psycho-oncology* 3: 39–46.

Morris, T. 1979. Psychological adjustment to mastectomy. *Cancer Treatment Reviews* 6: 41–61.

Munro, A. J., Biruls, R., Griffin, A. J. et al. 1989. Distress associated with radiotherapy for malignant disease: A quantitative analysis based on patients perceptions. *Br. J. Cancer* 60: 370–374.

Noyes, R. 1988. Beta-blocking drugs in anxiety disorders. In *Handbook of Anxiety Disorders*, eds. C. G. Last, M. Hersen, pp. 445–459, Pergamon Press, New York.

Noyes, R., Andreasen, N. J. C. & Hartford, E. 1971. The psychological reaction to severe burns. *Psychosomatics* 12: 416–422.

Noyes, R., Clancy, J., Hoenk, P. R. et al. 1978. Anxiety neurosis and physical illness. *Compr. Psychiatry* 19: 407–413.

Noyes, R., Garvey, M., Cook, B. et al. 1988. Benzodiazepine withdrawal: A review of the evidence. *J. Clin. Psychiatry* 49: 382–389.

Noyes, R., Holt, C. S. & Massie, M. J. In Press. Anxiety disorders. In Textbook of Psychooncology.

Noyes, R., Kathol, R. G., Debelius-Enemark, P. et al. 1990. Distress associated with cancer as measured by the Illness Distress Scale. *Psychosomatics* 31: 321–330.

Noyes, R., Wesner, R. B. & Fisher, M. M. 1992. A comparison of patients with illness phobia and panic disorder. *Psychosomatics* 33: 92–99.

Olafsdottir, M., Sjoden, P. O. & Westling, B. 1986. Prevalence and prediction of chemotherapy – related anxiety, nausea and vomiting in cancer patients. *Behav. Res. Ther.* 24: 59–66.

Ormel, J., Koeter, M. W. J., van den Brink, W. et al. 1991. Recognition, management, and course of anxiety and depression in general practice. *Arch. Gen. Psychiatry* 48: 700–706.

Öst, L-G., Lindahl, I. L., Sterner, U. et al. 1984. Exposure in vivo vs. applied relaxation in the treatment of blood phobia. *Behav. Res. Ther.* 22: 205–216.

Öst, L-G., Sterner, U. & Fellenius, J. 1989. Applied tension, applied relaxation and the combination in treatment of blood phobia. *Behav. Res. Ther.* 27: 109–121.

Ostrow, D. G., Monjan, A., Joseph, J. et al. 1989. HIV-related symptoms and psychological functioning in a cohort of homosexual men. *Am. J. Psychiatry* 146: 737–742.

Oswald, N. C., Waller, R. E. & Drinkwater, J. 1970. Relationship between breathlessness and anxiety in asthma and bronchitis: A comparative study. *Br. Med. J.* 2: 14–17.

Page, N. G. R. & Gresty, M. A. 1985. Motorists' vestibular disorentiation syndrome. *J. Neurol. Neurosurg. Psychiatry* 48: 729–735.

Papp, L. A., Weiss, J. R., Greenberg, H. E. et al. 1995. Sertraline for chronic obstructive pulmonary disease and comorbid anxiety and mood disorders. *Am J. Psychiatry* 152: 1531.

Peck, A. & Boland, J. 1977. Emotional reaction to radiation treatment. *Cancer* 40: 180–184.

Perdices, M., Dunbar, N., Grunsect, A. et al. 1992. Anxiety, depression, and HIV related symptomatology across the spectrum of HIV disease. *Aust. NZ J. Psychiatry* 26: 560–566.

Perry, S., Difede, J., Musngi, G. et al. 1992. Predictors of posttraumatic stress disorder after burn injury. *Am. J. Psychiatry* 149: 931–935.

Pollack, M. H., Kradin, R., Otto, M. W. et al. 1996. Prevalence of panic in patients referred for pulmonary function testing at a major medical center. *Am. J. Psychiatry* 153: 110–113.

Popkin, M. K., Callies, A. L. & Colon, E. A. 1990. Adjustment disorders in medically ill inpatients referred for consultation in a university hospital. *Psychosomatics* 31: 410–441.

Powers, P. S., Cruse, C. W., Daniels, S. et al. 1994. Posttraumatic stress disorder in patients with burns. *J. Burn Care Rehabilitation* 15: 147–153.

Pratt, R. T. C. & McKenzie, W. 1958. Anxiety states following vestibular disorders. *Lancet* 2: 347–349.

Quitkin, F. M., Harrison, W., Stewart, J. W. et al. 1991. Response to phenelzine and imipramine in placebo nonresponders with atypical depression. *Arch. Gen. Psychiatry* 48: 319–323.

Raj, A. & Sheehan, D. V. 1987. Medical evaluation of panic attacks. *J. Clin. Psychiatry* 48: 309–313.

Raskin, M., Bali, L. R. & Peeke, H. V. 1980. Muscle biofeedback and transcendental meditation. *Arch. Gen. Psychiatry* 37: 93–97.

Reich, P., DeSilva, R. A., Lown, B. et al. 1981. Acute psychological disturbance preceding life-threatening ventricular arrhythmias. *JAMA* 246: 233–235.

Renfroe, K. L. 1988. Effect of progressive relaxation on dyspnea and state anxiety in patients with chronic obstructive pulmonary disease. *Heart Lung* 17: 408–413.

Rickels, K., Amsterdam, J. D., Clancy, C. et al. 1991. Buspirone in major depression: A controlled study. *J. Clin. Psychiatry* 52: 34–38.

Robinson, D., Napoliello, M. J. & Schenk, J. 1988. The safety and usefulness of buspirone as an anxiolytic drug in elderly vs. young patients. *Clin. Ther.* 10: 740–746.

Roca, R. T., Spence, R. J. & Munster, A. M. 1992. Posttraumatic adaptation and distress among adult burn survivors. *Am. J. Psychiatry* 149: 1234–1238.

Rogers, M. P., White, K., Warshaw, M. G. et al. 1994. Prevalence of medical illness in patients with anxiety disorders. *Int. J. Psychiatry Med.* 24: 83–96.

Rosenbaum, J. F. & Pollack, M. H. 1991. Anxiety. In *Massachusetts General Hospital Handbook of General Hospital Psychiatry*, Third Edition, ed. N. H. Cassem, pp. 159–190, Mosby Year Book, St. Louis.

Roy-Byrne, P. P., Geraci, M. & Uhde, T. W. 1986. Life events and the onset of panic disorder. *Am. J. Psychiatry* 143: 1424–1427.

Ryle, J. A. 1948. Nosophobia. *J. Ment. Sci.* 94: 1–17.

Samet, C. M. & Geller, R. D. 1979. Anxiety associated with cardiovascular disorders: A study using lorazepam. *Psychosomatics* 20: 707–713.

Sartorius, N., Ustun, T. B., Lecrubier, Y. & Wittchen, H-U. 1996. Depression comorbid with anxiety: Results from the WHO study on psychological disorders in primary health care. *Br. J. Psychiatry* 168: 38–43.

Schiffer, R. B., Kurlan, R., Rubin, A. et al. 1988. Evidence for atypical depression in Parkinson's disease. *Am. J. Psychaitry* 145: 1020–1022.

Schulberg, H. C., Saul, M., McClelland, M. et al. 1985. Assessing depression in primary medical and psychiatric practices. *Arch. Gen. Psychiatry* 42: 1164–1170.

Schwab, J. J., McGinness, N. H., Marder, L. et al. 1966. Evaluation of anxiety in medical patients. *J. Chron. Dis.* 19: 1049–1057.

Schag, C. A. C. & Heinrich, R. L. 1989. Anxiety in medical situations: Adult cancer patients. *J. Clin. Psychology* 45: 20–27.

Sensky, T. 1993. Cognitive therapy in physical illness. In *Psychological Treatment in Disease and Illness*, eds. M. Hodes, S. Moorey, pp. 34–45, Gaskell, London.

Sensky, T., Dennehy, M., Gilbert, A. et al. 1989. Physicians' perceptions of anxiety and depression among their outpatients: Relationships with patients and doctors' satisfaction with their interviews. *J. Royal Col. Physicians (London)* 23: 33–38.

Sharer, A. U., Schreiber, S., Galai, T. et al. 1993. Posttraumatic stress disorder following medical events. *Br. J. Clin. Psychology* 32: 247–253.

Shavitt, R. G., Gentil, V. & Mandetta, R. 1992. The association of panic/agoraphobia and asthma: Contributing factors and clinical implications. *Gen. Hosp. Psychiatry* 14: 420–423.

Sherbourne, C. D., Jackson, C. A., Meredith, L. S. et al. 1996. Prevalence of comorbid anxiety disorders in primary care outpatients. *Arch. Fam. Med.* 5: 27–34.

Sherbourne, C. D., Wells, K. B., Meredith, L. S. et al. 1996. Comorbid anxiety disorder and the functioning and well-being of chronically ill patients of general medical providers. *Arch. Gen. Psychiatry* 53: 889–895.

Siemers, E. R., Shekhar, A., Quaid, K. et al. 1993. Anxiety and motor performance in Parkinson's disease. *Movement Dis.* 8: 501–506.

Singh, N. P., Despars, J. A., Stansburg, D. W. et al. 1993. Effects of buspirone on anxiety levels and exercise tolerance in patients with chronic airflow obstruction and mild anxiety. *Chest* 103: 800–804.

Smith, R. C., Greenbaum, R. B., Dean, H. A. et al. 1990. Psychosocial factors are associated with health care seeking rather than diagnosis in irritable bowel syndrome. *Gastroenterology* 98: 293–301.

Sommers-Flanagan, J. & Greenberg, R. P. 1989. Psychosocial variables and hypertension: A new look at an old controversy. *J. Nerv. Ment. Dis.* 177: 15–24.

Sparrow, D., Garvey, A. J., Rosner, B. et al. 1982. Factors in predicting blood pressure change. *Circulation* 65: 789–794.

Spiegel, D., Bloom, J. R. & Yalom, I. 1981. Group support for patients with metastatic cancer. *Arch. Gen. Psychiatry* 38: 527–533.

Spielberger, C. D., Gorsuch, R. C. & Lushene, R. E. 1970. *Manual for the State-Trait Anxiety Inventory*. Consulting Psychologists, Palo Alto, CA.

Starkman, M. N., Zelnik, T. C., Nesse, T. C., et al. 1985. Anxiety in patients with pheochromocytomas. *Arch. Intern. Med.* 145: 248–252.

Starkstein, S. E., Cohen, B. S., Fedoroff, P. et al. 1990. Relationship between anxiety disorders and depressive disorders in patients with cerebrovascular injury. *Arch. Gen. Psychiatry* 47: 246–251.

332   *Anxiety in the medically ill*

Stefanek, M. E., Shaw, A., DeGeorge, D. et al. 1989. Illness-related worry among cancer patients: Prevalence, severity, and content. *Cancer Invest.* 7: 365–371.

Stein, M. B., Asmundson, G. J. G., Ireland, D. et al. 1994. Panic disorder in patients attending a clinic for vestibular disorders. *Am. J. Psychiatry* 151: 1697–1700.

Stein, M. B., Heuser, I. J., Juncos, J. L. et al. 1990. Anxiety disorders in patients with Parkinson's disease. *Am. J. Psychiatry* 147: 217–220.

Sternbach, R. A. 1974. *Pain Patients: Traits and Treatment.* Academic Press, New York.

Stewart, W. S., Breslau, N. & Keck, P. E. 1994. Comorbidity of migraine and panic disorder. *Neurol.* 44 (Suppl. 7): 523–527.

Stewart, W. S., Linet, M. & Calentano, D. D. 1989. Migraine headaches and panic attacks. *Psychosom. Med.* 51: 559–569.

Stiefel, F. C., Breitbart, W. S. & Holland, J. C. 1989. Corticosteroids in cancer: Neuropsychiatric complications. *Cancer Invest.* 7: 479–491.

Storey, P. 1985. Emotional aspects of cerebrovascular disease. *Adv. Psychosom. Med.* 13: 71–84.

Stoudemire, A. & Fogel, B. S. 1995. Psychopharmacology in medical patients: An update. In *Medical-Psychiatric Practice*, eds. A. Stoudemire, B. S. Fogel, pp. 79–150, American Psychiatric Press, Washington, DC.

Stoudemire, A. & Moran, M. G. 1993. Psychopharmacologic treatment of anxiety in the medically ill elderly patient: Special considerations. *J. Clin. Psychiatry* 54 (Suppl. 5): 27–33.

Stoudemire, A., Strain, J. J. & Hales, R. E. 1989. DSM-IV issues for consultation psychiatry. *Psychosomatics* 30: 239–244.

Strain, F. & Ploog, D. 1988. Anxiety related to nervous system dysfunction. In *Handbook of Anxiety*, Vol. 2, eds. R. Noyes, M. Roth, G. D. Burrows, pp. 431–475, Elsevier, Amsterdam.

Strain, J. J., Liebowitz, M. R. & Klein, D. F. 1981. Anxiety and panic attacks in the medically ill. *Psychiatr. Clin. North Am.* 4: 333–350.

Sullivan, M., Clark, M. R., Katon, W. J. et al. 1993. Psychiatric and otologic diagnosis in patients complaining of dizziness. *Arch. Intern. Med.* 153: 1479–1484.

Taylor, C. B., King, R., Ehlers, A. et al. 1987. Treadmill exercise test and ambulatory measures in panic attacks. *Am. J. Cardiology* 60: 48J–52J.

Tesar, G. E. 1990. High-potency benzodiazepines for short-term management of panic disorder: The U.S. experience. *J. Clin. Psychiatry* 51 (Suppl. 51): 4–10.

Thompson, D. R. & Meddis, R. 1990. A prospective evaluation of in-hospital counseling for first time myocardial infarction men. *J. Psychosom. Res.* 34: 237–248.

Thompson, W. L. & Thompson, T. L. II. 1985. Psychiatric aspects of asthma in adults. *Adv. Psychosom. Med.* 14: 33–47.

Tiller, J. W. G., Dakis, J. A. & Shaw, J. M. 1988. Short-term buspirone treatment in disinhibition with dementia. *Lancet* 2: 510.

Tollefson, G. D., Luxenberg, M., Valentine, R. et al. 1991. An open label trial of alprazolam in comorbid irritable bowel syndrome and generalized anxiety disorder. *J. Clin. Psychiatry* 52: 502–508.

Triozzi, P. L., Goldstein, D. & Laszlo, J. 1988. Contributions of benzodiazepines to cancer therapy. *Cancer Invest.* 6: 103–111.

Trzepacz, P. T., McCue, M., Klein, I. et al. 1988. A psychiatric and neuropsychological study of patients with untreated Graves' disease. *Gen.*

Hosp. Psychiatry 10: 49–55.

Tyerman, A. & Humphrey, M. 1984. Changes in self-concept following severe head injury. *Int. J. Rehabil. Res.* 7: 11–23.

van Knippenberg, F. C. E., Duivenvoorden, J. H., Bouke, B. et al. 1990. Shortening the State-Trait Anxiety Inventory. *J. Clin. Epidemiol.* 43: 995–1000.

Victor, B. S., Lubetsky, M. & Greden, J. F. 1981. Somatic manifestations of caffeinism. *J. Clin. Psychiatry* 42: 185–188.

von Korff, M., Shapiro, S., Burke, J. D. et al. 1987. Anxiety and depression in a primary care clinic. *Arch. Gen. Psychiatry* 44: 152–156.

Walker, E. A., Katon, W. J., Jemelka, R. P. et al. 1992. Comorbidity of gastrointestinal complaints, depression, and anxiety in the epidemiologic catchment area (ECA) study. *Am. J. Med.* 92 (Suppl. 1A): 26S–30S.

Walker, E. A., Roy-Byrne, P. P. & Katon, W. J. 1990. Irritable bowel syndrome and psychiatric illness. *Am. J. Psychiatry* 147: 565–572.

Weiner, N. 1980. Norephedrine, ephedrine, and sympathomimetic amines. In *Pharmacological Basis of Therapeutics*, eds. A. G. Goodman, L. S. Goodman, A Gilman, p. 163, Macmillan, New York.

Weissman, M. M., Markowitz, J. S., Ouellette, R. et al. 1990. Panic disorder and cardiovascular/cerebrovascular problems: Results from a community survey. *Am. J. Psychiatry* 147: 1504–1508.

Wells, K. B., Godling, J. M. & Burnam, M. A. (1989a). Chronic medical conditons in a sample of the general population with anxiety, affective, substance use disorders. *Am. J. Psychiatry* 146: 1440–1446.

Wells, K. B., Golding, J. M. & Burnam, M. A. 1988. Psychiatric disorder in a sample of the general population with and without chronic medical conditions. *Am. J. Psychiatry* 145: 976–981.

Wells, K. B., Golding, J. M. & Burnam, M. A. 1989b. Affective, substance use, and anxiety disorders in persons with arthritis, diabetes, heart disease, high blood pressure, or chronic lung conditions. *Gen. Hosp. Psychiatry* 11: 320–327.

Williams, D. 1956. The structure of emotions reflected in epileptic experiences. *Brain* 79: 29–67.

Williams, J. B. W., Rabkin, J. G., Remien, R. H. et al. 1991. Multidisciplinary baseline assessment of homosexual men with and without human immunodeficiency virus infection. II. Standardized clinical assessment of current and lifetime psychopathology. *Arch. Gen. Psychiatry* 48: 124–130.

Wilson-Barnett, J. 1992. Psychological reaction to medical procedures. *Psychotherapy Psychosom.* 57: 118–127.

Winston, A., Pinsker, H. & McCullough, L. 1986. A review of supportive psychotherapy. *Hosp. Comm. Psychiatry* 37: 1105–1114.

Wood, P. 1941. Da Costa's syndrome (or effort syndrome). *Br. Med. J.* 1: 767–772, 805–811, 845–851.

World Health Organization (WHO) 1993. *The ICD-10 Classification of Mental and Behavioural Disorders: Diagnostic Criteria for Research*, World Health Organization, Geneva.

Yardley, L., Luxon, L. M. & Haacks, N. P. 1994. A longitudinal study of symptoms, anxiety and subjective well-being in patients with vertigo. *Clin. Otolaryngol* 19: 109–116.

Yellowlees, P. M., Alpers, J. H., Bowden, J. J. et al. 1987. Psychiatric morbidity in subjects with chronic airflow obstruction. *Med. J. Aust.* 146: 305–307.

Yellowlees, P. M., Haynes, S., Potts, N. et al. 1988. Psychiatric morbidity in

Anxiety in the medically ill

patients with life-threatening asthma: Initial report of a controlled study. *Med. J. Aust.* 149: 246–249.

Yeragani, J. K., Balou, R., Pohl, R. et al. 1990a. Decreased R-R variance in panic disorder patients. *Acta Psychiatr. Scand.* 81: 554–559.

Yeragani, J. K., Pohl, R., Balon, R. et al. 1990b. Risk factors for cardiovascular illness in panic disorder patients. *Neuropsychobiology* 23: 134–139.

Yeragani, J. K., Pohl, R., Berger, R. et al. 1993. Decreased heart rate variability in panic disorder patients: A study of power-spectral analysis of heart rate. *Psychiatry Res.* 46: 89–103.

Yingling, K. W., Watsen, L. R., Arnold, L. M. et al. 1993. Estimated prevalences of panic disorder and depression among conservative patients seen in an emergency department with acute chest pain. *J. Gen. Intern. Med.* 8: 231–235.

Zanbergen, J., Bright, M., Pols, H. et al. 1991. Higher lifetime prevalence of respiratory diseases in panic disorders. *Am. J. Psychiatry* 148: 1583–1585.

Zigmond, A. S. & Snaith, R. P. 1983. The Hospital Anxiety and Depression Scale. *Acta Psychiatr. Scand.* 67: 361–370.

Zung, W. W. K. 1986. Prevalence of clinically significant anxiety in a family practice setting. *Am. J. Psychiatry* 143: 1471–1472.

Index

335